WITHDRAWN
UTSA LIBRARIES

COUNSELING MUSLIMS

"*Counseling Muslims* is a valuable and outstanding contribution to the counseling literature on a timely topic. For a variety of reasons, Muslims in the United States and elsewhere have become an important ethnocultural and religious group that counselors and psychotherapists need to understand. The editors have assembled an outstanding group of scholars to provide a wonderful blend of scientific and clinically relevant information in a handbook format. It is an amazing resource and should become required reading in the field."

–Frederick Leong, PhD, Director,
Consortium for Multicultural Psychology Research, Michigan State University

"During this post-9/11 period in which the Islamophobia and the fear of terrorism pervade our society, there is a real need to understand Muslims, who represent 23% of the world's population. This book on counseling Muslims is an exceptional contribution that helps to provide this understanding. Mental health students and professionals, as well as the general public, will find it amazingly insightful, informative, engaging, and challenging."

–Stanley Sue, PhD, Professor and Director,
Center for Excellence in Diversity, Palo Alto University, California

"This is an innovative collection of writings from authors who are well versed in the field either as scholars or practitioners. Each chapter provides a depth of understanding into clinically useful ways of understanding mental health practice with Muslim patients; and the book provides most helpful guidance to practitioners, students, and scholars alike. I find it user friendly, accessible, and practical."

–John R. Graham, PhD, RSW, Murray Fraser Professor,
University of Calgary, Canada

"The need to address religion and spirituality in organizing and providing mental health services is becoming increasingly evident in most western countries. But there are few books that provide practical help for practitioners. This book provides mental health practitioners with a comprehensive text written specifically to help improve their services for Muslims whether through counseling and psychotherapy or more medically orientated psychiatric treatment. It covers a wide range of topics abundantly illustrated with case studies, and often includes direct practical advice. I think this book should be essential reading for mental health practitioners who deal with Muslim clients, but it could also interest educators and people involved in training mental health workers."

–Suman Fernando, Psychiatrist, Visiting Professor,
London Metropolitan University, UK

"This text teaches practitioners what words to use, techniques to implement, and how to judge the success of interventions with Muslim clients. It is a practical, useful source of information that represents an important contribution to the psychotherapy field."

–Harold G. Koenig, MD, Professor, Psychiatry and Behavioral Sciences; Director,
Center for Theology and Health, Duke University Medical Center

COUNSELING MUSLIMS

HANDBOOK OF MENTAL HEALTH ISSUES
AND INTERVENTIONS

EDITED BY
Sameera Ahmed and Mona M. Amer

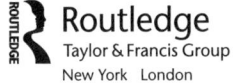
Routledge
Taylor & Francis Group
New York London

Routledge
Taylor & Francis Group
711 Third Avenue
New York, NY 10017

Routledge
Taylor & Francis Group
27 Church Road
Hove, East Sussex BN3 2FA

© 2012 by Taylor & Francis Group, LLC
Routledge is an imprint of Taylor & Francis Group, an Informa business

Printed in the United States of America on acid-free paper
Version Date: 20110708

International Standard Book Number: 978-0-415-98860-5 (Hardback)

For permission to photocopy or use material electronically from this work, please access www.copyright.com (http://www.copyright.com/) or contact the Copyright Clearance Center, Inc. (CCC), 222 Rosewood Drive, Danvers, MA 01923, 978-750-8400. CCC is a not-for-profit organization that provides licenses and registration for a variety of users. For organizations that have been granted a photocopy license by the CCC, a separate system of payment has been arranged.

Trademark Notice: Product or corporate names may be trademarks or registered trademarks, and are used only for identification and explanation without intent to infringe.

Library of Congress Cataloging-in-Publication Data

Counseling Muslims : handbook of mental health issues and interventions / edited by Sameera Ahmed, Mona M. Amer. -- 1st ed.
    p. cm.
Includes bibliographical references and index.
ISBN 978-0-415-98860-5 (hardback : alk. paper)
    1. Cross-cultural counseling. 2. Counseling--Religious aspects--Islam. 3. Psychiatry, Transcultural. I. Ahmed, Sameera. II. Amer, Mona M. III. Title.

BF636.7.C76C686 2011
158'.3088297--dc22   2011011251

Visit the Taylor & Francis Web site at
http://www.taylorandfrancis.com

and the Routledge Web site at
http://www.routledgementalhealth.com

Contents

Acknowledgments vii
Editors ix
Contributors xi
Foreword xv
Preface xvii

Part I Muslim Beliefs Within a Counseling Framework

1 Islam, Muslims, and Mental Health 3
   AMBER HAQUE and NAJEEB KAMIL

2 Conceptualizations of Mental Health, Illness, and Healing 15
   AISHA UTZ

3 Traditional Mental Health Coping and Help-Seeking 33
   OSMAN M. ALI and FRIEDA ABOUL-FOTOUH

Part II Models and Interventions

4 Mental Health Interview and Cultural Formulation 51
   FARAH TASLEEMA RAHIEM and HAMADA HAMID

5 Psychological Testing and Assessment 71
   OMAR M. MAHMOOD and SAWSSAN R. AHMED

6 Individual Psychotherapy/Counseling: Psychodynamic, Cognitive-Behavioral, and Humanistic-Experiential Models 87
   MONA M. AMER and BALAND JALAL

vi • Contents

7	Family Systems Therapy and Postmodern Approaches MANIJEH DANESHPOUR	119
8	Islamic-Based Interventions SABNUM DHARAMSI and ABDULLAH MAYNARD	135
9	Community-Based Prevention and Intervention NADIA S. ANSARY and RAJA SALLOUM	161

Part III   Service Settings

10	Inpatient Psychiatric Units SARAH MOHIUDDIN and SABA MAROOF	183
11	Home-Based Social Services ANEESAH NADIR and CHERYL EL-AMIN	197
12	University Counseling Centers MAJEDA HUMEIDAN	213

Part IV   Special Populations

13	Converts to Islam SAMEERA AHMED	229
14	Adolescents and Emerging Adults SAMEERA AHMED	251
15	Refugees SAMEERA AHMED and FRIEDA ABOUL-FOTOUH	281

Part V   Special Issues

16	Domestic Violence SALMA ELKADI ABUGIDEIRI	309
17	Sexuality and Sexual Dysfunctions AMAL KILLAWI	329
18	Substance Abuse LYNNE ALI-NORTHCOTT	355
	Index	383

Acknowledgments

The clinical depth and insights presented in this book would not have been possible without our clients, who have shared their lives with us over the years, and without our professional colleagues, who have influenced our development as clinicians and researchers. Countless colleagues and friends have contributed to this book by offering feedback, contacts, encouragement, and insights, and for that we are very grateful. We would like to thank our publisher, George Zimmar, for his constant patience, guidance, and support in the preparation of this book. We are moreover grateful to the publication staff at Routledge who were supportive throughout the process. We also appreciate the dedication and perseverance of the authors of this handbook, who invested countless days capturing their wisdoms on paper, even when there was very little in the published literature on which to depend. Thank you for your openness to guidance and criticism.

Sameera is thankful to the activists, religious scholars, and leaders, who have mentored, inspired, and exposed her to the complexities and variations within the Muslim community. They have served as religious resources, and provided her with the skills needed to cohesively integrate her mental health, sociocultural, and religious knowledge. I am also grateful to my colleagues, Syeda Mohammad, Hamada Hamid, Cynthia Arfken, and Mona Amer, for the support and advice they have provided over the years. I am indebted to my family and friends who have been patient with my shortcomings and supported me in numerous ways; your support has been humbling. To my children, who have sacrificed much for this book and continue to brighten my life with their smiles, energy, creativity, and good nature, thank you for reminding me to take breaks, appreciate life, and for constantly pushing me to be a better human being.

Finally, to my soul mate and beloved husband—this book would not have been possible without your continued support, encouragement, and personal sacrifices; your willingness to edit, review, and advise; as well as your wisdom, insight, and vision.

Mona is thankful to her mentors in multicultural psychology at the University of Toledo and Yale University School of Medicine for inspiring and guiding her growth, and for never wavering in their encouragement to develop this book. I recall the intellectual loneliness of my first few years developing cultural competence models for Muslims, so words cannot describe the appreciation I feel for the thriving network of colleagues—including my coeditor Sameera—who have invigorated this work with fresh insight. Most of all, my deepest appreciation goes to my family, whom I've missed dearly during the process of working on this book. You have been extraordinarily patient and have sacrificed immeasurably in accommodating my absences and inadequacies . . . without your unwavering support none of this would have been possible.

The Editors

Sameera Ahmed, Ph.D. is the director of the Family & Youth Institute (FYI), Canton, Michigan, as well as clinical assistant professor of psychiatry at Wayne State University, Detroit, Michigan. In addition, she is a Fellow at the Institute for Social Policy and Understanding (ISPU), an associate editor for the *Journal of Muslim Mental Health,* and has a private clinical practice. Dr. Ahmed has a Ph.D. in clinical psychology from Fairleigh Dickinson University, New Jersey and an M.S. in biology from Bowling Green State University, Ohio. Her areas of interest include risk behaviors and protective factors of Muslim adolescents and emerging adults, skills-based parenting and marital interventions to strengthen families, and promoting culturally and religiously meaningful psychotherapy. She has presented her research in sessions and workshops across the United States and Canada in both academic and community settings and has published numerous journal articles. In addition to her scholarly efforts, Dr. Ahmed has been involved in the Muslim community at both the local and national levels over the past 20 years and is intimately familiar with the heterogeneity and issues impacting Muslims in North America.

Mona M. Amer, Ph.D. is an assistant professor of psychology at the American University in Cairo, Egypt, where she was awarded the university's Excellence in Teaching Award. Dr. Amer has gained widespread recognition for developing cultural competence training curriculums for social service providers working with Muslims and Arabs, which she has presented in cities in the United States and the United Kingdom. For this work she was awarded the American Psychological Association's (APA) Award for Distinguished Graduate Student in Professional Psychology.

She was the editor-in-chief of the *Journal of Muslim Mental Health* and has consulted to local, state, and federal agencies regarding Arab American and American Muslim mental health post 9/11. Dr. Amer completed a Ph.D. in clinical psychology at the University of Toledo, Ohio and a postdoctoral fellowship specializing in racial/ethnic disparities in behavioral health at Yale University's Department of Psychiatry, New Haven, Connecticut. She was the sole recipient of APA's 2005–2007 minority postdoctoral fellowship in mental health and substance abuse services. In addition to teaching and research, she works as a psychotherapist in a private practice.

Contributors

Frieda Aboul-Fotouh, M.D. is a clinical fellow in psychiatry at Harvard Medical School and resident in child and adolescent psychiatry at Massachusetts General Hospital and McLean Hospital, Boston, Massachusetts. She obtained a B.A. in sociology from Rice University and completed her medical training at Baylor College of Medicine as a Presidential Scholar.

Salma Elkadi Abugideiri, M.Ed. is a licensed professional counselor who is certified in marriage and family therapy, and is the co-director of the Peaceful Families Project, Great Falls, Virginia. She is the co-author of *What Islam Says about Domestic Violence* and co-editor of *Change from Within: Diverse Perspectives on Domestic Violence in Muslim Communities.*

Sawssan R. Ahmed, Ph.D. is an assistant professor at the Department of Human Development, California State University, San Marcos, California. She holds a doctoral degree in clinical psychology from Wayne State University, Michigan. Her research focuses on the role of socio-cultural risk and protective factors in health disparities, with a special focus on Arab American adolescents.

Osman M. Ali, M.D. is a clinical assistant professor and director of the public and community psychiatry fellowship at the University of Texas Southwestern Medical Center, Dallas, Texas. He completed his psychiatry residency at Cornell University, New York and fellowship at Columbia University, New York. He is also a co-founder of Muslim Mental Health, Inc.

Lynne Ali-Northcott, M.Sc. is an addiction counselor at Nafas, a culturally-sensitive drug treatment center in London, England. Her clinical specialization is with clients from Muslim communities. She completed her M.Sc. in addiction psychology and counselling at London South Bank University, London, U.K.

Nadia Ansary, Ph.D. is an assistant professor of psychology at Rider University, Lawrenceville, New Jersey. She received her doctorate in developmental psychology from Teachers College, Columbia University, New York. Her research focuses on risk and resilience among vulnerable adolescent populations, particularly Muslim youth.

Manijeh Daneshpour, Ph.D. is the director of the marriage and family therapy Master and Certificate program at St. Cloud State University, St. Cloud, Minnesota, and works with individuals and families in private practice. Her research focuses on multicultural family therapy (including with Muslims), gender relations, social justice, and third-wave feminism.

Sabnum Dharamsi, B.A. Hons. is a counselor and trainer of Islamic counseling in London, Cambridge, and Birmingham, U.K. She is co-founder of the first U.K.-accredited Islamic counseling training programs, a partner at Stephen Maynard & Associates, Bedfordshire, U.K., and head facilitator for The Academy of Self Knowledge online self-development program.

Cheryl El-Amin, Ph.D. is a licensed social worker at the Office of School Social Work Service for Detroit Public Schools, Detroit, Michigan. She is the board secretary at the social service nonprofit organization Share-Detroit, one of the founding members of the International League of Muslim Women, Inc., and member of the Islamic Social Services Association-USA.

Hamada Hamid, D.O., M.P.H. is a clinical instructor of psychiatry and neurology at Yale School of Medicine, New Haven, Connecticut, and director of the Center for Global Health, Institute of Social Policy and Understanding, Clinton, Michigan. He is the founder and chief editor of the *Journal of Muslim Mental Health*.

Amber Haque, Ph.D. is an associate professor and director of the Master of Science program in clinical psychology at the Department of Psychology and Counseling, United Arab Emirates University, Al Ain, United Arab Emirates. He is the editor of the books *Psychology of Personality: Islamic Perspectives* and *Muslims in North America: Problems and Prospects*.

Majeda Humeidan, Ph.D. is a licensed psychologist and supervisor of student services at the Higher Colleges of Technology, Abu Dhabi, United Arab Emirates. She earned her doctorate in counseling psychology from Ball State University, and has worked in college counseling centers for 14 years. Her work focuses on developing counseling services for underserved students.

Baland Jalal is a psychology student and research assistant at the American University in Cairo, Cairo, Egypt, and a student of English at the University of Copenhagen, Copenhagen, Denmark.

Najeeb Kamil, M.S.W. is a child welfare worker for Alameda County's Department of Children and Family Services, Hayward, California. He obtained a diploma in Islamic studies from the Institute of Islamic Studies, Cairo, Egypt.

Amal Killawi, M.S.W. is a clinical social worker and research associate at the University of Michigan, Ann Arbor, Michigan. She obtained a master's degree in social work from the University of Michigan, and is currently pursuing a certification in sexual health. She also holds certifications in pre-marital and marital education.

Omar M. Mahmood, Ph.D. is a research scientist at the University of California, San Diego, and a neuropsychology fellow at the Veterans Administration San Diego Healthcare System, California. His clinical expertise is in the neuropsychological assessment of patient populations within the United States and Middle East.

Saba Maroof, M.D. is a child and adolescent psychiatry fellow at Wayne State University, Detroit, Michigan. She completed a B.A. in psychology from the University of North Carolina at Chapel Hill, a medical degree at Wayne State University, and an adult psychiatry residency at Henry Ford Health System, Detroit, Michigan.

Abdullah Maynard, M.A. is a counselor and trainer of Islamic counseling in London, Cambridge, and Birmingham for Stephen Maynard & Associates. He is co-founder of Islamic counseling training programs, founder of the Lateef Project, an Islamic counseling service, and author of the Department of Health scoping report on Muslim mental health, all in the U.K.

Sarah Mohiuddin, M.D. is director of the Consultation-Liaison Program and assistant training director of the fellowship program for child and adolescent psychiatry at University of Michigan Health System, Ann Arbor, Michigan. She received her psychology B.A. and medical doctorate from the University of Michigan.

Aneesah Nadir, M.S.W., Ph.D. is a social worker, diversity training and marriage/family life educator in private practice in Tempe, Arizona. She is the president of the Islamic Social Services Association-U.S.A. based in Tempe, Arizona.

Farah Tasleema Rahiem, M.D., M.P.H. is a psychiatry resident at the Department of Psychiatry, Yale University School of Medicine, New Haven, Connecticut. She received a B.S. in premedicine from Stetson University, a medical degree from the University of Miami, Florida, and a Master of Public Health from Johns Hopkins University, Maryland.

Raja Salloum, M.S.W. is a clinician specializing in individual, family, couple, and group therapy with Arab-American and Muslim clients at the Mental Health Association of Passaic County, Clifton, New Jersey. She is the co-founder of TANWEER: The Arab American Family Center of New Jersey, Inc., Clifton, New Jersey.

Aisha Utz (formerly Aisha Hamdan), Ph.D. is an assistant professor of clinical psychology at the College of Medicine, King Saud bin Abdulaziz University for Health Sciences, Riyadh, Saudi Arabia. She is author of *Nurturing Eeman in Children* and *Psychology from the Islamic Perspective*, and associate editor for the *Journal of Muslim Mental Health*.

Foreword

The timing of this publication is extremely important in mediating the actual and potential conflict and misunderstandings between Muslims and non-Muslims. This book provides the first comprehensive survey of the issues confronting clinicians or researchers attempting to understand the mental health issues that may impact Muslim clients. The book is unique in that it discusses clinical issues and interventions that have not been given previous attention in the literature, such as counseling for sexual and substance abuse issues, and the use of humanistic, home-based, and community interventions. The eighteen chapters were written by highly qualified authorities to present and discuss Muslim beliefs within a counseling framework while incorporating the latest literature and research on the topic. The editors and chapter authors recognized the absence of information needed to train counselors to be more religiously and culturally sensitive when working with Muslims, and this book was a response to that need. This book will increase the competence among readers working with Muslim clients.

Each chapter follows a uniform format with a balanced emphasis on both theory and practice. Each chapter acknowledges the diversity of views within the Muslim community while at the same time acknowledging the uniformity in basic beliefs. In addition, this book highlights the diversity and multicultural identities of the Muslim community living in Western nations, and leads the reader on a narrow path avoiding both the stereotypes of absolute uniformity and the chaos of total diversity. The result is a book that contextualizes the world views of Muslims across the topics likely to come up in counseling. While there are great differences between Islam and other religions, there are also similarities. Likewise, Muslims share many similarities but among Muslims there are also many cultural variations. The authors acknowledge the importance of these within-group and between-group differences. All behaviors are learned and/or displayed in a cultural context. Consequently accurate assessment, meaningful understanding, and appropriate intervention require us to consider the cultural context of a client's behavior before we attempt to change the client's behavior.

There are several main ideas in this book which the reader might consider. First, the book attacks the damaging negative stereotypes of Muslims that may be particularly hurtful to clients. Second, the authors describe spiritual perspectives of mental health, which distinguishes their approach from other mental health literature and may be helpful in understanding the clients' worldview and conceptualization of their illness. Third, the book includes a balanced emphasis on theory and practice. Fourth, almost all chapters include case studies that help to illustrate the kinds of cases encountered and are useful in the classroom. Fifth, both within-group and between-group differences are included to give a broad representation of the various Muslim cultures present in Western nations. These differences may be ethnographic, demographic, or related to social status and affiliations. Sixth, clinical, medical, and educational applications are included. The authors of this book have contributed significantly to the literature for counselors, researchers, and educators at a time when those contributions are extremely important.

My own experiences have helped me see the value of this book in many ways. From 1970 to 1980 I was a counselor in the International Students Advisor's Office at the University of Minnesota where I had considerable contact with Muslim students and faculty. I taught at Nommensen University in Sumatra, Indonesia, the University of Malaya, Malaysia, and at Taiwan universities for a total of more than seven years abroad, with considerable contact with the Muslim community. In addition, I have written or co-authored 45 books and several hundred articles on multicultural counseling. Through contact with providers and consumers from other cultures including Muslims, we will succeed in making multiculturalism a "fourth force" to supplement psycho-dynamic, humanistic, and behavioral systems.

In conclusion, the reader of this book can expect to become better prepared to deal with issues involving the Muslim community in specific ways. Misinformation and prejudices towards Muslims have increased over the years. This book is the foundation for counselors, researchers, and educators seeking common ground across cultural differences.

Paul Pedersen
Professor Emeritus, Syracuse University
Syracuse, New York

Preface

> Do you not see how God has given the example of a good word? It is like a good tree, whose root is firmly fixed, and whose branches reach the sky, ever yielding its fruit in every season with the leave of its Lord. God gives examples for mankind that they may take heed. (Quran 14:24–25).

Much of the work of mental health practice involves conveying meaning through words. When a practitioner's words are rooted in cultural awareness, knowledge, and sensitivity, they have the potential to stimulate positive growth like the tree described in this verse. Words can have a powerful and far-reaching impact, even beyond the lives of the immediate clients.

Unfortunately, when working with Muslim clients, practitioners are often unsure of what words to use, what techniques to implement, or how to judge the success of interventions. They are mystified when trying to understand why well-intentioned efforts do not produce the intended results. Searching for answers or guidance can be difficult. Postgraduate training textbooks do not include information on Muslims, and thus even Muslim practitioners may be at a loss as to which theories or interventions are better suited to Muslim clients. The popular media is tainted with misconceptions and prejudice, and the scholarly literature is only now beginning to emerge, with numerous gaping holes to fill.

The availability of culturally competent practitioners has not kept pace with the growing number of Muslims in the West who are seeking formal mental health services. This increase in service utilization can be largely attributed to struggles coping with acculturation challenges, stressors ensuing from the sociopolitical climate of the post-9/11 world, and increasing mental health awareness. The fact that Muslims are bypassing significant cultural stigma and shame to access mental health services indicates not only a need for such services, but also a greater trust in mental health professionals. Unfortunately, there is a lack of practical, useful sources of information for this population.

This handbook aims to be a resource for mental health professionals in guiding them to provide religio-culturally competent care, thereby fulfilling their clients' trust. It also compiles the latest research as a resource for scholars. It goes beyond previous publications on this topic (which focus mostly on introducing the reader to the Islamic faith and Muslims' cultures) by providing specific recommendations and examples for effective mental health service provision. Authors have painstakingly synthesized the latest research literature with their own clinical wisdoms as well as the feedback of their clients and communities. This has produced unique and powerful insights on the conceptualization and implementation of mental health interventions for Muslim clients.

This book is distinct in its scope, content, and format. Previous mental health literature conflated Muslim and Arab communities, or emphasized heavily the experiences of immigrants and refugees. Instead, this book offers relevance to the realities of the heterogeneous and multicultural Muslim community, including persons born in the West, converts to Islam, and those from smaller ethnic minorities. Moreover, unlike the previous discourse, which has been largely limited to individual psychotherapy, chapters in this book reflect interventions at various levels of ecological analysis, ranging from the individual to the wider community.

Issues and interventions discussed in this book are diverse and multifaceted. The book introduces topics that have been virtually ignored in the literature such as assessment interviewing, psychological testing, humanistic-experiential therapies, sex therapy, substance abuse counseling, university counseling, and community-based prevention.

The book begins by contextualizing the faith and worldviews of Muslims by exploring Islamic beliefs and practices, religious and cultural mental health concepts, and traditional coping and help-seeking behaviors. The second section details various interventions and approaches that may be effective with Muslim populations. This section reviews case formulation and psychological assessment, in addition to individual, family, and community-level models. The third section addresses the diverse needs of Muslims in different service settings, specifically inpatient, home-based, and college counseling centers. Fourth is a section focused on segments of the Muslim community that are often misunderstood, namely converts, youth, and refugees. Finally, the fifth section highlights sensitive issues needing attention, specifically the topics of domestic violence, sexual dysfunction, and substance abuse.

Readers of this book, whether they are practitioners, researchers, service administrators, or students, will find the material straightforward and easy to follow. Chapters integrate tables, lists, and suggested phrasing for practitioners; these are all aimed at presenting the concepts in a useful manner. Most distinct to this book, however, are the embedded case studies that are used by the authors to help illustrate concepts and potential interventions. These cases challenge the reader to think more deeply about the material as well as how to reframe psychological concepts and techniques in a religiously meaningful manner.

It is the sincere hope of the editors and the authors that this book enables mental health professionals to use the immense power of words to stimulate positive growth and development in the tree of humanity.

PART I
Muslim Beliefs Within a Counseling Framework

CHAPTER 1
Islam, Muslims, and Mental Health

AMBER HAQUE and NAJEEB KAMIL

Muslims constitute approximately 23% of the world's population and serve as a majority in approximately 50 countries around the globe (Miller, 2009). Although Islam dates back more than 1,400 years and has roots in Western nations for many centuries, interest in Islam and Muslims prior to the 9/11 incidents in America was minimal. However, 9/11 and the subsequent attacks in Madrid and London led to an increased visibility of Muslims and an interest in Islam. These events, in addition to the growing diversity and multicultural awareness in Western countries, has resulted in increased curiosity about Islam, how Muslims conduct their daily lives, and what the Qur'an preaches. Despite the increased interest in Islam, the average person has very little knowledge about the religion and its followers (Pew, 2007).

Lack of knowledge about the beliefs and values of a religious group that is under continuous scrutiny can be problematic within a clinical setting, especially in light of the potential importance spirituality may have for a client. The spiritual perspective posits that one of the main sources of clients' strengths is their spirituality, which can be used to help clients face their problems and obstacles (Sermabeikian, 1994). The spiritual perspective complements well the strengths perspective in which clients' personal and environmental strengths are emphasized in the recovery process (Hodge, 2001). Therefore, it is important for mental health practitioners to have knowledge about the basic beliefs and practices of Islam. In addition, they should be aware of common misconceptions about Islam and their impact on the psychological well-being of Muslims. This would increase and strengthen the therapeutic relationship between the client and the practitioner, thus forming the foundation from which the therapeutic process can progress. Knowledge of Islam can also bring to the forefront any biases a practitioner may have and decrease the negative impact of transference or countertransference. Lastly, it is important for the practitioner to realize that Muslims range in religious adherence, much like followers of other religions.

This chapter begins by presenting the basic tenets of Islam to orient the clinician about beliefs and practices that may be integral to clients' lives and potentially be incorporated in treatment. Second, the importance of psychology in Islam will be highlighted in order to provide a starting point for clinicians working with Muslim clients. Third, some basic demographic information is presented regarding Muslims living as minorities in the West so that clinicians can be aware of the possible cultural issues intermixed with the religious issues facing Muslims. Finally, a discussion of important contemporary issues facing Muslims in the West and the clinical ramifications will be presented.

Basic Tenets of Islam

Islam comes from the Arabic root word meaning peace. The word *aslama* is derived from these letters and refers to the one who has submitted to Allah, Arabic for God. The name Allah was a term used to refer to God even before the Qur'an, the Muslim holy book, was revealed and continues to be used today by Arabic-speaking Jews and Christians.

Islam is a monotheistic religion and asserts that since the beginning of time, Allah has sent to nations numerous prophets or messengers who brought the message of *tawhid*, or the Oneness of God. Examples of earlier prophets include Solomon, David, Noah, Moses, Abraham, Ismail, and Jesus. Muslims not only believe and are taught to respect previous prophets, they are also instructed not to deny the Truth in other religions sent to humankind. Islam preaches the same principles given by Abraham, and therefore is one of the three *Abrahamic* religions, which also includes Christianity and Judaism.

There are six basic beliefs in Islam. The first is to have faith in Allah. According to Islamic beliefs, Allah created everything and is All-Powerful. The second belief is the existence of angels who also obey Allah. The third belief is in the prophets and messengers of God and that Prophet Muhammad was the last prophet. Muslims also believe in all the religious texts revealed by God such as the Bible, Torah, and the Qur'an. However, they also believe that additions and deletions were made to the previous religious texts by their followers. As such, the Prophet Muhammad was sent to spread the final Message, which is considered to be the same, word-for-word, as it was 1,400 years ago. Thus, the Qur'an is the book of guidance for Muslims. The fifth belief is the existence of the Day of Judgment when individuals will be resurrected in front of God and be judged according to their deeds. The last basic belief is the belief in *Al-Qadr,* or predestination. Muslims believe that God knows what will happen to an individual, but at the same time the individual has free will. This last belief in predestination is important for the clinician as it could undermine a Muslim client's willingness and ability to engage in the change process. Free will is a major component of this belief, which Muslim clients may not acknowledge, and the clinician can highlight. In addition, understanding the beliefs of Muslims will enable clinicians to avoid making misdiagnoses, as in the case of a patient's mention of the presence of angels, which could be interpreted as a psychotic delusion.

In addition to the main beliefs, there are five pillars, or essential practices, in Islam. The *Shahadah,* or the belief that there is only one God and Muhammad is the last messenger, is the central pillar. The second pillar is *salah,* performing the five daily prayers. The third is *sawm,* or fasting, refraining from eating or drinking from dawn to sunset, during the month of Ramadan. The fourth pillar is *zakat,* giving charity to the poor and needy. The last pillar is *hajj,* performing pilgrimage to the holy city of Makkah, if one is able to financially and physically. Religious practices can influence treatment. For example, patients may not be able to schedule sessions at certain times because of conflicts with prayer times. In addition, some rituals can be incorporated into the client's treatment plan, such as praying or reading the Qur'an to relieve stress or fast to overcome negative desires that may contribute to depression. It is important to mention here that Muslims, like any other followers of a religion, have varied levels of religiosity, and it is critical for a clinician to explore the role and importance of Islam to the individual client during the intake assessment.

Sources of Muslim Legal Code

Understanding the Islamic legal code and process of legislation will help the clinician appreciate how Muslims may arrive at different perspectives and practices on a particular issues. For example, there are various views held by Islamic scholars on issues such as conflict management, divorce, parenting, and the roles and responsibilities of spouses. During a counseling session, different family members can present conflicting views that may be confusing if the sources of legal code are not understood. The clinician can assist them in understanding each other's perspective or coming to a compromise without being confused by the apparent conflict in religious perspectives.

In order to act in accordance with Islamic beliefs, Muslims turn to the Qur'an, the Muslim Book of Guidance, and the *hadith*, sayings of the Prophet Mohammad, which provide the basic structure of the laws of human conduct, also known as *Shariah* or Divine Laws. The literal meaning of *shariah* is "to introduce" or "prescribe." *Shariah* is more than just rules about religious rituals, and civil and criminal matters—it also includes ethical and moral principles. Unfortunately, *shariah* is discussed in negative terms by ideologues and propagated through the different media outlets, and is described as a set of laws that Muslims want to enforce on the world regarding criminal punishments.

Islamic jurisprudence or *fiqh* is based on *shariah* or Divine Laws. These laws cover ways of worship, right and wrong, and dealings in one's everyday lives, including business transactions, family issues, societal issues, etc. Although all prophets preached the same faith, the Divine Laws each prophet brought were suited for their specific time and helped to build a civilized and moral society. Muslims believe that Muhammad, as the last prophet of Allah, brought the final version of the Divine Laws, which apply to all of humanity and for all times. Islamic jurisprudence is derived primarily from the Qur'an and *Sunnah* and is dynamic in nature because individual and societal considerations are taken into account. The Qur'an is considered the Word of Allah, and is understood to have stronger proofs than the *sunnah*, or the sayings, actions, and attitudes of Prophet Muhammad. The details of the application of Islam in everyday life may not always be explained in the Qur'an. As such, Muslims rely on the Prophet's *Sunnah* for such guidance. As a result, there is much attention dedicated to the verification and authentication of sayings and actions of Prophet Mohammad, and depending on the scholar and the importance given to the different criteria for authentication, one can find more than one opinion on an issue.

For matters that fall beyond the direct orders written explicitly in the Qur'an or espoused by the Prophet's sayings, actions, and attitudes, Islamic scholars use juristic consensus (*ijma*) or analogy (*qiyas*). *Ijma* refers to a consensus on an issue by Islamic scholars. *Qiyas* refers to laws that are made by analogy. For example, wine is forbidden in Islam due to its intoxicating effects, so by *analogy* other intoxicating drugs are also forbidden by Islamic law. When other jurists do not agree on *qiyas*, one can follow juristic preference (*istihsan*) between two analogies, which can also result in differing scholarly interpretations on a particular issue. At certain times, Islamic rulings can be made in the interest of the society, balancing individual and collective rights. Islamic law also allows for the inclusion of local social norms and customs into consideration, as long as the local norms and customs do not contradict the principles of the Qur'an and *Sunnah*.

In addition to rules on dealing with one's everyday life, Islamic jurisprudence also covers mental health. Islamic law governing mental illness and insanity dates back to the seventh and eighth centuries. Islamic laws also address patient confidentiality, insanity defense, involuntary hospitalization and treatment, mental competencies, family laws related to the mentally handicapped, child custody issues, child abuse and child witness, etc. A book by Chaleby (2001) covers citations of original sources in detail, and Haque (2002) covers its critical review.

Historical Perspective

It may be helpful for the clinician to understand the historical context from which Muslims have obtained their code of conduct, how the advent of Islam in Arabia caused a moral conflict, and what Muslims find inspiring in the history of Islam. In addition, allowing Muslim clients to speak about the history of Islam from their perspective promotes a "shedding the cloak of the expert who knows best" and provides the clinician critical information about the beliefs and values of the client (Brandell, 2010).

Muhammad was born in Mecca in 570 A.D., and it was in his 40th year that he started receiving his revelations and preaching Islam. As a result of conveying the message of Islam, Muhammad was tortured by his tribesmen, who tried to kill him on many occasions. He preached monotheism and perfecting one's character while in Mecca. After 13 years of persecution, Muhammad migrated to Medina where he established the first Muslim community. In Medina, Prophet Muhammad continued to teach Islam to people. Much of the *shariah* was revealed in Medina, and Muhammad elaborated on the rituals in Islam for the Muslim community. It was also in Medina that Muhammad began to teach people general concepts of justice, freedom, tolerance, and understanding. He made treaties with nearby tribes and groups that consisted of people of other faiths. The Arabs from Mecca fought battles with the Muslims on multiple occasions in an effort to eradicate Islam in its infancy stage, but were not successful. By the time he died in 633 A.D., the entire Arabian Peninsula had adopted Islam (al-Mubarkpuri, 2002).

After the Prophet's death, a political difference emerged over views on who should become the successor of Prophet Muhammad. The Muslims at the time were divided into two different groups. The first group believed that the caliphate, or successor, should have remained within the Prophet's family (Shi'a). The second group believed that the caliph should be chosen through an elective process (Sunni). Modern-day Sunni and Shi'a share basic Islamic beliefs but differ in their interpretation of Islamic jurisprudence.

Contributions to Psychology

Muslim scholars have made major contributions to the arts and sciences, especially in the area of psychology (Haque, 2004b; Badri, 2000). Muslims were pioneers in specializations such as child development, social psychology, psychotherapy, and cognitive psychology. For example, Abu Zaid Al-Balkhi, a cognitive psychologist, was the first to differentiate between neuroses and psychoses and came up with a treatment approach similar to Joseph Wolpe's reciprocal inhibition. Abu Bakr Mohammad Ibn Zakariya al-Razi (Rhazes), an early psychologist, promoted psychotherapy and was a master of psychological, psychosomatic, and organic disorders (Haque, 2004b). Ibn Sina, also known as Avecenna, wrote about the mind and its relationship to the body by linking physical and psychological illnesses, and used psychological techniques to treat his patients (Haque, 2004b). Islamic psychology differs from contemporary psychology as it incorporates religion and studies the soul of an individual (Haque, 2004b).

Islam has a long and deep legacy in the field of psychology. It is necessary for clinicians to be aware of these historical contributions to psychology, as clinicians may come across Muslim clients who are resistant to the idea of therapy and counseling, believing that it is something foreign and of no value. A clinician can incorporate in therapy some of the terminology used by historical Muslim psychologists. For example, a clinician may utilize specific terms such as *qalb*, or heart, to delve into how clients are feeling and why they are feeling this way. Another term that can be used is *irada*, or will, to investigate where a client is in the process of change. Incorporating these terms in sessions can also help a clinician solidify the clinician–client relationship and provide important insights into the client's issues.

Demographics of Muslims Living in Western Countries

There are approximately 1.57 billion Muslims living in 232 countries around the world, representing 23% of an estimated 2009 world population of 6.8 billion (Pew Research Center, 2009). Table 1.1 provides a more detailed description of the Muslim population distributed in major Western nations.

Considering that Muslims reside in 232 countries around the world, they constitute a multitude of ethnicities, and Muslims in Western countries are ethnically diverse. In addition, Muslims have a long history in Western countries. There are records that reveal early Muslim arrivals in the United States starting from the 10th century (Nyang, 1999). Enslaved Muslims from Africa are documented to be the first Muslim community in the United States (Diouf, 1998). A large wave of Muslim immigration to the United States took place in the second half of the 19th century,

Table 1.1 Demographics of Muslims Living in Western Countries

Country	Muslim Population
Australia	340,000
Belgium	500,000
Bulgaria	920,000
Denmark	200,000
Canada	657,000
France	3,554,000
Germany	4,026,000
Netherlands	946,000
Sweden	325,000
United Kingdom	1,647,000
United States	4,000,000

Source: Pew Research Center, 2009.

primarily from the Middle East for economic reasons. Muslims from other backgrounds immigrated throughout the 1900s. Muslim emigration to Europe began as early as the seventh century starting with Spain, through invasion and trade. Another large wave of Muslim immigration to Europe was in the 1960s and 1970s from European colonies.

There are stark differences in the socioeconomic makeup of Muslims in Europe and the United States. Muslims in Europe are mainly of South Asian, Arab, or Turkish origin and are more likely to be laborers working in low-paying jobs (Open Society Institute [OSI], 2005, 2010). They report discrimination with regard to employment, education, and the criminal justice system (OSI, 2010). As a result, there appears to be greater resistance by European Muslims toward assimilating into their respective country's culture, while American Muslims appear to have assimilated to a greater degree and have adopted the American outlook, values, and attitudes (Pew Research Center, 2007). In addition, Muslim Americans are mainly of middle-class socioeconomic status, although there are significant populations that are underserved (Pew Research Center, 2007).

Contemporary Issues Facing Muslims in the West

Since the September 11, 2001, terrorist attacks, numerous misconceptions and attacks on Muslims and Islam have been propagated by the media and various political figures. It is important for the clinician to be aware of these misconceptions as they may have a negative impact on the Muslim psyche, especially on children and adolescents who are already struggling with identity issues. In addition, understanding these misconceptions can help clinicians to be aware of biases they may have and prevent possible misinterpretations of Muslim clients' behaviors. This section will highlight some of the major issues facing Muslims in the West today including Islamophobia, women in Islam, and *jihad*.

Islamophobia

The 9/11 attacks, and those in London and Madrid, have increased the social phenomenon called "Islamophobia." Such developments have led some Western governments and politicians to consider the Islamic belief system and practices as a threat to the Western lifestyle. The attacks have instilled fear and negativity toward Muslims by those living in the West as manifested by increased hate crimes, discrimination, and profiling (Ghazali, 2002). The media has also played a major role in creating negative attitudes toward Muslims by providing a forum to Islamophobes and disseminating misconceptions about Islam (Sheridan, 2006). Misinformation and stereotyping has led to discriminatory actions and policies that have negatively affected Muslims (Haque, 2004a; Berlin, 2002). Inayat (2002) found that post 9/11, British Muslims reported feelings of loss and confusion about their own faith and a need to be different from the perpetrators of the 9/11 attacks. In addition, other studies have found Muslims reporting decreased self-esteem and increased psychological stress post 9/11 (Moradi & Hasan, 2004). Therefore, it is critical for clinicians to explore and understand the social, cultural, and political context of Muslim clients when conducting a psychosocial assessment during intake.

Women in Islam

Given the misinformation about Islam and women, it is helpful for clinicians to understand the notions of gender equity in Islam, particularly because of its relevance when working in couple or marital counseling, as well as to identify possible bias or assumptions the clinician may unconsciously maintain.

In pre-Islamic Arabia, women were considered of low status and giving birth to a girl was considered dishonorable. Islam introduced a paradigm shift in the way women were viewed in society. The Qur'an teaches humankind that God created men and women from a single soul (Qur'an 4:1) and that it is not the gender, but the acts of righteousness and faith, that will determine their status with God (Qur'an 49:13).

Although men and women are equal, their innate differences give rise to occasional different social roles or rules as evidenced by familial financial responsibility, inheritance laws, and clothing requirements. For example, males are financially responsible for their family, whereas females are not and may use their wealth however they choose. However, as a result men may receive a greater inheritance than a female, depending on the relationship to the deceased kin and the presence of other relatives. In Islam, a woman enjoys absolute equality with regard to civil and criminal laws. A woman's life, honor, and property are as sacred and sacrosanct as that of a man. If a woman is wronged she receives the same compensation as that of a man.

A related issue regarding the status of women in Islam is marriage. Monogamy is the norm in Muslim marriages, but polygamy is allowed in Islam under certain conditions, such as in war-torn regions where men have been killed, or to have children when one's wife is sterile. This kind of marital arrangement provides the woman her individual needs including cohabitation, family support, the ability to raise her own family, and fulfillment of her emotional and sexual needs. However, if such a family arrangement is made, the man is required to be able to provide financially, emotionally, sexually, etc., equally, which is difficult. In Western societies, polygamous marriages are uncommon but do exist. However, these marriages are often not legal and are viewed negatively by society.

It is important to realize that while Islam demands respect for all women, the influences of personalities, local customs, and cultures may lead to practices that are often in violation of Islamic laws.

Jihad and Terrorism

Many, including some Muslims, misunderstand the notion of jihad in Islam. Jihad is a term that has been used synonymously with Islamic extremism and thus translated as a "holy war" (a term synonymous with the Crusades in Christianity). Jihad is not holy war but a "struggle" in the most comprehensive sense, beginning with the self. Jihad can refer to controlling selfish wishes and desires for the purpose of enhancing the level of one's *nafs* or desires. For example, when a person experiences depression the challenge of changing their negative cognitions may be considered jihad. The Qur'an permits Muslims to defend themselves from aggression, but it also prohibits Muslims from being the aggressors. It is important to point out that fighting and warfare was a very small part of jihad (Armstrong, 1993). Prophet Muhammad informed his followers that the "greater jihad" is the struggle against one's desires and committing sins. Consequently, if clients are religious, the clinician can help them reframe their presenting problem as a personal jihad.

A related issue is that of Muslims using suicide bombings. Taking an innocent life, including one's own, is prohibited in Islam, as evidenced by the following verse:

> Because of this did We ordain unto the children of Israel that if anyone slays a human being—unless it be [in punishment] for murder or for spreading corruption on earth—it shall be as though he had slain all mankind; whereas, if anyone saves a life, it shall be as though he

had saved the lives of all mankind. And, indeed, there came unto them Our apostles with all evidence of the truth: yet, behold, notwithstanding all this, many of them go on committing all manner of excesses on earth. (Qur'an 5:32)

Muslims in a Post-9/11 World

Muslims living in the West, especially those who are immigrants and refugees, may face issues of alienation, identity, and nostalgia of homeland, which may challenge their ability to acculturate into society. The 9/11 terrorist attacks have exacerbated these challenges because Muslims no longer feel safe and wanted (Ghazali, 2002). Terrorism has increased hostility toward Muslims in many Western countries, as evidenced by an increase in hate crimes, and Muslims have started to reassess the meaning of their presence (Ghazali, 2002). They are beset with psychological issues that are varied and complex. Muslims that appear to be Arab or South Asian are treated with suspicion, and some have been arrested based on vague claims, such as possibly intending to commit acts of terrorism without direct evidence (Zaal, Salah, & Fine, 2007). Consequently, many youth are confused as they try to reconcile what appears to them to be contradictory identities (Balsano & Sirin, 2007). Clinicians may encounter this type of identity crisis in younger children as well as older Muslims. A thorough exploration of how different environments may affect a Muslim's psyche (family, friends, neighborhood, community, and country) should occur.

Conclusion

Clinicians have traditionally approached clients from a "faith blind" perspective, but spirituality and religion are often powerful client strengths. The ecological perspective consists of five domains: historical, environmental, cultural, family, and individual (Pardeck, 1996). Spirituality and religion play key roles in how a client views these domains and how each domain interacts with the other. It is important for clinicians to understand a client's spirituality because it may provide relevant information regarding the client's worldview (Hodge, 2005). As Muslim populations in the West continue to grow, the challenge of providing Muslim clients with culturally appropriate mental health services needs to be addressed. Clinicians can overcome this challenge by educating themselves about the influence of an Islamic worldview on the mental health of Muslim clients in the context of present-day society. In addition, utilizing Islam and resources in the Muslim community can provide more positive outcomes for clinicians working with Muslim clients.

References

Al-Mubarkpuri, S. (2002). *The sealed nectar: Biography of the noble Prophet.* Houston, TX: Dar-us-Salam Publications.
Armstrong, K. (1993). *Muhammad: A biography of the Prophet,* Harper: San Francisco.
Badri, M. (2000). *Contemplation: An early psychospiritual study.* London: UK: Cambridge University Press.
Balsano, A.B. and Sirin, S.R. (2007). Commentary on the Special Issue of ADS Muslim Youth in the West: "collateral damage" we cannot afford to disregard. *Applied Development Science,* 11, 3, 178–183.
Berlin, F. T. (2002). *Muslims in the USA after 9/11.* Unpublished manuscript, American Council on Germany, New York.
Brandell, J. R. (2010). *Theory and practice in clinical social work.* Thousand Oaks, CA: Sage Publications.
Bunglawala, I (2002). British Muslims and the media, in Muslim Council of Britain, *The Quest for Sanity,* pp 43–52.
Chaleby, K. (2001). *Forensic psychiatry in Islamic jurisprudence.* Herndon, VA: International Institute of Islamic Thought.
Diouf, S. (1998). *Servants of Allah: African Muslims enslaved in the Americas.* New York, NY: New York University Press.
Ghazali, A. S. (2002). *Post 9/11 challenges: Hate crimes and discrimination.* Council on American-Islamic Relations. www.cair.org.
Haque, A. (2002). Review on *Forensic psychiatry in Islamic jurisprudence* by Kuteba Chaleby, *American Journal of Islamic Social Sciences,* 19(3), 111–114.
Haque, A. (2004a). Islamophobia in North America: Confronting the menace. In P. Batelaan and B. Van Driel (Eds.), *Islamophobia in educational settings.* pp. 1–8. London, UK: Trentham House.
Haque, A. (2004b). Psychology from an Islamic perspective: Contributions of early Muslim scholars to psychology and the challenges to contemporary Muslim psychologists. *Journal of Religion and Health,* 43(4), 367–387.
Hodge, D. R. (2001). Spiritual assessment: A review of major qualitative methods and a new framework for assessing spirituality. *Social Work,* 46(3), 203–214.
Hodge, D. R. (2005). Spirituality in social work education: A development and discussion of goals that flow from the profession's ethical mandates. *Social Work Education,* 24(1), 37–55.
Miller, T. (2009). *Mapping the global Muslim population: A report on the size and distribution of the World's Muslim population.* Pew Research Center, www.pewresearch.org.
Moradi, B. and Hasan, N.T. (2004). Arab American persons' reported experiences of discrimination and mental health: The mediating role of personal control. *Journal of Counseling Psychology,* 51, 4, 418–428.
Nyang, S. S. (1999). *Islam in the United States of America.* Chicago, IL: ABC International Group, Inc.
Open Society Institute (OSI) (2005). *Muslims in the UK: Policies for engaged citizens. EU Monitoring and Advocacy Program.* Hungary: QED Publishing.
Open Society Institute (OSI) (2010). *A report on 11 EU cities. At Home in Europe Project.* Hungary: QED Publishing.

Pardeck, J. T. (1996). *Social work practice: An ecological approach.* Westport, CT: Greenwood Publishing Group.
Pew Research Center (2007). *Muslim Americans: Middle class and mostly mainstream.* www.pewresearch.org.
Pew Research Center (2009). *Mapping the global Muslim population.* www.pewresearch.org.
Sermabeikian, P. (1994). Our clients, ourselves: The spiritual perspective and social work practice. *Social Work, 39*(2), 178–183.
Sheridan, L. P. (2006). Islamophobia pre and post September 11th, 2001. *Journal of Interpersonal Violence, 21,* 317–336.
Zaal, M., Salah, T., & Fine, M. (2007). The weight of the hyphen: Freedom, fusion, and responsibility embodied by young Muslim-American women during a time of surveillance. *Applied Development Science, 11*(3), 164–177.

CHAPTER 2
Conceptualizations of Mental Health, Illness, and Healing

AISHA UTZ

In recent years, there has been a growing interest within the mental health professions regarding the link between religiosity/spirituality and mental health. Research that has been conducted thus far indicates that those who are more religious or spiritual tend to have better mental and physical health. Numerous studies have found a significant positive association between religiosity/spirituality and better mental health and well-being, defined as having more hope, optimism, purpose, and meaning in life; greater marital satisfaction and stability; and higher levels of social support. Religiosity has also been associated with less depression and faster recovery from depression, less anxiety, lower suicide rates, and less substance abuse (Koenig, 2008; Koenig, McCullough, & Larson, 2001).

Although most of this research has been conducted with Christian populations in the West, two recent literature reviews of a mounting body of evidence with Muslim populations suggests that religiosity/spirituality also benefits the mental health of Muslim adherents (Abu-Raiya & Pargament, 2010; Hamdan & Oman, submitted for publication). The general conclusion from these studies is that Muslims who are religious/spiritual and practice their faith experience higher levels of happiness, well-being, life satisfaction, and marital satisfaction, and have a reduced likelihood of depression, anxiety, death anxiety, antisocial behavior, and suicide.

Abu-Raiya and Pargament (2010) concluded that the Islamic faith provides comfort, meaning, identity, spirituality, and community for its followers. Two factors, positive religious coping and intrinsic religiosity, were noted to be consistently and positively linked to well-being outcomes. According to the research, Muslims commonly use religious coping during tribulations and times of stress (Hamdan & Oman, submitted for publication). Religious coping is generally defined as the "process that people engage in to attain significance and meaning in stressful circumstances" (Pargament, 1997, p. 90). It may provide meaning to the tribulation and provide explanations for such concepts as suffering, good versus evil, and guilt. The more stressful the situation, the more likely people are to use religion to cope.

This chapter presents Muslims' conceptualizations of mental health and illness. It begins with a discussion of the causal explanations and purposes of mental illness, which covers a variety of issues. Prevention, healing, and treatment are considered with emphasis on clinical applications. Some attention is given to cultural variations in Muslims' explanations and treatment for mental health concerns. Finally, an illustrative case study is presented to demonstrate and highlight key points.

View of Physical and Mental Health

Effective coping can be influenced by an individual's understanding of the meaning of health and illness. From the perspective of Islam, physical and mental health is considered to be a bounty from Allah[1] and a trust that should be preserved. The Prophet Muhammad (peace and blessings be upon him) said, "There are two blessings which many people lose: [They are] health and free time for doing good" (Al-Bukhari, Book 74, no. 2091 as cited in Az-zubaidi, 1996, p. 981).[2]

It is also understood in Islam that Allah may test humans through various trials, including physical and/or psychological illnesses. It is believed that the purpose of these tests is to determine if the afflicted person will be patient, rely upon Allah in times of distress, and/or view the experience as an opportunity for spiritual growth and purification. In this regard, mental illness is not distinct from physical illness, although it tends to have a greater cultural stigma attached to it. It is also not uncommon in the Muslim world to find psychological ailments manifested as physical symptoms (i.e., somatization), which may be related to attempts to avoid the stigmatization of mental illness (Al-Krenawi & Graham, 2000).

---

[1] Allah is the Arabic word for God, which will be used throughout this chapter.
[2] Hadith are the sayings of the Prophet Muhammad (peace and blessings be upon him), which are second to the Qur'an as a source of legal textual evidence. For that reason they are cited frequently throughout this chapter.

Causes of Mental Illness

There are various conceptualizations as to the causes of mental illness in the Islamic framework. These may include biological, psychological, environmental, spiritual, or supernatural. Each of these will be discussed in some detail with relevant supporting evidence provided. More emphasis will be given to spiritual and supernatural explanations as the others are more widely known. Further information will be provided in a later section as to how these beliefs may impact the Muslim client's attitudes, beliefs, and approach to mental health.

Biological, Psychological, and Environmental Theories

Some mental illnesses may be purely biological in nature or may be triggered or exacerbated by stressful life events, negative thinking, or environmental circumstances (e.g., poverty). In Islam, scientific exploration and inquiry are encouraged and, as such, these theories are plausible explanations that may be incorporated into the Islamic conceptualization of mental illness. In fact, historical accounts of 13th- and 14th-century Muslim scholars indicate that they proposed biological causes for some mental disorders (Philips, 1997, p. 92).

The Prophet Muhammad (peace and blessings be upon him) alluded to biological, psychological, and environmental attributions to disease in several of his sayings. He said, "There is no disease that Allah has sent down except that He also has sent down its treatment" (Al-Bukhari, Vol. 7, Book 76, no. 5678 as cited in Khan, 1997, p. 326). He also said, "Every illness has a cure, and when the proper cure is applied to the disease, it ends it, Allah willing" (Muslim as cited in al-Jauziyyah, 2003, p. 24). These and other sayings of the Prophet (peace and blessings be upon him) are general and may refer to various types of diseases, including mental illness. The sayings point to the notion that there may be biological or psychological causes for diseases for which Allah has sent down a cure. It is upon human beings to discover the cure and apply it to the appropriate cases.

There are several examples of environmental or situational factors in the Qur'an and *ahadith*. A famous story involves that of Prophet Joseph (Yusuf, peace be upon him) and his younger brother, Benjamin (Binyamin). At a young age, Joseph's older brothers had intended to kill him because of their jealousy of him, but decided instead to place him in a well, and a caravan of travelers found him who took him to Egypt. His father, Prophet Jacob (Yacub), was deeply saddened by this loss and questioned the brothers' story that a wolf had indeed eaten Joseph. Years later, Benjamin was also taken away. Jacob's reaction to the loss of Binyamin is related in the Qur'an: "And he turned away from them (the older brothers who related the story) and said, 'O, my sorrow over Joseph,' and his eyes became white (he lost his sight) from grief, for he was [of that] a suppressor" (Qur'an 12:84). This verse indicates that when Prophet Jacob thought he had lost his second son, it brought back memories of the first son (Joseph). He was overcome by grief to such an extent that he lost his sight. He did not express the intensity of his grief or anger, but was patient and relied on Allah for help. This story illustrates the strong influence of situational factors in a human's life that may lead to psychological distress (or mental illness). Many Muslim patients will believe in environmental influences, and it may be an important consideration during the treatment process.

Spiritual Disease

Muslims may believe that mental illness is related to spiritual disease or distancing from Allah. This does not necessarily mean that everyone who suffers from mental illness is morally deficient, but detachment from Allah may increase the likelihood of difficulties. For example, a person with weak faith may struggle with understanding certain stressful life events or be more easily affected by the influence of the *jinn*.[3] Allah mentions the effect of turning away from Him: "And whoever turns away from My remembrance—indeed, he will have a depressed [i.e., difficult] life, and We will gather [i.e., raise] him on the Day of Resurrection blind" (Qur'an 20:124).

Those who turn away from the remembrance of Allah may experience an onerous life. This refers to the many types of difficulties that a human may experience such as depression, anxiety, and grief, as well as various stressful events. Ibn Kathir[4] explains this verse as meaning that the individual's life will be difficult in this world. He or she will not find tranquility, but rather his or her heart will be constrained due to misguidance. Even if he or she appears to others to be at ease and in comfort, he or she will not be happy inside as his or her heart will lack pure certainty and guidance. He or she will be in agitation, bewilderment, confusion, and doubt. This is from the greatest hardships of life (Ibn Kathir, 2000, p. 406). This does not imply that all individuals who are distanced from Allah will suffer from mental illness, but it does increase the likelihood. On the other hand, those who are close to Allah reflect upon His Mercy and the bounties that He has bestowed upon the individual, are less likely to have negative thoughts about self, others, or the future, and are less likely to experience depression or anxiety.

---

[3] *Jinn* are a type of creation of Allah distinct from humans and angels. They are discussed in more detail later in the chapter.

[4] Ibn Kathir was a well-known 12th-century Islamic scholar. His explanation of the Qur'an, Tafsir Ibn Kathir, is believed to be the most widely used explanation of the Qur'an in the modern world.

Supernatural Explanations

Various verses in the Qur'an and the Hadith mention the existence of supernatural beings. As such, Muslims may attribute their mental illnesses to supernatural forces. There are four possible methods by which Muslims may feel they have been influenced: whispering, magic, evil eye, and possession. These effects are thought to occur through the influence of evil *jinn* or through humans working with the evil *jinn*. The *jinn* are a type of being, distinct from humans and angels, who were created from fire. This is mentioned several times in the Qur'an including the following verse: "And We created the jinn from a smokeless flame of fire" (Qur'an 55:15). *Jinn* are believed to live in a world of their own, but may interact with and influence the world of humans. They are considered to have some characteristics like humans, including the ability to reason and to choose between good and evil (al-Ashgar, 1998, p. 5). For this reason, there are Muslim *jinn* who submit to Allah, as well as evil *jinn* who disobey Allah and are involved in the harming of humans.

Whispering (Waswaas) Muslims believe that one of the primary ways by which the evil *jinn* influence humans is through whispering and affecting their thoughts and feelings. It was the whispering of Satan (who is a *jinn*) that led Adam to disobey Allah's command: "Then Satan whispered to him; he said, 'O Adam, shall I direct you to the tree of eternity and possession that will not deteriorate?'" (Qur'an 20:120). In addition to whispering from the *jinn*, whispering may also come from the soul itself. The purpose of the whispering is to mislead humans to engage in negative behaviors and to avoid acts of worship. Some Muslims may attribute symptoms of obsessive-compulsive disorder, for example, to the whisperings of *jinn*.

Magic (Sihr) Magic (*sihr*) is believed to involve spoken or written incantation, or actions that will affect the body, heart, or mind of the bewitched individual without making contact with him or her (Philips, 1997, p. 98). This may be caused by evil *jinns* and includes sorcery, witchcraft, and divination. Some Muslim patients may attribute their mental health or life problems to the effects of magic carried out against them by other people. Muslim scholars believe in the existence of magic as evidenced in the following Qur'anic verse.

> And they followed [instead] what the devils had recited during the reign of Solomon. It was not Solomon who disbelieved, but the devils disbelieved, teaching people magic and that which was revealed to the two angels at Babylon, Harut and Marut. But they [i.e., the two angels] do not teach anyone unless they say, "We are a trial, so do not disbelieve [by practicing magic]." (Qur'an 2:102)

Evil Eye (Al-'Ayn or Nazr) and Envy (Hasad)   Another means by which some Muslims believe the *jinn* may psychologically influence humans is through the use of the evil eye (*al-'ayn* or *nazr*). The concept of evil eye involves a process in which the envious glance of one person causes harm to another, primarily due to envy *(hasad)* or desiring that which is possessed by another. Some Muslims believe that the harmful effect is due to the evil *jinn*, not the eye itself (Philips, 1997, p. 108). The envying individual may also act upon his or her feelings and do something harmful to the one whom he or she envies. It should be mentioned that envy is more general than evil eye. All those who look with an evil eye are envious, but every envier does not put the evil eye on the envied person. The existence of this concept is mentioned in the following verse of the Qur'an: "And I seek refuge from the evil of an envier when he envies" (Qur'an 114:5). The Prophet (peace and blessings be upon him) also said, "The effect of the evil eye is real for if there were anything which could overtake destiny, it would have been [the effect of] the evil eye" (Al-Bukhari and Muslim as cited in Philips, 1997, p. 108).

Possession by Jinn   Clients who present for therapy may attribute their symptoms to *jinn* possession. Although there is a difference of opinion among religious scholars regarding the existence and validity of *jinn* possession, those who believe that *jinns* are capable of possession often cite the Qur'anic verse (2:275) as well as *hadiths* to support their belief. One *hadith* that describes this phenomenon is an incident in which the Prophet was passing a mother whose son suffered from "fits." She informed the Prophet of her son's affliction and requested his assistance. The Prophet (peace and blessings be upon him) said,

> "Give him to me." So she lifted him up to the Prophet. He then placed the boy between himself and the middle of the saddle, opened the boy's mouth and blew in it three times, saying, "In the name of Allah; I am the slave of Allah. Get out, enemy of Allah!" (Ahmad and al-Hakim as cited in Philips, 1997, pp. 81–82)

The Prophet was ordering the *jinn* to leave the boy, and after this incident, the boy no longer experienced fits.

As noted in this *hadith*, epileptic fits represent one possible physical manifestation of *jinn* possession (although most epilepsy is organic in nature). Other physical symptoms attributed to *jinn* possession may include unusual strength, catatonic symptoms, voice changes, anesthesia to pain, and psychosomatic pains (Philips, 1997, pp. 144–145). Symptoms may also be psychological in nature. In fact, the word *majnoon* in Arabic, literally meaning insane or a mad person, suggests that such a person is possessed by the *jinn*, as both words come from the same linguistic root. Some of the psychological symptoms attributed to *jinn* possession by Muslims may include changes in personality or behavior (e.g., mood swings, depression, uncontrollable laughing or crying, isolation), cognitive changes (clouding of consciousness, speaking an unfamiliar language or meaningless speech, nightmares, insomnia) (Philips, 1997, pp. 144–145). There may also be spiritual changes due to *jinn* possession, such as abandonment of religious practices and/or negative reactions to the recitation of the Qur'an (Philips, 1997, p. 145).

Clinical Implications Related to Supernatural Beliefs   Due to evidence from religious texts, many Muslims continue to believe in the effects of whispering, magic, the evil eye, and *jinn* possession and the harm that they may bring to people. Magic, for example, may be attributed to physical or psychological symptoms and cause sicknesses, marital or relationship problems, and other misfortunes in life. Clients participating in counseling may be reluctant to discuss these beliefs with a non-Muslim clinician, but they should be explored due to their potential influence on the therapeutic process and treatment outcomes. It is important to note that many Muslims may attribute their symptoms to supernatural causes, even when they are unrelated to the condition and evidence for biological or environmental factors are clearly present (e.g., a case of depression due to marital problems).

Cultural Variations in Explanations of Mental Illness
There is limited research on Muslim patients' explanations of mental illness in Western nations. Within the worldwide population of Muslims, there is a substantial amount of cultural variation, which is also manifested in explanatory models for mental illness and treatment approaches. Some of the similarities and differences will be discussed in the following section, but this is not meant to be an exhaustive representation of the topic.

It is interesting to note that although biological and psychosocial theories have advanced in modern times, Muslims may continue to adhere to the "supernatural" explanations for mental illness. These beliefs may be less common in Muslim groups living in Western countries, depending on the level of acculturation (Ismail, Wright, Rhodes, Small, & Jacoby, 2005). For example, in a recent qualitative study of Muslims in Britain, Weatherhead and Daiches (2010) reported that the majority of participants attributed mental illness to life events (e.g., stress). Religious causes, such as punishment from Allah or supernatural influences (witchcraft or *jinn*) were also mentioned, but were less prominent. However, these results have not always been consistent. In a study of Muslims in New York City, 84% of the sample stated belief in devil possession of the mentally ill person and 98% of the same sample agreed that life stressors were a test of faith (Abu-Ras, Gheith, & Cournos, 2008). Similarly, in a qualitative study of beliefs about epilepsy among South Asians in England, all informant groups (people with epilepsy, caregivers, and community groups) believed that epilepsy was caused by *jinn* possession, which may be a common belief among particular groups of Muslims living in the United Kingdom (Ismail et al., 2005).

In Western countries there are many Muslim immigrants and refugees; therefore, understanding the common cultural beliefs of country of origin could be helpful for the clinician. Arab patients, for example, may view the causes of psychiatric or psychological problems as external to themselves rather than biomedical in nature. This may include the influence of supernatural forces, such as the *jinn*, or the work of humans with the help of *jinn* through evil eye or magic. These beliefs do not seem to be related to educational level (Al-Krenawi & Graham, 2000; El-Islam & Abu-Dagga, 1992).

In a study of 45 faith healers[5] in Saudi Arabia, Al-Habeeb (2004) reported that faith healers recognized the psychological symptoms caused by evil eye, magic, or *jinn* possession. The most common symptoms associated with the spiritual disorders were anxiety, obsessions, and fear/doubt of developing disease. Other psychological symptoms reported included insomnia, depressive ideas, marital discord, hyperactivity, seizure-like states, psychotic disturbance, altered consciousness, abnormal movements, and somatic complaints (Al-Habeeb, 2004).

In a study of beliefs about mental illness in Malaysia, Razali, Khan, and Hasanah (1996) reported that 53% of 134 Malay patients (mainly Muslims) with mental illness attributed their illness to supernatural agents, the most common being witchcraft and possession by evil spirits. The belief in supernatural causes was not significantly associated with age, gender, level of education, or occupation of the patients. Haque (2005) noted that Malays also believe that psychological symptoms may be due to loss of "semangat" or soul substance, which leads to physical weakness and confusion. This is more of a cultural belief than a religious-based belief, although it may be related to the general belief that mental disorders are due to abandoning or neglecting Islamic values and practices. Another culturally-based belief among Malays is that gas in the stomach, nerves, and blood vessels contributes to hallucinations and delusions (Haque, 2005).

---

[5] Individuals who use prayers and rituals in order to bring about healing.

Purpose of Mental Illness

In Islam, mental illness may serve a function in this life whether or not humans are able to ascertain that purpose. The various purposes may include Allah testing the individual, expiation for sins, an opportunity for rewards, punishment or reminder, and/or purification of the soul. These concepts are often interrelated and are discussed in the following section.

Test and Trial from Allah

Muslims may believe that life consists of tests and tribulations intermingled with times of ease and enjoyment. Allah mentions in the Qur'an, "You will surely be tested in your possessions and in yourselves" (Qur'an 3:186). From this perspective, each test experienced has a purpose and a lesson by which to attain spiritual growth and purification. As mentioned earlier, mental illness may be one such test. Within this understanding, the individual can choose to be patient and seek Allah's assistance or to become defiant, ungrateful, and obstinate. An understanding of the purpose of this test is important for effective coping and treatment.

Expiation for Sins/Increase in Rewards

The pain or suffering of mental illness that an individual may face in this life may be contextualized within a religious framework as a cause for expiation of sins or result in an increase in good deeds and rewards. In either case, there is some benefit that is gained by the sufferer. The Prophet Muhammad (peace and blessings be upon him) said, "No fatigue, nor disease, nor sorrow, nor sadness, nor hurt, nor distress befalls a Muslim, even if it were the prick he receives from a thorn, but that Allah expiates some of his sins for that" (Al-Bukhari, Vol. 7, Book 75, no. 56451, 5642 as cited in Khan, 1997, p. 75). In relation to the Hereafter, tribulations in this world are considered advantageous for the human being because they can save him or her from the Hellfire or raise his status in Paradise. What humans may perceive as an evil affliction or torment can be viewed as a portion of Allah's mercy. This particular aspect may be used in psychotherapy to reframe the client's difficulty in a positive manner.

Punishment/Reminder from Allah

Those who have engaged in religiously prohibited behaviors may believe that their mental illness is a punishment or it may serve as a reminder to call the individual back to the "Straight Path."⁶ This belief is based on the following verse in the Qur'an:

> Corruption has appeared throughout the land and sea by [reason of] what the hands of people have earned so He [i.e., Allah] may let them taste part of [the consequence of] what they have done that perhaps they will return [to righteousness]. (Qur'an 30:41)

Such a reminder can also be viewed as a mercy from Allah, as it provides the opportunity for repentance and returning to Him. In addition, Muslims believe that the punishment in this life is less severe than that of the Hereafter. This belief is based on the Qur'anic verse, "And We will surely let them taste the nearer punishment short of the greater punishment that perhaps they will return [i.e., repent]" (Qur'an 32:21). The nearer punishment in this verse could be understood to refer to the tribulations and calamites of this life, which may include mental illness.

Spiritual Growth and Purification

Muslims may view mental illness as contributing to the purification of the individual's soul. Many Muslims believe that humans have various tendencies and weaknesses that may hinder their complete and sincere submission to Allah and impede the development of their relationship with Allah (Zarabozo, 2002, pp. 393–403). Life's trials and tribulations may be viewed as enhancing the process of purification by overcoming weaknesses and augmenting the person's obedience to Allah, resulting in a firm and close relationship with Him. It is actually through this relationship with Allah that peace and happiness can be found.

Prevention, Healing, and Treatment

From an Islamic perspective, healing is in the realm of possibility. For the person suffering from mental illness, as well as family members, an element of hope and optimism can be very helpful. Some Muslims believe that Allah is capable of producing a cure if the individual (and/or his or her family) sincerely turns to Him for assistance. As mentioned earlier, for every disease on this earth, Allah has sent down a cure. The following topics will be covered in this section: prevention, patience and reliance upon Allah, clinical applications, and *ruqya* (supplications). It should be noted that many of these concepts may be integrated into the counseling process, particularly with religious clients.

---

⁶ In Islam, it refers to the path ordained for humans by Allah in order to achieve success in this life and in the Hereafter. It includes the various beliefs and practices of Muslims as well as details of what is lawful and what is prohibited.

Importance of Prevention

Islam values prevention, and as such has various injunctions in place to protect the individual from potential physical and psychological harm, some of which will be explored in the following. These injunctions are meant to protect the individual from harm through a number of means and methods. It is believed that submitting to and obeying Allah's commands in one's life can serve as preventative measures. Prevention within the Islamic framework includes refraining from harmful substances (e.g., alcohol, drugs) and activities (e.g., gambling, risk-taking behavior), leading a balanced life of moderation, taking care of both the mind and the body as they are considered trusts from Allah, and seeking education about particular topics (e.g., marriage, parenting).

Patience and Reliance upon Allah

Because the Hereafter is considered an important goal for Muslims, understanding the Islamic conceptualization of this life and the tests that come with it will assist them to be patient with and even grateful to Allah. The remembrance of the temporal nature of this world and the rewards that will be obtained can help ease the burden of psychological distress. According to Islamic beliefs, the trials and tribulations that are experienced benefit the individual if he or she is patient and demonstrates reliance upon Allah. From this perspective, the person will have the hope of earning reward from Allah for submitting to Him and the events that He has planned. As a result of a test, individuals' faith may increase, they may become closer to Allah, and their mental illness may be lifted. They will obtain the benefits if they are patient and rely upon Allah to ease the burden.

Allah mentions in the Qur'an,

> And We will surely test you with something of fear and hunger, and a loss of wealth and lives, and fruit, but give glad tidings to the patient, Who, when disaster strikes them, say, "Indeed, we belong to Allah and indeed to Him we will return." Those are the ones upon whom are blessings from their Lord and mercy. And it is those who are the [rightly] guided. (Qur'an 2:155-157)

During one's lifetime, the individual will either be in a state of gratitude to Allah or a state of patience.

The Prophet (peace and blessings be upon him) said,

> The affair of the believer is amazing in that it is always good for him and this is true only for a believer. If something joyful comes to him, he gives thanks and that is good for him. If something harmful comes to him, he is patient and that is good for him. (Muslim, Book 68, no. 2092, as cited in Al-Mundhiri, 2000, p. 1117)

In response to the test, the human is instructed to rely upon Allah. Allah says,

> And whoever relies upon Allah—then He is sufficient for him. Indeed, Allah will accomplish His purpose. Allah has already set for everything a [decreed] extent. (Qur'an 65:3)
>
> Rely upon Allah; and sufficient is Allah as Disposer of affairs. (Qur'an 33:3)

From an Islamic perspective, reliance upon Allah does not mean abandoning the means to achieve an end, nor should an individual abandon hope in Allah's Mercy (and rely upon oneself or the means alone), although clients may believe this. Both personal action and trust in Allah must be combined together for maximum benefit. Action entails taking the means created by Allah in order to achieve a certain desired outcome. In the case of mental illness, the steps may include medication, counseling, and psychotherapy, and the desired outcome may result in a cure or reduction of symptoms. At the same time, Muslims are encouraged to trust and depend upon Allah and that He will actually bring about the cure as it is only He who has that ability. The medicine, therapy, and doctors are thought to be the means by which the cure is achieved, but they are not considered the primary cause. Relying upon Allah in this way is believed to lead to beneficial results, both in this life and in the Hereafter.

Reliance upon Allah may also be connected to the belief in His *qadar* (divine will and predestination). Allah mentions,

> No disaster strikes upon the earth or among yourselves except that it is in a register before We bring it into being—indeed that, for Allah, is easy—In order that you not despair over what has eluded you and not exult [in pride] over what He has given you. (Qur'an 57:22-23)

The concept of *qadar* may help clients who suffer from mental illness to accept their reality and trust in Allah's plan and wisdom.

Clinical Applications of Islamic Concepts

In contemporary psychology, there has been a growing acknowledgment of the important role of religiosity and spirituality in the psychotherapeutic process (Pargament, Murray-Swank, & Tarakeshwar, 2005). Some researchers have termed this integration of spiritual issues into the therapeutic process as "theistic psychotherapy" or religious psychotherapy (Richards & Bergin, 2005).

Some efforts have been made to develop a religious psychotherapy approach specifically for Muslims that integrates some of the above-mentioned key Islamic concepts of mental health and healing. Thus far, five studies have found beneficial results for religious psychotherapy in the treatment of anxiety, depression, or bereavement with Muslim patients (Azhar & Varma, 1995a, 1995b; Azhar, Varma, & Dharap, 1994; Razali, Aminah, & Khan, 2002; Razali, Hasanah, Aminah, & Subramaniam, 1998). In each of these studies, participants in the religious psychotherapy group responded significantly faster than those receiving conventional treatment. This may have been due to the fact that the religious psychotherapy matched the clients' religious-cultural belief systems. In the religious psychotherapy, unproductive beliefs were identified and modified or replaced with beliefs derived from Islam, using a modification of cognitive therapy (Azhar, Varma, & Dharap, 1994; Azhar & Varma, 1995b). Other goals of Islamic religious psychotherapy are to revive spirituality and religious practice in order to cope with mental illness or stressful life events. Such approaches have strong potential in terms of intervention for mental illness, which requires further consideration and development.

Treatment with Ruqyah

Ruqyah is one of the prescribed treatments that may be utilized by Muslims who are suffering from mental illness. It involves the recitation of various Qur'anic verses or supplications in order to cure the afflicted person. The belief is that the cure comes from Allah. The specific verses or supplications read will depend on the particular cause of the disease. The cure for magic, for example, will be different from that for envy or possession. *Ruqyah* may be used alone for cases with a purely spiritual or supernatural cause and may be used in combination with medical or psychological treatments for other causes. These processes require an experienced and knowledgeable religious person. It is actually best for individuals to do *ruqyah* for themselves, but this may not always be possible, depending on the severity of the case and the person's knowledge of the Qur'an.

CASE STUDY

Religion and religiosity have a profound impact upon Muslims in relation to mental health, as discussed throughout this chapter. A case study is presented here to highlight some of the issues and concepts discussed in previous sections. Identifying information about the client has been changed for purposes of confidentiality.

Zainab is a 20-year-old female student who studies at a university in the United States and resides in the campus dormitories. The Department of Academic Affairs refers her to the on-campus student counselor due to poor grades. If her performance does not improve, she will be forced to withdraw from the university. The counselor does a complete intake assessment and determines that Zainab suffers from anorexia nervosa, purging type. Her weight has significantly declined in the past year, she reports amenorrhea for the past four months, and she indicates body image dissatisfaction despite obvious thinness. She eats small amounts of food daily (apple, carrot, water, diet soda), exercises excessively (2 to 3 hours per day), and regularly purges following consumption of food. Due to her condition, she has fainted on several occasions. Her parents, who live in another country, come to campus to meet with the counselor and medical doctors. Zainab's parents are very concerned about her health and express their support of efforts by the university to assist her. While observing the interaction of Zainab with her family, it becomes evident to the clinician that Zainab makes use of her illness in attempts to control her family, particularly her wealthy father.

For several months, the counselor attempts to approach the problem from a psychosocial perspective, utilizing a cognitive-behavioral strategy. Zainab's maladaptive thoughts around weight, eating, and the ideal body are challenged and tested. Family issues and dynamics are discussed as these obviously contribute to her problem. Due to the distance, it is not possible to conduct therapy with the family. Zainab is very resistant to treatment, manipulative throughout the process, and makes little progress.

During one session, Zainab shares with the counselor that she believes her problem is caused by magic, which is prevalent in her home country. She was afraid to mention it previously, as she thought that the Western-educated counselor would consider her to be ignorant and foolish. It is suggested by the therapist that an imam be contacted to assess this possibility. A local imam is contacted and he agrees to complete the assessment. He determines that Zainab has been affected by magic and recommends various Qur'anic chapters, verses, and supplications of the Prophet (peace and blessings be upon him) for treatment. He himself conducts *ruqya* for her over several sessions. The counseling sessions also continue and focus on relevant psychological, social, and academic issues. Over a period of two months of psychotherapy and sessions with the imam in the masjid, Zainab begins to improve. She experiences fewer obsessions with weight and body image and is able to eat a larger quantity of food without concerns over gaining weight. It is indicated from this case that the therapist's respect for Zainab's beliefs and openness to including the imam in the process contributed to her significant improvement.

Conclusion

This chapter presented an overview of Muslims' beliefs regarding mental health, illness, and healing. It is important to note the diversity of beliefs within the Muslim community, while at the same time understanding religious conceptualizations and background for these beliefs. The challenge ultimately arises in the application of this knowledge during clinical work. It may be difficult, for example, to determine the difference between *waswaas* and auditory hallucinations or to discriminate between cases with a biological cause from those with a more supernatural basis. Likewise, clinicians would need to be familiar with Islamic cultural beliefs to determine if beliefs or behaviors are beyond what may be considered "normal" within religious or cultural normative beliefs. Knowledge is the key to the effective integration of these principles within the counseling process, which is a main goal of this chapter.

Cases with a supernatural etiology do not necessarily automatically rule out the need for clinical or counseling interventions, as such cases often tend to be complex with a combination of supernatural, social, and psychological factors. It should be noted, however, that psychotherapeutic techniques are less likely to be effective in situations attributed to supernatural influences. In cases in which a clinician is uncertain or confused by the presentation, it would be advisable to consult either with a Muslim mental health professional who has knowledge and insight regarding these issues or a religious leader (i.e., imam or sheikh) who has some training and experience with mental-health-related concerns. Larger Muslim communities often have these types of resources available.

It is hoped that this chapter provides mental health professionals with a better understanding of the perspectives of their Muslim clients. The ultimate purpose is to encourage culturally relevant treatment approaches in order to achieve more effective outcomes.

References

Abu-Raiya, H., & Pargament, K. I. (2010). Empirically based psychology of Islam: Summary and critique of the literature. *Mental Health, Religion & Culture* 14(2), 93–115.

Abu-Ras, W., Gheith, A., & Cournos, F. (2008). The imam's role in mental health promotion: A study at 22 mosques in New York City's Muslim community. *Journal of Muslim Mental Health, 3,* 155–176.

Al-Ashgar, U. S. (1998). *The world of the jinn and devils.* (J. Zarabozo, Trans.). Boulder, CO: Al-Basheer Company for Publications and Translations.

Al-Habeeb, T. A. (2004). Pilot study of faith healers' views on the evil eye, *jinn* possession, and magic in Saudi Arabia. Retrieved March 3, 2010 from www.daarussalaam.com/A-STRARAGIES/A15mass/09PilotStudy.pdf

Al-Jauziyyah, I. Q. (2003). *Healing with the medicine of the Prophet* (J. Abual Rub, Trans.). Riyadh, Saudi Arabia: Darussalam Publishers and Distributors.

Al-Krenawi, A., & Graham, J. R. (2000). Culturally sensitive social work practice with Arab clients in mental health settings. *Health & Social Work, 25*(1), 9–22.

Al-Mundhiri, Z. A. (2000). *The translation of the meanings of summarized Sahih Muslim*. Riyadh, Saudi Arabia: Darussalam Publishers and Distributors.

Azhar, M. Z., & Varma, S. L. (1995a). Religious psychotherapy in depressive patients. *Psychotherapy and Psychosomatics, 63*, 165–168.

Azhar, M. Z., & Varma, S. L. (1995b). Religious psychotherapy as management of bereavement. *Acta Psychiatrica Scandinavica, 91*(4), 233–235.

Azhar, M. Z., Varma, S. L., & Dharap, A. S. (1994). Religious psychotherapy in anxiety disorder patients. *Acta Psychiatrica Scandinavica, 90*(1), 1–3.

Az-Zubaidi, Z. A. A. (1996). *The translation of the meanings of summarized Sahih Al-Bukhari*. Riyadh, Saudi Arabia: Darussalam Publishers and Distributors.

El-Islam, M. F., & Abu-Dagga, S. I. (1992). Lay explanations of symptoms of mental ill health in Kuwait. *The International Journal of Social Psychiatry, 38*(2), 150–156.

Hamdan, A., & Oman, D. (2011) *Religiosity, spirituality, and mental health: Review of research with Muslim populations, explanatory mechanisms, and future directions*. Manuscript submitted for publication.

Haque, A. (2005). Mental health concepts and program development in Malaysia. *Journal of Mental Health, 14*(2), 183–195.

Ibn Kathir. (2000). *Tafsir ibn Kathir* (J. Abualrub, N. Khitab, H. Khitab, A. Walker, M. Al-Jibali, & S. Ayoub, Trans.). Riyadh, Saudi Arabia: Darussalam Publishers and Distributors.

Ismail, H., Wright, J., Rhodes, P., Small, N., & Jacoby, A. (2005). South Asians and epilepsy: Exploring health experiences, needs and beliefs of communities in the north of England. *Seizure, 14*, 497–503.

Khan, M. M. (1997). *The translation of the meanings of Sahih Al-Bukhari*. Riyadh, Saudi Arabia: Darussalam Publishers and Distributors.

Koenig, H. G. (2008). *Medicine, religion, and health: Where science and spirituality meet*. West Conshohocken, PA: Templeton Foundation Press.

Koenig, H. G., McCullough, M. E., & Larson, D. B. (2001). *Handbook of religion and health*. Oxford, UK: Oxford University Press.

Pargament, K. I. (1997). *The psychology of religion and coping: Theory, research and practice*. New York, NY: Guilford Press.

Pargament, K. I., Murray-Swank, N. A., & Tarakeshwar, N. (2005). An empirically based rationale for a spiritually integrated psychotherapy. *Mental Health, Religion and Culture, 8*(3), 155–165.

Philips, A. A. B. (1997). *The exorcist tradition in Islaam*. Sharjah, United Arab Emirates: Dar Al Fatah.

Razali, S. M., Aminah, K., & Khan, U. A. (2002). Religious–cultural psychotherapy in the management of anxiety patients. *Transcultural Psychiatry, 39*(1), 130–136.

Razali, S. M., Hasanah, C. I., Aminah, K., & Subramaniam, M. (1998). Religious-sociocultural psychotherapy in patients with anxiety and depression. *Australian and New Zealand Journal of Psychiatry, 32*(6), 867–872.

Razali, S. M., Khan, U. A., & Hasanah, C. (1996). Belief in supernatural causes of mental illness among Malay patients: Impact on treatment. *Acta Psychiatrica Scandinavica, 94*(4), 229–233.

Richards, P. S., & Bergin, A. E. (2005) *A spiritual strategy for counseling and psychotherapy* (2nd ed.). Washington, DC: American Psychological Association.

Weatherhead, S., & Daiches, A. (2010). Muslim views on mental health and psychotherapy. *Psychology and Psychotherapy: Theory, Research and Practice, 83*, 75–89.

Zarabozo, J. M. (2002). *Purification of the soul: Concept, process, and mean.* Denver, CO: Al-Basheer Company for Publications and Translations.

CHAPTER 3
Traditional Mental Health Coping and Help-Seeking

OSMAN M. ALI and FRIEDA ABOUL-FOTOUH

Like their non-Muslim counterparts, many Muslims with mental or behavioral health problems may never see the inside of a mental health professional's office. Yet the professional should appreciate what coping strategies and help-seeking behaviors Muslims may have already utilized or what interventions may be suggested as alternatives or augmentations to traditional clinical interventions.

Muslims experiencing difficulties in their social situation, pained by psychological distress, or struggling with mental health symptoms may engage several strategies to cope with their problems. Muslims turn to the Qur'an and *hadith* as primary sources to find solace from their difficulties, to seek guidance, and to implement strategies that will prevent further difficulties (Haque, 2004). Indeed, Muslims use religious coping (Amer, Hovey, Fox, & Rezcallah, 2008) for symptoms of depression (Loewenthal, Cinnirella, Evdoka, & Murphy, 2001), as well as for non-mental-health symptoms (Abu Raiya & Pargament, 2010). Typically, the imam or other respected religious scholar (e.g., mufti, alim) may be consulted (Ali, Milstein, & Marzuk, 2005). Sometimes the intervention is based on what the individual views as the cause of his or her distress. For example, Muslims may engage traditional healers or wise men/wise women (e.g., *hakims*,[1] *pirs*[2]) to address concerns about spirit possession

---
[1] Practitioner using herbal medicine of Greco-Arabic tradition.
[2] A term for spiritual guide used by South Asians.

(Dein, Alexander, & Napier, 2008). As Islam emphasizes respect for the elderly and parents, the family often plays a powerful role in mediating difficulties (Ahmed & Reddy, 2007; Daneshpour, 1998).

Although some writers have begun to describe problem- and emotion-focused coping strategies used by a Muslim population (Khawaja, 2008) as well as help-seeking behaviors toward professional counseling or psychiatric care (Aloud & Rathur, 2009; Khan, 2006), that is not the focus of this chapter. Rather, we categorize the coping behaviors associated with Muslim tradition and culture generally and present case scenarios addressing the following three coping strategies: (a) strengthening essential Islamic practices, (b) diminishing supernatural causes, and (c) seeking sage guidance.

The fictionalized case scenarios presented in this chapter serve as education tools and should not be construed as medical advice or clinical supervision. Case scenarios are useful teaching tools but carry the risk of creating or propagating stereotypes in the minds of clinical and nonclinical individuals. Readers should remain aware of this and be cautious not to make assumptions about their clients or patients. Muslims are diverse in their ethnic, cultural, and social backgrounds, and their identities and practices can vary tremendously. Some of what is presented here may apply to one subgroup of Muslims wholly while being completely irrelevant to another subgroup of Muslims. It is important to appreciate that, regardless of their degree of internalized or outwardly expressed religiosity, Muslims may perceive the causes of their problems differently and may utilize diverse strategies independent of religiosity.

Strengthening Essential Islamic Practices: Faith, Prayer, Reflection, and Supplication

CASE A: "FORGETTING THE FUNDAMENTALS"
Case A, Part 1

> The university counselor calls the next individual to her office. Rashid is a 22-year-old never-married international graduate student who lives off campus alone. He states that he needs a "psych evaluation" in order to obtain a leave of absence from school. His advisor has decided not to graduate him because he seems unable to elucidate basic concepts, let alone show mastery in his thesis topic. He continues to miss several extended deadlines, becoming irritated and unappreciative when more opportunities to make up his work are provided. The counselor notes that he is minimally talkative, and his soft speech and poor eye contact make him appear almost dismissive of the counselor's questions. He

looks sleep deprived, thin, and seems not to have shaven for several days. He does not admit to feeling "down" or depressed but does admit to having had headaches and difficulty sleeping, and he is particularly concerned with trouble with his memory.

- What possible diagnoses are you considering at this point?
- How should the counselor interpret Rashid's soft speech and poor eye contact?
- What ought to be the priority for the counselor at this time?

Discussion of Case A, Part 1 The counselor appreciates that in many ways, this individual is no different than anyone else who presents with symptoms suggestive of a mental disorder. Medical and substance use contributions are definitely a priority and should be ruled out through lab work and medical evaluation. Although Rashid does not present with statements of depressed mood, his irritability and restricted affect could be appreciated as part of a mood disorder. Missing deadlines may be due to concentration problems stemming from a depressive disorder. It is possible he lacks psychological awareness and familiarity with the concept or language of mood disorders. Therefore, he may be more apt to discuss physical symptoms. Even though medications might be appropriate, the stigma against mental illness may inhibit willingness to take medications. The individual may be more open to discussing the underlying issues and a problem-solving approach (Soheilian & Inman, 2009). Attempts to educate about the value of cognitive-behavioral therapy techniques would likely be much better received than attempts to encourage acceptance of Freudian psychodynamic principles.

Cultural beliefs about mental illness, as well as lack of familiarity with it, can inhibit the utilization of professional mental health services (Aloud & Rathur, 2009). There is some evidence to suggest that Muslims are more likely to believe in the efficacy of religious coping and less likely to seek professional help (Loewenthal et al., 2001). Therefore, an approach that validates religious coping as well as discusses professional interventions may be more effective in promoting resiliency and recovery among religiously oriented clients (Bhui, King, Dein, & O'Connor, 2008).

At least equally as important as making an accurate diagnosis is establishing rapport with Rashid and educating him about the nature of the evaluation. It is important for him to be informed about the degree of confidentiality of the evaluation as well as discuss possible misconceptions he may have regarding the intent of the counselor. This may be of particular concern to immigrants who may be concerned about whether the evaluation results could have an impact on their immigration status. Muslims in the United States may have immigration concerns that confound psychiatric presentations and should not be confused with paranoia. Clearly this would not apply to the many Muslims who are born and raised in the United States. In addition to these concerns, Rashid may have been raised in a country in which the opposite sexes have little direct interaction. If that is the case, the lack of eye contact and lack of openness to the interaction may be a reflection of discomfort with an unfamiliar situation, rather than evidence of pathology, poor social skills, or a personality disorder. Making direct eye contact would be seen as religiously and culturally disrespectful, and being alone with a woman who is not a family member may be unfamiliar or uncomfortable to him if he believes it to go against his religion.

Case A, Part 2

Rashid indicates that it is religiously acceptable for him to meet with the counselor alone since this a professional setting rather than a social one. He states that he is concerned that what he says will be used against him or be given to immigration officials. The counselor explains that this evaluation is confidential and only in the case of imminent safety risk could confidentiality be breached. She explains that only if he signs a consent form will she communicate in general terms with his department in order to determine his eligibility for a medical leave of absence. As she talks to him she learns that he has recently lost his uncle back in his native country, but he does not cry when mentioning it. He seems more preoccupied than sad, and then mutters something in another language under his breath. The counselor inquires about his lack of shaving and he describes it as intentional as he wants to become more identified with his religion. He has begun attending the campus mosque more frequently and states that he has been taking public transport to the city's nearest mosque, where he states that he sits, reflects, and contemplates deeply.

- How might Rashid use his faith to understand his uncle's death?
- Would it be appropriate for the counselor to suggest that Rashid is having a crisis with religion or identity as a Muslim?
- Would spending time at the mosque lead to improvements or problems in Rashid's ability to do his work?

Discussion of Case A, Part 2 Although it may lead to sadness and tearfulness, many Muslims seek solace and acceptance in the fact of death by reciting the verse from the Holy Qur'an (2:156): "Verily, unto God do we belong and, verily, unto Him we shall return." When Rashid was muttering he was actually reciting this verse when the topic of his uncle's passing away was raised, as a means of self-reassurance. If a Muslim unexpectedly recites a verse softly to him or herself, this should not be mistaken for responding to internal stimuli or "talking to oneself." This can be a sign of Faith and submitting to Allah's[3] Will, and believing that only He knows what is best and only He is most Powerful. Through the Islamic perspective all life events are a result of God's Will. Therefore, not only psychosocial stressors, but also the suffering that follows, are understood in the context of God's Will (Al-Krenawi & Graham, 1999). Faith facilitates acceptance, an important psychological part of the grieving process. Faith helps Muslims accept their circumstances and that they are not in control (Basit, 2007).

Rashid's increased mosque attendance in the face of his uncle's death can therefore be understood as a positive coping mechanism. Many individuals experience spiritual growth and maturity in the face of adversity. Rashid is not having a crisis of faith or identity; rather, he has become more cognizant of faith's role in his life after he experienced the loss of a loved one.

In addition to the family member's death, what may disturb Rashid is that he is now considered the primary breadwinner for the home, which includes an extended family. His preoccupation may be related to concern that he is still a student and unable to send money to his family. Without his financial support, other family members must work, which could make him feel humiliated for not fulfilling his understood responsibility to his family. When Rashid reports that he goes to the mosque to contemplate, it is important for the counselor to be curious about his thoughts. Although suicide is against Islamic beliefs, the term "contemplate" in mental health often precedes the term "suicide." Anyone with a serious mental illness is susceptible to suicidal thinking and this should be explored carefully. The counselor should be aware that first-generation immigrants may perceive suggestions that they have thought about suicide as an insult to their level of faith. Questions about suicide can begin with an acknowledgment that these are important questions that must be asked of all clients.

However, if Rashid is spending time at the mosque in contemplation of life and its meaning, and Allah and His Greatness, this could be seen as a positive coping mechanism (Dover, Miner, & Dowson, 2007). He may be seeking solace and performing supplication, as Muslims believe that if you pray sincerely and ask from Allah, He will provide what you ask for, if it is best for you. Affiliation with a peer group at the mosque and identification with one's Islamic heritage and background may be a means for Rashid to feel closer to his community and thus his family from whom he is separated. In fact, distance from one's faith may sometimes be perceived as the

---

[3] "Allah" is the Arabic word for God.

cause for mental illness (Cinnirella & Loewenthal, 1999). Muslims value prayer as being helpful for managing mood difficulties, and many believe it to be more helpful than medical treatments (Loewenthal, 1999). Religious coping has positive effects for Muslims dealing with losses (Aflakseir & Coleman, 2009).

Diminishing Supernatural Causes: Black Magic, Evil Eye, *Jinn* Possession

CASE B: "KEEPING AN EYE OUT"
Case B, Part 1

A mother brings her 18-year-old daughter, Sakina, to a primary care physician reporting that her daughter is presenting for a routine evaluation. During the visit the mother begins to ask the physician several questions and suggests that maybe her daughter needs vitamins. She says that her daughter has been failing her classes in the past six months and it is unlike her because she is normally very intelligent. The mother then states that she believes her daughter may not be trying hard enough, and at times is oppositional and uninvolved with her schoolwork or family. The physician finds no medical causes for these symptoms but notes that Sakina is an attractive young woman with an odd affect, wearing loose-fitting black string bracelets and some amulets on a necklace with foreign writings and a peculiar design. When the physician asks to see Sakina alone, her mother refuses, stating that she has always been present during her daughter's evaluations and there are no secrets between them. The daughter bursts into tears and yells at her mother to leave the office and states that she wishes her mother and father would "stop doing all of these weird things to me!"

- What do you think about the closeness of the relationship between the mother and daughter?
- Do you think the physician should dismiss the mother from the office and call child protective services at this time?
- What diagnoses are you considering and how might you go about addressing them?

Discussion of Case B, Part 1 Traditionally, disrespecting one's mother is not acceptable in most Muslim cultures, and Muslims believe in the well-known *hadith*[4] that Heaven lies at the feet of one's mother (meaning

---

[4] Hadith refers to a practice or saying of the Prophet Muhammad (peace be upon him).

one should always respect one's mother). However, with the intercultural gap between first-generation immigrant mothers and their second-generation daughters, it is common for young people to be less cognizant of these traditional boundaries. It is culturally appropriate for relationships between parents and children to be very close; therefore, it should not be viewed as "enmeshed." With regard to the mother's unwillingness to leave the room, it is common for mothers to be protective of their daughters. The mother may be particularly anxious about a male physician who is asking to examine her teenage daughter alone. Whenever possible, Muslim females should be given the option of having female providers. Because of the close relationship, the mother may be surprised if asked to leave the room, and allowing her to stay, at least initially, could build rapport. This rapport will be necessary to engage the mother as well as the daughter in conventional interventions (Haboush, 2007).

Although one might respect the familial closeness often seen in Muslims (Carolan, Bagherinia, Juhari, Himelright, & Mouton-Sanders, 2000), in this situation it is very important that the daughter and mother be interviewed separately given that there is a concern of abuse, although a call to protective services would be premature. Without more information it is too early to make assumptions about what exactly is occurring. Sakina could have a depressive disorder or a covert drug or alcohol problem, or she could have normal adolescent angst and feel that her mother is overprotective. It is concerning that Sakina quickly becomes so emotional when the mother refuses to leave the room and exclaims that something "weird" is being done to her.

Case B, Part 2

The physician asks the mother to speak with the social worker at the clinic that day about what is happening. When the mother sits down with the social worker she reveals that she actually has been quite concerned about the fact that her daughter has begun to exhibit odd behaviors including talking to herself when no one is in the room. The mother states that she knows of no abuse that her daughter is facing from either the mother herself or her husband. However, the mother states that Sakina's comment about "weird things" may be referring to the parents' reading of religious phrases and then blowing upon her, as well as having Sakina wear amulets to ward off the evil eye and black magic that may have been cast upon her in jealousy.[5] The mother also reports that they have been taking Sakina to someone who claims he

---

[5] The evil eye or black magic is a common cultural belief that some people have the power of inflicting injury or bad luck by envious or evil gazes or by witchcraft.

can exorcise her soul of evil *jinn*.[6] Sakina's parents have been quite concerned about Sakina's irrational thinking, particularly when she gets extremely agitated, unpredictably, over seemingly small things at home to the point that it frightens her younger siblings. The parents deny any family history of mental illness and have now exhausted other interventions except a referral to a psychiatrist.

When alone with the social worker, Sakina reports a similar history, stating that she is tired of the strange people she has been taken to, the incense, the rituals and prayers that are read to her or read upon what she eats or drinks. She believes that they may be poisoning her by doing this and that they are extracting her thoughts and broadcasting them on the radio so that people on the bus will know what she is thinking. She has been very distracted by these thoughts and has been unable to focus on regular daily activities.

- Are Sakina's thoughts within the norms of her cultural and religious backgrounds?
- Is it possible that Sakina actually does have a family history of mental illness?
- What can the physician and social worker do to increase the chances that Sakina sees a psychiatrist?

Discussion of Case B, Part 2   Sakina's worries about being poisoned and having her thoughts broadcasted are not part of any cultural worldview. Rather, they are evidence for a thought disorder or psychotic process. Sakina's first presentation with psychosis could be the product of a mood disorder or drug use, or may be the beginning of schizophrenia. When discussing with the family, it is important to be aware that it is devastating for family members to be told that their son or daughter may have a serious mental illness, such as schizophrenia. The family members may feel shame and guilt, and parents may become frustrated and desperate to find cures in vitamins or naturopathic supplements. Families may have no genuine awareness of severe mental illness in their relatives as members living in less-developed countries may have either never been diagnosed or fared well despite a predisposition (Hopper, Harrison, Janca, & Sartorius, 2007). Or they may be so concerned about stigma that they are quick to deny the presence of family mental illness. While causes for the psychosis should be explored, if the diagnosis is schizophrenia, the family should be provided with referrals for community advocacy and support groups as

---

[6] In Islamic belief, *jinn* are spirits that are capable of assuming human or animal form and exercising supernatural influence over people.

well as reliable psychoeducation materials (e.g., www.healthyminds.org), preferably in their native language.

However, it is possible that the family may not accept these references and instead turn to religion to try to manage mental illness. Compared to other religious groups, Muslims may be even more prone to turn to faith practices to counter illness (Cinnirella & Loewenthal, 1999). Muslims may turn to several sources on the Internet for information including Islamic sites and chat rooms. It is important to counter false information that is rampant on the Internet. Although well meaning, many people, including Muslims, may present unsound information, providing false hope at best and harmful treatments at worst (Dein & Sembhi, 2001). Many also believe that mental illness could be the result of *jinn* possession (Khalifa & Hardie, 2005). The Qur'an mentions the existence of beings in parallel worlds, or *jinn*, that mostly do not overlap the human world. Muslims interpret that *jinn* exist as unseen beings and can possess human beings in rare circumstances. It is therefore important to support the family in their belief system regarding the unseen. However, the family can be approached with the following strategy that respects both religious and scientific points of view: There are proximate and ultimate causes for illness. In this context, the biochemical alterations in the functions of mental circuitry would be considered proximate causes, while Allah's Will would be considered an ultimate cause. The health professional provides interventions geared toward the proximate causes. If the family believes that their faith explains the ultimate cause, then there is no conflict with the professional's explanation. In addition, a discussion can ensue about how addressing both proximate and ultimate causes is most likely to enhance the person's chances for recovery. Alternatively, the therapist might emphasize that what is understood religiously as unseen could refer to the unconscious, psychological aspects that exist in human beings outside of their own awareness. Helping the family incorporate both a medical and religious model of understanding will strengthen the alliance and increase the likelihood of engagement in treatment.

Seeking Sage Guidance: Respected Family Elders, Community Elders, and Imams

CASE C: "SEEKING SUPPORT"
Case C, Part 1

A police officer comes to a home where neighbors report yelling. When the officer arrives he quickly ascertains that there is a domestic disturbance between an interracial husband and wife. He notes no physical injury and the two young children appear unaffected by the commotion. After briefly questioning both adults about their safety the officer suggests that they keep the noise to a minimum and seek counseling. Several days later, the wife calls her mother stating that her husband is verbally abusive especially when he drinks alcohol, is intimidating to her, and she does not know what to do. When the husband finds out about the phone call, he calls the wife's mother and reports that their problems began when his wife began to work. He states that in the past few weeks his wife has been staying up all hours of the night obsessively engaged in work activities. Furthermore, he accuses her as being verbally abusive to him, and states that he is going to divorce her if she does not stop disrespecting him by flirting with men from work. After several arguments between the couple's parents about who is right and who is wrong, both sides of the family eventually decide to sit down and discuss the matter together before any decisions about a possible divorce are made.

- Who, if anyone, do you think may have a mental health problem?
- How should the wife's allegation of abuse be addressed?
- Is this family meeting a form of psychotherapy?

Discussion of Case C, Part 1   It is not possible to make a diagnosis at this time. Although intermittent explosive disorder and alcohol abuse come to mind for the husband and obsessive-compulsive disorder or hypomania come to mind for the wife, the real issues may only be maladaptive coping skills or personality issues. The immediate question in this case is about safety. If the wife reported to a provider that the husband had been verbally abusive, the question becomes how to approach this topic in a culturally sensitive way (Kiely-Froude & Abdul-Karim, 2009). Any form of abuse is unacceptable Islamically. A distinction of roles between husband and wife does not imply an imbalance of power. This should be emphasized to the couple if they present to treatment. The Imam may also be recruited to reinforce this to the couple.

The family intervention is not a form of psychotherapy. It is more of an arbitration to determine the social causes of the problems and determine fair solutions. It is common for a family intervention to occur in the case of significant marital problems. The Qur'an recommends that Muslim families attempt to resolve issues between couples in order to avoid divorce. Elders are also an important source for counsel. Sometimes the immediate needs of the individuals are sacrificed in order to keep the peace within the family or for the sake of children.

Case C, Part 2

During the family meetings the wife's side of the family is shocked to hear about the husband's alcohol use while the husband's side of the family reports that the wife drove him to drink by going to work. The husband denies regular drinking and states that it will not be a problem for him to stop. The families also decide that the husband's mother will help care for the children if the wife must work, but suggest that it is in the best interest of the couple that the wife discontinues working.

- What will determine the likelihood that the husband will stop drinking?
- What are some advantages and disadvantages with the proposed interventions?

Discussion of Case C, Part 2 It is naive to think that substance abuse can stop without intervention if it has been a problem. Prior drinking history is important to determine the likelihood that the husband will stop. The fact that he drinks, despite it being prohibited in Islam and outside of his family culture, suggests that either he is not very adherent to his religion or he finds it difficult to stop. People under stress have used alcohol in predominantly Muslim countries (Mohamad, 2009), so it is not surprising that in countries where there is no prohibition of alcohol Muslims may use it (Burazeri & Kark, 2010). Muslims may face additional challenges when seeking substance abuse treatment including social stigma, as well as cultural and language barriers (Arfken, Berry, & Owens, 2009).

One problem with the proposed intervention is that it assumes that the wife's work is the cause of their troubles, whereas it may be related more to the husband's perception of her work as a problem. Yet, the clinician should be careful not to impose the view that the wife must have the same career desires as her non-Muslim counterparts (Carolan et al., 2000).

Case C, Part 3

The couple decides that they would rather not have the mother-in-law provide daycare for the children after all, and several months after the wife has stopped working the couple's arguments have escalated. At another family meeting the husband reports to the elders that he has stopped drinking. The family strongly encourages the couple to seek advice from the imam about the Islamic jurisprudence regarding divorce. The couple presents to the imam after Friday prayers. Although the imam asks that they return during his marriage counseling designated hours, they insist that it is important and that he make time for them as soon as possible. The imam tells them he must meet with each spouse individually first.

- What counseling training and experience do imams have that could be helpful in this type of case scenario?
- Is it common for a Muslim family to seek help from the imam in this type of situation?
- Why is it important for clinicians who treat Muslim clients to establish contacts with imams?

Discussion of Case C, Part 3 Although some Muslims will be inhibited by fear of social stigma and damaging the family honor by sharing private matters with an imam, many will seek out imams as a source of support in the case of interpersonal and family conflict (Ali et al., 2005). Although it is typical for imams to be asked about marriage concerns, it is atypical that imams would have the mental health expertise to draw out potential diagnoses of a mood disorder, let alone relate past experiences to current maladaptive psychological coping mechanisms and behaviors. Despite their lack of training, imams have begun to see increasing numbers of people who present with problems with discrimination, anxiety, and financial difficulties, especially after 9/11 (Ali et al., 2005). Some Muslim communities cannot afford to hire an imam, and in such cases volunteers, without mental health or social work experience, become prayer and community leaders and play the imam's role. In many Western countries the imam is often an immigrant and an elder, which means that he may give advice from a different cultural perspective than the congregant.

Despite these challenges, congregants, particularly those who are used to identifying their religious leaders as sources of counseling support, may rely heavily on the imam to guide them both spiritually and psychologically. Although the imam may choose to play the role of counselor, he also has a religious role to fill by informing the couple about Islamic jurisprudence in situations such as divorce. The imam may reference verses from the Qur'an showing that both husband and wife have rights, roles, and responsibilities to each other and to their families.

Many Muslims may feel more encouraged by Muslim mental health providers or at least those that the imam has found to be culturally sensitive enough to provide support that does not disrespect their religion. While imams do not have a robust referral base for Muslim mental health providers, recent evidence suggests that they would utilize such support if made available to them (Ali & Milstein, in press), and they would support religious coping, as well as psychotherapy and medication management, to help people with mental health problems (Abu-Ras, Gheith, & Cournos, 2008). Regardless of how the issue is ultimately dealt with for the couple, the mosque's role in working with this couple may be a strong determinant of the outcome for this couple, as well as for their children.

Conclusion

This chapter focused on coping strategies that Muslims may traditionally employ in challenging times. Three case scenarios were given in order to demonstrate different coping help-seeking behaviors employed by Muslims. These individuals may never seek out a mental health professional, but their stories highlight common themes that may be part of Muslim clients' presentations. The focus on faith in times of strife is coping and help-seeking is not unique to Islam and is a common way Muslims are taught to manage stresses. Muslims may understand the cause of some stressors to be from the unseen, and the practitioner's awareness and acknowledgment of this can be immensely helpful to the alliance. The unique psychosocial context of Muslims' mental health problems should be appreciated. Finally, utilizing the community resources of extended family, elders, and the imam is a common method of managing personal difficulties.

The previous discussions are not exhaustive, but the cases are intended to elicit discussion among Muslim mental health professionals, clinicians, and students interested in this area of study. Knowing more about Muslims' coping behaviors helps clinicians to adjust their own interventions and behaviors so that they are more likely to develop and maintain a relationship that yields the most therapeutic benefit to the client or patient (Hamdan, 2007; Hodge, 2005). If mental health professionals appreciate Muslims' attitudes toward mental health and help-seeking behaviors, strategic outreach and engagement can be improved.

References

Abu Raiya, H., & Pargament, K. I. (2010). Religiously integrated psychotherapy with Muslim clients: From research to practice. *Professional Psychology: Research and Practice, 41*(2), 181–188.

Abu-Ras, W., Gheith, A., & Cournos, F. (2008). The imam's role in mental health promotion: A study at 22 mosques in New York City's Muslim community. *Journal of Muslim Mental Health, 3*(2), 155–176.

Aflakseir, A., & Coleman, P. G. (2009). The influence of religious coping on mental health of disabled Iranian war veterans. *Mental Health, Religion and Culture 12*(2), 175–190.

Ahmed, S., & Reddy, L. A. (2007). Understanding the mental health needs of American Muslims: Recommendations and considerations for practice. *Journal of Multicultural Counseling and Development, 35*(4), 207–218.

Ali, O. M., Milstein, G., & Marzuk, P. (2005). The Imam's role in meeting the counseling needs of Muslim communities in the United States. *Psychiatric Services, 56*(2), 202–205.

Ali, O. M., & Milstein G. (in press). United States' imams' recognition of mental illness and their willingness to refer. *Journal of Muslim Mental Health*, Fall 2001.

Al-Krenawi, A., & Graham, J. R. (1999). Social work and Koranic mental health healers. *International Social Work, 42*(1), 53–65.

Aloud, N., & Rathur, A. (2009). Factors affecting attitudes toward seeking and using formal mental health and psychological services among Arab Muslim populations. *Journal of Muslim Mental Health, 4*(2), 79–103.

Amer, M., Hovey, J., Fox, C., & Rezcallah, A. (2008). Initial development of the Brief Arab Religious Coping Scale (BARCS). *Journal of Muslim Mental Health, 3*(1), 69–88.

Arfken, C. L., Berry, A., & Owens, D. (2009). Pathways for Arab Americans to substance abuse treatment in southeastern Michigan. *Journal of Muslim Mental Health, 4*(1), 31–46.

Basit, A. (2007). An Islamic perspective on coping with catastrophe. *Southern Medical Journal, 100*(9), 950–951.

Bhui, K. D., King, M., Dein, S., & O'Connor, W. (2008). Ethnicity and religious coping with mental distress. *Journal of Mental Health, 17*(2), 141–151.

Burazeri, G., & Kark, J. D. (2010). Alcohol intake and its correlates in a transitional predominantly Muslim population in southeastern Europe. *Addictive Behavior, 35*(7), 706–713.

Carolan, M., Bagherinia, G., Juhari, R., Himelright, J., & Mouton-Sanders, M. (2000). Contemporary Muslim families: Research and practice. *Contemporary Family Therapy, 22*(1), 67–79.

Cinnirella M., & Loewenthal, K. M. (1999). Religious and ethnic group influences on beliefs about mental illness: A qualitative interview study. *British Journal of Medical Psychology, 72*(4), 505–524.

Daneshpour, M. (1998). Muslim families and family therapy. *Journal of Marital & Family Therapy, 24*(3), 355–368.

Dein, S., Alexander, M., & Napier, A. D. (2008). Jinn, psychiatry and contested notions of misfortune among East London Bangladeshis. *Transcultural Psychiatry, 45*(1), 31–55.

Dein S., & Sembhi, S. (2001). The use of traditional healing in South Asian psychiatric patients in the UK: Interactions between professional and folk psychiatries. *Transcultural Psychiatry, 38*(2), 243–257.

Dover, H., Miner, M., & Dowson, M. (2007). The nature and structure of Muslim religious reflection. *Journal of Muslim Mental Health, 2*(2), 189–210.

Haboush, K. L. (2007). Working with Arab American families: Culturally competent practice for school psychologists. *Psychology in the Schools, 44*(2), 183–198.

Hamdan, A. (2007). A case study of a Muslim client: Incorporating religious beliefs and practices. *Journal of Multicultural Counseling and Development, 35*(2), 92–100.

Haque, A. (2004). Religion and mental health: The case of American Muslims. *Journal of Religion and Health, 43*(1), 45–58.

Hodge, D. R. (2005). Social work and the House of Islam: Orienting practitioners to the beliefs and values of Muslims in the United States. *Social Work, 50*(2), 162–173.

Hopper, K., Harrison, G., Janca, A., & Sartorius, N. (2007). *Recovery from schizophrenia: An international perspective.* A report from the WHO Collaborative Project, The International Study of Schizophrenia. New York, NY: Oxford University Press.

Khalifa, N., & Hardie, T. (2005). Possession and *jinn. Journal of the Royal Society of Medicine, 98*(8), 351–353.

Khan, Z. (2006). Attitudes toward counseling and alternative support among Muslims in Toledo, Ohio. *Journal of Muslim Mental Health, 1*(1), 21–42.

Khawaja, N. (2008). An investigation of the factor structure and psychometric properties of the COPE Scale with a Muslim migrant population in Australia. *Journal of Muslim Mental Health, 3*(2), 177–191.

Kiely-Froude, C., & Abdul-Karim, S. (2009). Providing culturally conscious mental health treatment for African American Muslim women living with spousal abuse. *Journal of Muslim Mental Health, 4*(2), 175–186.

Loewenthal, K. M. (1999). Beliefs about the efficacy of religious, medical and psychotherapeutic interventions for depression and schizophrenia among women from different cultural-religious groups in Great Britain. *Transcultural Psychiatry, 36*(4), 491–504.

Loewenthal, K. M., Cinnirella, M., Evdoka, G., & Murphy, P. (2001). Faith conquers all? Beliefs about the role of religious factors in coping with depression among different cultural-religious groups in the UK. *British Journal of Medical Psychology, 74*(3), 293–303.

Mohamad, M. S. (2009). Daily hassles, coping strategies, and substance use among Egyptian manufacturing workers. *Journal of Muslim Mental Health, 4*(1), 17–29.

Soheilian, S., & Inman, A. G. (2009). Middle Eastern Americans: The effects of stigma on attitudes toward counseling. *Journal of Muslim Mental Health, 4*(2), 139–158.

PART II
Models and Interventions

CHAPTER 4
Mental Health Interview and Cultural Formulation

FARAH TASLEEMA RAHIEM and HAMADA HAMID

This chapter is intended to provide general guidelines for the mental health interview and case formulation of Muslim clients. It is not intended to replace the essential process of formal and supervised training. Mental health professionals, as well as pastoral care counselors, imams, and Islamic chaplains, will find this chapter to be a pragmatic reference when caring for a Muslim client. It is important to note that there is no monolithic Muslim culture and there is no formulaic approach to "the Muslim client." Muslim individuals differ in socioeconomic background, level of religiosity, acculturation, and cultural identity. There is no single personality structure, coping style, or defense mechanism that Muslims share as a group. However, there are some cultural norms and forces that inform the client's experience. Many Muslims, across different ethnicities, share common existential beliefs about the role of God (or Allah), morality, and emotional health that are distinct from other religious traditions. Many Muslims also share social stressors that are closely tied to their religious identity.

Throughout the chapter the authors will draw from the principles laid out in the Diagnostic and Statistical Manual of Mental Disorder IV–Text Revision Cultural Formulation (DSM-IV TR) as a model. To review, the mental health interview is the means by which information about a client is gathered. The formulation process entails concisely organizing that interview data in order to create a hypothesis as to "causes, precipitants, and maintaining influences" of the client's psychological distress (Eells, 2007, p. 4). This formulation, in turn, will help with diagnosis and can

Table 4.1 Components of the Cultural Formulation

Cultural identity of the individual
Cultural explanations of the individual's illness
Cultural factors related to the psychosocial environment
Cultural elements of the relationship between the individual and the clinician
Cultural elements of disease manifestations
Overall cultural assessment for diagnosis and management options

be used to tailor treatment options. The *cultural* formulation highlights the cultural influences upon the client's symptomatology (Table 4.1). This chapter takes its readers through important components of the interview and cultural formulation of a Muslim client. Readers may also find reviewing published cultural formulations of Muslim cases to be helpful (e.g., Hasan & Kuluva, 2006; Varma, 2008).

The Culturally Informed Mental Health Interview

The first step in the initial interview is explaining the interview process and assessing the client's language preference. In cases where the clinician and client do not share the same language, the use of a translator will be necessary. Although the subtleties of language often preclude a word-for-word translation, it is important to instruct the translator not to paraphrase the client's report as important information may be missed. Once the literal meaning of the client's report is translated, the language interpreter may also function as a cultural informant, providing guidance with idioms, appropriateness of content, and, in some cases, general practices of the client's culture. Utilization of the translator as a cultural informant should ideally be reserved for a meeting with the interpreter after the interview. After the assessment of linguistic needs, the clinician should discuss issues of confidentiality with the client. The clinician should ensure the client that all mental health records will be kept in the strictest confidence and this information will only be "released with the authorization of the [client] or under proper legal compulsion" (Sadock & Sadock, 2008, p. 710). A discussion about privacy is particularly important for Muslim immigrants, who may not be familiar with the legal ramifications of the clinician–client privilege. Any client concerns about privacy should be thoroughly discussed at this time, as establishing an environment of trust and comfort is essential in setting the ambience for the interview.

Cultural Identity of the Individual

The cultural identity can be ascertained in the context of gathering demographic information. The interviewer should not impose any assumptions about the client's cultural identity based on appearance. During the course of the initial interview and later encounters, the multiple levels of the client's identity may emerge.

Common terminology used to define one's identity includes race, ethnicity, and culture. For clarification, these terms will be defined, with the understanding that they may hold an entirely different meaning when used in other contexts. Race will be described as the phenotypical similarities of a group that affect interpersonal and institutional interactions and that could lead to a hierarchical status designation within society (Pinderhughes, 1989). Ethnicity will be defined as an individual's sense of belonging to a group with whom he or she may share a common ancestry, history, kinship, or language (Lim, 2006). Culture will be used as a more general term that may include the client's race and ethnicity, as well as religious affiliation, gender, profession, nationality, political affinity, sexual orientation, and family role (Lu, Lim, & Mezzich, 1995).

For instance, a Muslim who was born and raised in the United States, but whose parents are of Guyanese-Indian origin, may see him or herself as racially Indian and ethnically Guyanese—but culturally as a Muslim American of Guyanese Indian descent who is a second-generation immigrant. Gathering such information during the initial interview and future sessions may be useful in elucidating the dynamic and multifaceted nature of the client's cultural identity.

Religiosity Assessment

As suggested previously, religious affiliation can be a defining feature of a client's cultural identity. In addition to having differing sectarian affiliations, such as Sunni or Shi'a, Muslim clients may also have varying degrees of identification with Islam. Questions pertaining to the level of socialization with other Muslims and the client's religious practices should be asked, but in a nonjudgmental fashion. One valuable point to consider is that the religious commitment of some Muslims could be the result of external (societal or familial) pressure, internal commitment, or some combination of the two. Other topics that could be explored include the client's perceived religious discrimination, the level of religious exploration prior to "owning" Islam as the client's religion of choice, the extent to which religious beliefs may promote or interfere with help-seeking behaviors, changes in religious perspectives over time, the parents' religious background(s), and any stress resulting from differences between the religious preference of the client and that of parents, spouse, siblings, and friends (Caraballo et al., 2006; Puchalski, 2006; Sadock & Sadock, 2008). Delving into these aspects of the patient's life may give the clinician insight into religiously oriented psychological stressors or coping mechanisms.

Sample questions clinicians may consider using include

- Do you consider yourself a religious person? How so? If asked what religion you practice, what would you say? Is this the religion of your parents? How did you come to incorporate religion into your life?
- How do your religious beliefs affect your day-to-day life? Do you find comfort in prayer and/or fasting?
- Do you have friends who practice your religion? Do you feel comfortable around them?
- Are you involved in any religious groups in your community? Do you find this to be a source of support or distress?
- Do you find that your connection with religion is distressing to you? How so?
- Do you find that your religious connection is helpful to you in dealing with stress? How so?
- Are there any aspects of your religious beliefs that have helped you come in to see me today? Are there any aspects of your religious beliefs that may have prevented you from coming to see me or from getting treatment?

There may be a developmental component to the client's perception of religion. During childhood and adolescence, the individual typically internalizes the values—critiques or praises—of the caregivers (McWilliams, 1994). The experiences with the caregivers and their levels of religiosity may shape the client's perception of religion as a whole. For example, if the client was raised by a religious and critical father but a less religious and more accepting mother, the client may grow to associate religion with criticism. Clinicians could inquire about the level of religiosity of caregivers and the caregivers' influence on the client by asking questions such as

- Which parent did you identify with more?
- Do you believe that has affected your perception of Islam or your level of religiosity?

Immigration History

Another essential element of the client's background is his or her immigration history. Of note, mistakenly assuming that a native-born client is from another land, with opening questions such as, "So what country are you from?" may be insulting and create barriers between the client and clinician. Many European and American Muslims are second-/third-generation immigrants or converts to Islam who are well settled and view themselves as natives. A less presumptive line of questioning would be,

"Where were you born? Where did you grow up?" If the client is an immigrant, important questions to ask include (Caraballo et al., 2006)

- Was there a reason you immigrated? (Typical reasons include the pursuit of economic or educational opportunities and escape from war and persecution.)
- Who came with you?
- What did you leave behind? (This includes relatives, belongings such as a home, profession, and social circle.)
- When did you immigrate? Was time spent in a displaced location such as a refugee camp? What was that experience like?
- Any future plan of returning to your country of origin?
- Are there any difficulties revolving around your immigration status?

Immigration status is a sensitive subject that should be approached with caution, as the client may be illegally living in the country and thus apprehensive about providing such information (Caraballo et al., 2006).

Acculturative Stress Assessment

Acculturative stress is closely tied to the cultural experience of immigrants. Acculturation is defined as the dynamic process in which beliefs, values, and social behavior are exchanged between both host culture and that of the client (Mavreas, Bebbington, & Der, 1989). The clinician should explore the client's identification with the host culture as well as with his or her culture of origin, in an effort to identify potential stress resulting from this possible intrapsychic negotiation. For example, if the client has difficulty with the language of the host culture, this may cause a problem in adjusting to the host culture and should be asked about in a sensitive fashion. Also, if the client was able to obtain employment, but secured a job that is lower paying or of lower social standing than what he or she had in his or her country of origin, this may be a source of distress. Other possible problems include feelings of guilt resulting from a perceived dissociation from the culture of origin when adjusting to the host culture, difficulty adapting to the host culture for fear of losing one's native cultural values, familial conflicts due to the role reversal of parents and children or husbands and wives, and perceived discrimination (McGoldrick, Giordano, & Garcia-Preto, 2005). Sample questions to ask the client, based on Lim's (2006) suggestions, include

- Do you have any friends who are from [the client's culture of origin]? How frequently do you see them? Do you feel comfortable around them? How do you relate to them? Are you involved with any community group associated with [the client's culture of origin]?

- Do you have friends who are not from [the client's culture of origin]? How do you relate to those individuals? Do you feel comfortable around them?
- Which group of friends would you say you relate to better?
- Do you find that adapting to your newer environment has been difficult or easy? How so?
- Have you felt in any way discriminated against in your newer culture? How has this affected you?

Explanatory Model of the Individual's Illness

The client's explanatory model of his or her problem is an essential component of any mental health interview. Although a psychiatrist or psychotherapist may draw from the medical, psychodynamic, cognitive-behavioral, and other models in understanding the causes of emotional distress and interpersonal problems, the client may hold a completely different belief system. Although explanatory models of mental health can be classified in varying ways, the authors have chosen to divide them into five broad categories, namely medical, psychological, social, moral, magical, and spiritual/religious. The medical model attributes mental illness to biologically driven processes that shape an individual's emotional state, perception, cognition, and behavior. It relies on psychotropic medications, surgery, electroconvulsive therapy, and other medical procedures for intervention.

A psychological understanding of distress attempts to address how individuals perceive, process, understand, and react to the world around them. Psychologists, psychiatrists, psychotherapists, and counselors alike employ variations of psychodynamic, cognitive-behavioral, humanistic, and interpersonal techniques to address a client's psychological needs. According to the social model, the central cause of distress is "everyday" life stress, such as economic strain, loss of employment, loss of housing, physical impairment, limited social supports, and access to services. Moral explanatory models attribute personal defects such as laziness, selfishness, or unethical behavior as the source of personal woes. Formal (such as social workers, occupational therapists, chaplain, religious authority, life coach) and informal (family and friends) resources are important in addressing both social and moral needs. Magical explanatory models are seen in every culture and can present as superstition, witchcraft, and sorcery. In some Muslim cultures, black magic, the "evil eye," or *jinn* (a specific type of spirit described in the Islamic tradition) possessions may be blamed for life's problems (Al-Issa, 2000). Muslims may go to traditional healers, community elders, or imams to address these issues (Aloud & Rathur, 2009). The spiritual and religious explanatory model posits that problems are due to weakness of faith, abandonment of religious rituals, or misunderstandings of religious teachings—including reasons why Allah (God) has placed one in the world.

Muslims often have multiple explanatory models that act in concert. For instance, among a sample of New York City Muslims, 88% believed in the use of both Qur'anic healing and medication/Western psychotherapy for the treatment of the mentally ill (Abu-Ras, Gheith, & Cournos, 2008). Mental health practitioners should ask Muslim clients about their explanatory models in a nonjudgmental way. Recommendations on how to word such a question are

- What do you believe has caused these symptoms you are experiencing?
- Many Muslims believe in the evil eye, black magic, or *jinn*; did that play a role in your current situation?

If a Muslim client believes in the role of a magical explanatory model, then it is important to explore the events and circumstance that led to that narrative. If the person visits a traditional healer, imam, or religious authority, offering the client to work with those resources may greatly strengthen the therapeutic alliance.

Cultural Components of the Psychosocial Environment

The client's psychosocial environment is a vast milieu that includes, but is certainly not limited to, family, ethnic community, cultural and religious institutions, occupation, and social network. The specific psychosocial settings of family and religious community are discussed in this section. In Muslim cultures, generally speaking, the family is regarded as the basic unit of society. Qur'anic verses and traditional teachings emphasize the importance of maintaining kinship ties, particularly those with one's parents. Islamic tradition also places great importance on one's relationship with the Muslim spiritual community. A Muslim client's family and the religious community may contribute greatly to the psychosocial environment (Hamid, 2008; Muslim, 2009a).

Family Psychosocial Factors

Probing into family-based psychosocial stressors should include questions about the level of the family's involvement in the client's life, the amount of influence family authority figures have over the client's decisions, which members of the family are seen as the authority figures, the role the client plays in the family power dynamic, and the client's familial responsibilities. Many Muslim societies have hierarchical family structures that promote authoritarian and collectivist environments (Dwairy, 2006). This is of particular importance to immigrants living in Western countries who have maintained close relationships with their cultures of origin. In collective systems, priority is given to the goals of the group and interpersonal responsibilities, rather than the goals and freedoms of the individual. As a result, there can be significant psychological, economic, and social interdependence of family members. To the clinician, it may appear that the familial authority figures micromanage the lives of other family members—having influence over their choices of dress, food, friends, and major life decisions such as career path and spouse. This involvement is typically not restricted to the nuclear family, but can also involve cousins, uncles, aunts, and grandparents. The clinician must keep in mind that what may appear to the Western-trained clinician as a family being enmeshed could actually be quite normative and may not be a source of psychological distress. It should also be noted that while such a familial system lends itself to much individual sacrifice and responsibility to the family, the familial network may also provide significant emotional, economic, and other support, especially in times of personal crises. As can be imagined, however, such a closely knit family structure can also be the source of substantial distress. Asking the client about familial interactions in an open-ended manner is thus essential. The family may be a central aspect of the client's psychosocial well-being and family cohesion may be highly valued. When offering interventions, clinicians should be mindful that compromising that individual–family relationship could lead to the client discontinuing treatment (Dwairy, 2006).

Clinicians should also be aware that a common feature of collective families is an authoritarian child-rearing style. As noted by Dwairy (2006), corporal punishment tends to be commonly accepted as a part of authoritarian parenting (Al-Kittani, 2000; Al-Mahroos, 2001; Al-Shqerat & Al-Masri, 2001; Qasem, Mustafa, Kazem, & Shah, 1998; Saif El-Deen, 2001). Although clinicians must be very careful not to condone or promote physical abuse, they should remain keen to the nuances of authoritarian parenting styles. Some studies of children exposed to either authoritarian parenting or corporal punishment have shown that it may be detrimental to the child's mental health (Gershoff, 2003; Mulvaney & Mebert, 2007). However, other studies suggest that the cultural and environmental context should be considered. For instance, a study involving 431 Arab adolescents raised in Israel found no significant correlations between authoritarian parenting styles and poor mental health outcomes (Dwairy, 2004). Researcher Marwan Dwairy (2006) argues that authoritarian parenting, when applied to the authoritarian Muslim society, does not have the negative outcomes that are associated with authoritarian approaches in Western populations. In fact, studies show that Arab youth are generally content with authoritarian parenting styles and experience that style as an expression of care and concern on the part of their parents (Hatab

& Makki, 1978). That being said, the clinician should still remain alert for any accounts of excessive physical punishment.

Community-Based Psychosocial Factors

Islamic traditions and beliefs foster a communal worldview in which Muslims view each other as brothers and sisters who all constitute a larger Muslim community, or *ummah* (Ramadan, 2007). The Prophet Muhammad metaphorically compared the Muslim community to that of one human body, saying that if there is an illness in one member of the body, then the whole body responds to the illness by becoming sick (Muslim, 2009b). Prophetic traditions also remind Muslims of the strength in unity (Ramadan, 2007). Community-oriented practices such as the breaking of the Ramadan fast together, group prayer, public religious celebrations, and mosque-based activities serve to nurture and reinforce this communal sentiment. Thus, many Muslims are closely tied to their Muslim communities and mosques, and use them as a source of psychological support. A study involving 102 Muslims and 22 Imams in post-9/11 New York City found that 59% of participants sought advice from the imam (religious leader) as a result of the distress of 9/11 (Abu-Ras et al., 2008). Furthermore, the study reported that 94% of participants viewed the imam as a counselor. Other studies have found that the community is frequently the first line of support of some Muslims (Graham, Bradshaw, & Trew, 2008; Al-Issa 1990; Al-Krenawi & Graham 2000; Hodge, 2005). Exploration of these community connections as both sources of support and psychosocial stress is thus critical for Muslim clients.

The Concept of Self in a Collective Culture

Inextricably bound to the understanding of a client's psychosocial vulnerabilities is a strong grasp of his or her concept of self. Margaret Mahler described a commonly accepted model for childhood development in her four phases of separation-individualization (Mahler, Pine, & Bergman, 1975). The process of individualization is critical for the development of a cohesive sense of self and for developing healthy attachments with others. A break or disruption in this process may result in characterological problems such as borderline and narcissistic disorders and even psychosis. Mahler described the "transition object" as an inanimate object such as a blanket or teddy bear as a tool children use to self-soothe as parents have limited time to spend with their child. Contemporary psychoanalytic theorist Salman Akhtar argues that, although Mahler's developmental model is very important, it must be historically and culturally placed (Akhtar, 1999). He argues that Mahler's observations were based on privileged, white New York City babies in the 1960s. The development and notion of self may take on a completely different process in Eastern cultures with large, extended family systems, in which there is little separation of babies from adult arms. In densely populated urban areas such as Cairo and Karachi, a baby may be passed on from mom to aunt to sister to cousin without ever separating from an adult figure. Interestingly, transition objects are not known to be existent in these cultures. The sense of self and sense of family bond takes on a different meaning in such contexts (Akhtar, 1999)

Difficult Topics of Discussion: Sex, Drugs, and Suicide

The three subjects of substance abuse, sexual issues, and suicide may produce some discomfort in both the clinician and the patient during the initial interview. The Qur'an and Prophetic traditions discuss these topics quite bluntly and extensively; however, within many Muslim communities these subjects are sensitive topics of discussion—especially among individuals who have just met.

Tobacco, Drugs, and Alcohol

Knowing about the client's use of tobacco, alcohol, other illicit drugs, and (overuse of) prescribed medications is critical. However, asking questions such as, "Have you ever used any drugs/tobacco in the past?" may not elicit a response that fully reflects a Muslim client's substance use. Many Muslims may not perceive some substances as harmful or addictive. For instance, *khat* is a psychostimulant used commonly in Yemen and East Africa (Al-Hebshi & Skaug, 2005). Clients may not report using khat, as it may not be viewed as a drug of abuse. Likewise, water-pipe smoking (a tobacco-smoking practice otherwise known as hooka or sheesha) has been gaining noteworthy popularity among teenagers and adolescents. Water-pipe smoking is associated with an increased risk of malignancy, decreased pulmonary function, and the spread of infectious diseases such as tuberculosis (Knishkowy & Amitai, 2005). Asking specifically about the use of these substances during the interview may be useful.

In the Islamic tradition, the use of alcohol and recreational drugs is explicitly forbidden. Many Muslims are likely to hide their substance abuse habits from their family and communities, as a considerable amount of social stigma exists within communities with regard to substance abuse (Arfken, Berry, & Owens, 2009; Tahboob-Schulte, Ali, & Khafaji, 2009). The stigma is generally directed toward substance *use* itself, as well as abuse (Arfken et al., 2009). The moderate use of some substances, such as alcohol, may be normative for non-Muslim populations. However, for the Muslim client, even in moderate amounts, alcohol use may be looked down upon as a failure to live up to Muslim cultural and religious standards. Inquiry into the client's perceptions of how substance use has affected his or her relations with family and community members may give the clinician a clearer picture of the client's experience. Reassurance of clinician–client confidentiality is key during this component of the interview. Substance use could also be addressed after establishing a stronger clinician–client rapport.

Suicide

Clinicians should also consider religious and cultural factors when assessing suicide risk. In Islam, committing suicide or attempting to do so is considered sinful. The Qur'an states, ". . . and kill not one another nor yourselves. Lo! Allah is ever Merciful unto you" (Qur'an 4:29). Thus, suicide may be regarded by the Muslim client as a weakness of faith and is associated with a significant amount of social stigma. As such, a Muslim client could exhibit some resistance to disclosing such information. A more natural and less direct method of inquiring about suicide is to fit it into the context of assessing for mood and anxiety symptoms.

Sexual Activity

Another sensitive discussion topic for many Muslims is sexual activity. It is common for a Muslim's first romantic relationship to be with his or her spouse. In Islamic law, having a significant premarital romantic relationship is prohibited. The religious tradition is that an unmarried man and woman should not be secluded together, unless there is a third party (Muslim, 2009c). Such standards usually preclude boyfriend/girlfriend relationships commonly seen in Western cultures. The degree of social stigmatization against premarital romantic relationships varies depending on the views of the client, his or her family, and the Muslim community. Generally, however, premarital sex tends to be a source of considerable shame, especially in the case of females. If it is disclosed that a particular Muslim client has engaged in premarital sex, not only is that individual's reputation at stake, it may undermine the reputation of the family and also negatively affect the client's ability to find a spouse within the community.

Remaining chaste until marriage and being loyal to one's spouse during marriage are considered to be duties incumbent upon a Muslim. Thus a Muslim client may view premarital or extramarital sex as a laxity of his or her Islamic responsibilities. Such beliefs, compounded with community and familial stigma, could result in a significant amount of guilt and conflicted feelings. Therefore, counselors should be very cautious regarding how they address a client's sexual impulses and practices.

Cultural Elements of the Relationship between the Individual and the Clinician

Cultural elements inevitably affect the relationship between a clinician and a client. Some questions for clinicians to ask themselves when dealing with all clients are

- Do I feel comfortable with my knowledge of the normative practices and values of the client's culture?
- Are what I label as "signs and symptoms" actually acceptable beliefs within the client's culture?
- How do my personal beliefs and worldviews affect how I engage with the client?
- How does the client's perception of me affect how the client engages me?

Clinicians should be knowledgeable about the normative practices and values of their clients' cultures. Acceptable beliefs and behaviors within a client's culture should not be mislabeled as "signs and symptoms." A clinician should also be aware of how his or her personal beliefs and worldviews affect how he or she engages the client.

The clinician should be conscious of intercultural and intracultural transference and countertransference. Although it is not possible to enumerate or describe all of the possible ways that ethnicity and religion shape transference and countertransference, several different possible scenarios are provided.

Intercultural Considerations

Intercultural considerations consist of both interethnic (when clinician and client are from different ethnicities) and inter-religious (when clinician and client are from different religious traditions) transference and countertransference.

Transference   Interethnic transference may result from a perceived power differential between the client and the clinician. For instance, a client from an ethnic minority culture may be overly eager to please a clinician from the dominant ethnicity. In this case, the clinician from the dominant ethnicity may be viewed as an authority figure, or as a member of an institution (e.g., hospital, clinic, government, or the dominant ethnicity in general) that has authority. Interethnic transference may also manifest as distrust toward the therapist. This could be the result of past negative interactions that the client may have had with individuals from the clinician's ethnicity. Other common interethnic themes listed by Comas-Díaz and Jacobsen (1991) are the client's denial of the importance of ethnic factors in his or her life and being ambivalent about obtaining treatment.

One inter-religious transference theme is the Muslim client hesitating to share information with the clinician for fear of being stereotyped. A hypothetical scenario is a domestically abused Muslim woman who is uncomfortable telling the non-Muslim clinician about the abuse, for fear of reinforcing stereotypes that Muslim women are oppressed or commonly beaten by their husbands. Other inter-religious transference topics are feeling frustrated by the clinician's lack of understanding of Islamic cultural norms, being distrustful of the non-Muslim clinician who may be perceived as one who dislikes Muslims, and feeling the need to represent Muslims to the non-Muslim therapist and thus hiding information from the non-Muslim clinician in order to give a more positive view of Islam.

Countertransference   One instance of interethnic countertransference is a clinician from the dominant ethnicity feeling guilty about social injustices that a minority client may have to endure. This could result in the clinician being more shy and apprehensive when interviewing the client. Another interethnic countertransference theme is questioning the client about elements of his or her culture based solely on the clinician's personal interest and not on the clinical situation (Comas-Díaz & Jacobsen, 1991).

Inter-religious countertransference could be due to clinicians harboring negative feelings toward their Muslim clients. If a therapist has Muslim friends or colleagues, those relationships may consciously or unconsciously shape how the therapist thinks and feels about Muslims. A poll of 1,003 American adults found that 41% of people reported being acquainted with a Muslim, 38% had a negative view of Islam, and 35% believed Islam is more likely than other religions to encourage violence (Pew Forum on Religion and Public Life, 2010). Another countertransference theme is the clinician attributing harmful practices—such as domestic violence—to being within the realm of Islamic cultural norms. Other inter-religious countertransference themes parallel the interethnic countertransference themes mentioned previously. For example, the clinician may feel guilty about the social injustices suffered by the Muslim client and be less bold during the interview. The clinician may also feel insecure about his or her knowledge about Islam and ask the Muslim client questions about religious issues that are not relevant to the clinical situation. This scenario may prompt the client to play the role of the "representative Muslim." Furthermore, clinicians may feel less competent about their abilities to incorporate the clients' religion into therapy; as such they may avoid delving into religious topics at all (Henning & Tirrell, 1982). Clinicians may also avoid religious topics because of apprehensions about imposing their value systems upon their clients (Henning & Tirrell, 1982).

Intracultural Considerations

Transference   Transference can be as potent in intraethnic situations as it is in interethnic encounters. Clients who share the same ethnic background as their clinicians may idealize them. Also, clients who have antagonistic relationships to their own ethnic heritages may have negative thoughts about the therapist. They may even assume that the therapist is less skilled than a clinician from the dominant ethnicity. Additionally, clients with different levels of acculturation compared to their clinicians may view the clinicians as having "sold out" to the dominant ethnicity (Caraballo et al., 2006; Comas-Díaz & Jacobsen, 1991).

Some Muslim clients who share the same religion as their clinicians may not discuss situations in which the client has acted in a fashion that is contradictory to Islamic norms. For example, a Muslim client who drinks alcohol may not feel comfortable telling this to a Muslim clinician, for fear of being judged. Furthermore, if the Muslim client views mental health problems as stemming from a deficiency of faith, the client may feel insecure about his or her level of religiosity. Thus, the client may emphatically display outward signs of religious commitment when dealing with the clinician.

Countertransference Examples of intraethnic countertransference, as stated by Comas-Díaz and Jacobsen (1991) and later mentioned by Caraballo and colleagues (2006), are defensive distancing by the clinician, becoming angry because of greater demands from the client, feelings of guilt concerning the clinician's socioeconomic circumstances versus that of the client, and over-identification with the client. Also, clinicians who share the same ethnicity as their clients may feel a sense of "tribal" responsibility to better the condition of the client because he or she is one of "our own." In such situations, the clinician may find him or herself having difficulty drawing boundaries.

The concept of "tribal" responsibility also extends to the relationship between clients and clinicians who share the same religious background. A Muslim clinician may feel more obligated to assist a Muslim client than a non-Muslim client, and thus may encounter difficulties with maintaining appropriate boundaries. Also, the Muslim clinician may assume that he or she completely understands the way the Muslim client views the world, when actually, despite sharing the same religious traditions, they may have differing ideas about Islam. Additionally, the Muslim clinician may have negative feelings about Islam and could project these on the Muslim client.

Cultural Elements of Disease Manifestations

Many clinicians trained in Western society are taught about signs and symptoms of diseases, such as depression, as if they were objective findings and universal to all humans around the globe. More recently, cultural influences have gained wider acceptance as substantial modifiers of the symptoms of psychiatric disease (Smart & Smart, 1997). The clinician must keep in mind that the content of complaints and clinical relevance are culturally influenced. One example of this is the case of a Javanese Muslim woman who was admitted to a mental hospital in Java secondary to "slamming doors and loudly expressing resentment and suspicion." This kind of behavior was regarded as particularly abnormal in the region of Java where she resided, as the native people pride themselves on having a tranquil affect (Browne, 2001). If this same patient were to be evaluated in a different cultural setting, her symptoms may not have been viewed as pathological, and consequently a mental health practitioner may not have even seen her. The authors are not in any way implying that such a patient does not have underlying psychological problems, but that the manifestations may vary depending on the cultural context. Another example is a Muslim client who claims that he or she knows something to be true because God revealed it in a dream. In the Islamic tradition it is believed that dreams are a means by which Allah (God) may disclose information to an individual (Muslim, 2009d). Therefore, the previously stated claim may not be a delusion. Mental health practitioners should remain aware that a delusion should be distinct from culturally held values (Sadock & Sadock, 2008). The effect of culture on disease manifestation can be quite substantial and clinicians should not hesitate to request a "cultural consultation" from a mental health professional, imam, or community leader who is competent in the client's cultural needs.

Cultural Formulation, Overall Assessment, and Management Options

Clinicians should list relevant cultural factors that may affect the client's symptoms and clinical course, making sure to address the following categories:

1. The client's cultural identity
2. The client's cultural explanation of the symptoms
3. Cultural components of the psychosocial environment
4. Cultural elements of the relationship between the individual and clinician
5. Cultural elements of disease manifestation

Then, a series of possible hypotheses pertaining to the role of culture on the client's illness should be generated. Final considerations should include the following:

- How does the cultural formulation affect management (i.e., interventions offered by the clinician)?
- Which type of psychotherapy (if indicated) is most appropriate for the client's case?

- What are the response rate and side effects of psychotropics in the racial group of the client?
- Should other supports such as family, community, and traditional healers be incorporated into interventions?

Clients from collective cultures may be more interested in family therapy, which could involve the extended family as well. On the other hand, people from individualistic societies may be more amenable to individualized expressive psychodynamic psychotherapy (Caraballo et al., 2006).

The type of treatment recommended for the client should also take into account the client's explanation for the illness. For instance, clients who are prescribed medications, but do not believe in a biological basis for their symptoms, may not take them. Other issues that could affect adherence to medications in Muslim clients specifically include

1. The use of medications containing alcohol, gelatin (denatured collagen which is frequently derived from pigs), and other pork products
2. The use of medications during Ramadan (the Islamic holy month of fasting)

The religious regulations regarding medication use in these circumstances are quite complex and differ on a case-by-case basis (Ibn Adam al-Kawthari, 2005). Therefore, a cultural consultation from a learned imam—possibly multiple imams—should be sought in such instances. These issues cannot be addressed, however, unless clinicians remember to inquire into what might prevent a client from adhering to a treatment regimen.

Conclusion

When interviewing a Muslim client and constructing a cultural formulation, such salient elements as the patient's cultural identity, explanation for the symptoms, cultural factors related to the psychosocial environment, clinician–client relationship, and treatment options must be considered. An emphasis should be placed on establishing a therapeutic alliance in which the client feels understood. Maintaining an open mind, asking the client to explain aspects of the interview that were not understood, and consulting experts with more knowledge about the client's culture, such as imams or community leaders, are essential to promoting an environment of empathy and acceptance. Clinicians should keep in mind that parts of the mental health interview can be revisited during later sessions. Components of the cultural formulation and the therapeutic relationship itself will evolve over time, as the client and clinician become more familiar with each other.

References

Abu-Ras, W., Gheith, A., & Cournos, F. (2008). The imam's role in mental health promotion: A study at 22 mosques in New York City's Muslim community. *Journal of Muslim Mental Health, 3*(2), 155–176.

Akhtar, S. (1999). *Immigration and identity: Turmoil, treatment, and transformation.* Northvale, NJ: Jason Aronson Press.

Al-Hebshi, N., & Skaug, N. (2005). Khat (*Catha edulis*)—An updated review. *Addiction Biology, 10*, 299–307.

Al-Issa, A. (1990). Culture and mental illness in Algeria. *International Journal of Social Psychiatry, 36*, 230–240.

Al-Issa, I. (Ed.). (2000). *Al-junun: Mental illness in the Islamic world.* Madison, CT: International Universities Press.

Al-Kittani, F. (2000). *Al-ittijahat al-walideyah fi al-tanshia'a al-ijtima'ayah [Parents' approaches in socialization].* Amman, Jordan: Dar Al-Shurooq.

Al-Krenawi, A., & Graham, J. R. (2000). Islamic theology and prayer: Relevance for social work practice. *International Social Work, 43*, 289–302.

Al-Mahroos, F. (2001, October). Rasd thaherat soo'a al-moa'amalah fil Bahrain [Observations on abuse in Bahrain]. Abstract of the conference on child abuse, Baharini Society for Child Development, Bahrain, October, 20–22.

Aloud, N., & Rathur, A. (2009). Factors affecting attitudes toward seeking and using formal mental health and psychological services among Arab Muslim populations. *Journal of Muslim Mental Health, 4*(2), 79–103.

Al-Shqerat, M. A., & Al-Masri, A. N. (2001). Al-isaa'a al-laftheyah ded al-atfal [Verbal abuse against children]. Majallat al-tofoolah al-'arabiah [Journal of Arab Childhood], 2(7), 33–45.

American Psychiatric Association. (2010). Outline for cultural formulation and glossary of culture-bound syndromes. In *Diagnostic and statistical manual of mental disorders* (4th ed., Appendix I). doi: 10.1176/appi.books.9780890423349.7060

Arfken, C. L., Berry, A., & Owens, D. (2009). Pathways for Arab Americans to substance abuse treatment in southeastern Michigan. *Journal of Muslim Mental Health, 4*(1), 31–46.

Browne, K. O. (2001). Cultural formulation of psychiatric diagnoses *sakit jiwa*, *ng(amuk)*, and schizoaffective disorder in a Javanese woman. *Culture, Medicine and Psychiatry, 25*, 411–425.

Caraballo, A., Hamid, H., Lee, J. R., McQuery, J. D., Rho, Y., Kramer, E. J., Lim, R. F., & Lu, F. G. (2006). A resident's guide to the cultural formulation. In R. F. Lim (Ed.), *Clinical manual of cultural psychiatry* (pp. 243–265). Arlington, VA: American Psychiatric Publishing Inc.

Comas-Díaz, L., & Jacobsen, F. M. (1991). Ethnocultural transference and countertransference in the therapeutic dyad. *American Journal of Orthopsychiatry, 61*(3), 392–402.

Dwairy, M. (2004). Parenting styles and mental health of Palestinian-Arab adolescents in Israel. *Transcultural Psychiatry, 41*(2), 233–252.

Dwairy, M. (2006). *Counseling and psychotherapy with Arabs and Muslims.* New York, NY: Teacher's College Press.

Eells, T. D. (2007). *Handbook of psychotherapy case formulation*. New York, NY: The Guilford Press.

Gershoff, E. T. (2003). Corporal punishment by parents and associated child behaviors and experiences: A meta-anaytic and theoretical view. *Psychological Bulletin, 128*(4), 539–579.

Graham, J. R., Bradshaw, C., & Trew, J. L. (2008). Social worker's understanding of the immigrant Muslim client's perspective. *Journal of Muslim Mental Health, 3*(2), 125–144.

Hamid, H. (2008). A brief introduction. In S. Akhtar (Ed.), *The crescent and the couch: Cross currents between Islam and psychoanalysis* (pp. 5–19). Lanham, MD: Rowman & Littlefield Publishers, Inc.

Hasan, A., & Kuluva, J. (2006). Arranged marriage: A socially acceptable form of migration? Case report and cultural formulation. *Journal of Muslim Mental Health, 1*(1), 65–75.

Hatab, Z., & Makki, A. (1978). Al-solta el-abawia wa al shabab *[Parental authority and youth]*. Beirut, Lebanon: Ma'had al-Inma'a al'Arabi.

Henning, L. H., & Tirrell, F. J. (1982). Counselor resistance to spiritual exploration. *The Personnel and Guidance Journal, 61*(2), 92–95.

Hodge, D. (2005). Social work and the house of Islam: Orienting practitioners to the beliefs and values of Muslims in the United States. *Social Work, 50*, 162–174.

Ibn Adam al-Kawthari, M. (2005). Using unlawful medication, question ID 4039. (Online). October 28, 2010. Sunnipath the online Islamic academy. Retrieved from http://qa.sunnipath.com/issue_view.asp?HD=1&ID=4039&CATE=233

Knishkowy, B., & Amitai, Y. (2005). Water-pipe (Narghile) smoking: An emerging health risk behavior *Pediatrics, 116*, e113–e119.

Lim, R. F. (2006). *Clinical manual of cultural psychiatry*. Arlington, VA: American Psychiatric Publishing Inc.

Lu, F. G., Lim, R., & Mezzich, J. E. (1995). Issues in the assessment and diagnosis of culturally diverse individuals. In J. Oldham & M. Riba (Eds.), *Review of psychiatry* (Vol. 14, pp. 477–510). Washington, DC: American Psychiatric Press.

Mahler, M.S., Pine F., & Bergman A. (1975). *The psychological birth of the human infant*. New York, NY: Basic Books.

Mavreas, V., Bebbington, P., & Der, G. (1989). The structure and validity of acculturation: Analysis of an acculturation scale. *Social Psychiatry and Psychiatric Epidemiology, 24*(5), 233–240.

McGoldrick, M., Giordano, J., & Garcia-Preto, N. (Eds.). (2005). *Ethnicity and family therapy* (3rd ed.). New York, NY: The Guilford Press.

McWilliams, N. (1994). *Psychoanalytic diagnosis: Understanding personality structure in the clinical process*. New York, NY: The Guildford Press.

Mulvaney, M. K., & Mebert, C. J. (2007). Parental corporal punishment predicts behavior problems in early childhood. *Journal of Family Psychology, 21*(3), 389–397.

Muslim, S. (2009a). Translation of Sahih Muslim, Book 32, Chapter 1, Number 6180, the book of virtue, good manners and joining of the ties of relationship. (Online). October 17, 2010. University of Southern California Center for Muslim Jewish Engagement. Retrieved from http://www.usc.edu/schools/college/crcc/engagement/resources/texts/muslim/hadith/muslim/032.smt.html#032.6180

Muslim, S. (2009b). Translation of Sahih Muslim, Book 32, Chapter 15, Number 6260, the book of virtue, good manners and joining of the ties of relationship. (Online). October 17, 2010. University of Southern California Center for Muslim Jewish Engagement. Retrieved from http://www.usc.edu/schools/college/crcc/engagement/resources/texts/muslim/hadith/muslim/032.smt.html#032.6260

Muslim, S. (2009c). Translation of Sahih Muslim, Book 7, Chapter 72, Number 3110, the book of pilgrimage. (Online). October 18, 2010. University of Southern California Center for Muslim Jewish Engagement. Retrieved from http://www.usc.edu/schools/college/crcc/engagement/resources/texts/muslim/hadith/muslim/007.smt.html#072.3110

Muslim, S. (2009d). Translation of Sahih Muslim, Book 29, Chapter 1, Number 5621, the book of vision. (Online). October 28, 2010. University of Southern California Center for Muslim Jewish Engagement. Retrieved from http://www.usc.edu/schools/college/crcc/engagement/resources/texts/muslim/hadith/muslim/029.smt.html#029.5621

Pew Forum on Religion and Public Life. (2010). *Public remains conflicted over Islam*. Philadelphia, PA: Pew Global Attitudes Project. Retrieved from http:pewforum.org/Muslim/Public-Remains-Conflicted-Over-Islam.aspx

Pinderhughes, E. (1989). *Understanding race, ethnicity, and power: The key to efficacy in clinical practice*. New York, NY: The Free Press.

Puchalski, C. (2006). Spirituality assessment in clinical practice. *Psychiatric Annals, 36*(3), 150–155.

Qasem, F. S., Mustafa, A. A., Kazem, N. A., & Shah, N. M. (1998). Attitude of Kuwaiti parents towards physical punishment of children. *Child Abuse and Neglect, 22*, 1189–1202.

Ramadan, T. (2007). *In the footsteps of the Prophet: Lessons from the life of Muhammad*. New York, NY: Oxford University Press.

Sadock, B. J., & Sadock, V. A. (2008). *Kaplan & Sadock's concise textbook of clinical psychiatry* (3rd ed.). Philadelphia, PA: Wolters Kluwer Health, Lippincott Williams.

Saif El-Deen, A. (2001, October). Soo'a al-moa'amalah wa ihmal al-atfl *[Abuse and neglect of children]*. Abstract of the conference on child abuse, Bahrain, October 20–22.

Smart, D. W., & Smart, J. F. (1997). DSM-IV and culturally sensitive diagnosis: Some observations for counselors. *Journal of Counseling & Development, 75*, 392–398.

Tahboob-Schulte, S., Ali, A. Y., & Khafaji, T. (2009). Treating substance dependency in the UAE: A case study. *Journal of Muslim Mental Health, 4*(1), 67–75.

Varma, S. (2008). Clozaril and Allah—A patient's journey into wellness: A case report and cultural formulation. *Journal of Muslim Mental Health, 3*(1), 89–97.

CHAPTER 5

Psychological Testing and Assessment

OMAR M. MAHMOOD and SAWSSAN R. AHMED

Given that Muslims in Western countries come from a multitude of ethnic and linguistic backgrounds, the psychological assessment of clients in Muslim communities shares many of the same challenges as that of other minority groups. In addition to the influences of cultural norms and traditions, religious beliefs and practices may also be important considerations for any clinician conducting an assessment with a Muslim client. Despite these challenges, the psychological assessment of cognitive function, personality, and mood symptoms is important and necessary in addressing the mental health needs of Muslims. With appropriate consideration and accommodation for cultural and religious factors relevant to Muslims, clinicians who are mindful of client and family expectations, testing procedures, and the interpretation of results can effectively carry out such assessments.

The tools of psychological assessment, including psychometric measures, cognitive tests, self-report questionnaires, and other instruments employed by clinicians to form a representation of a client's psychological profile, are potentially susceptible to bias effects that could result in the mischaracterization of Muslim clients. Tests that are developed using standardization samples in Western countries tend to reflect the predominant values, knowledge, language, and cultural experiences of people within those societies. Thus, an individual who comes from a nondominant cultural group may produce scores representing something other than what the test-maker originally intended (Padilla, 2001). Potential problems when assessing members of a cultural minority can be minimized when clinicians take into consideration a cultural framework that addresses the individual-difference factors that could influence the examination (Butcher, Nezami, & Exner, 1998).

This chapter provides an overview of potential considerations for the mental health professional who wishes to conduct a psychological assessment with a Muslim client. First, we discuss factors relating to the demographics and cultural norms of Muslims that may be relevant when the clinician initially prepares for the assessment. Next, we highlight aspects of the testing session itself that may require special attention or adjustment for some Muslim clients. This includes recommendations for specific domains of functioning and the measures used to assess those domains. Finally, we present some advice for the clinician when interpreting the findings, writing a report, and providing feedback after the assessment. Notably, this chapter is most relevant to the kind of assessment of a client or patient who is typically referred to a clinical psychologist or other mental health professional in a hospital or clinic setting. We focused primarily on three major areas of assessment that are frequently addressed in such settings to aid in diagnosis: cognitive ability, personality, and emotional functioning. Other types of assessment procedures that may incorporate broader sources of clinical information across multiple settings such as in schools or occupational settings (e.g., assessments of behavioral or social functioning, developmental inventories, or measurements of workplace effectiveness) are beyond the scope of this chapter. However, many of the concepts presented here are still relevant to a wide variety of referral questions that clinicians working with Muslims may encounter. We conclude with a case example to illustrate how the points discussed in this chapter can be applied to an actual client.

Factors to Consider when Assessing a Muslim Client

In preparation for the assessment, the clinician should bear in mind that the client may have unique characteristics requiring some modifications to the assessment that depart from standard procedure. These cultural qualities will dictate the kind of interaction that takes place between the clinician and client during the assessment. In the following we discuss the levels of interaction that are affected, including how clinician and client communicate (language), how they learn about each other (mutual understanding of the presenting problem), and how they eventually collaborate (forming the goals of the assessment).

Language

Language is a potentially integral factor that a clinician must be aware of when assessing a Muslim client. In some cases, the evaluation may not directly present with language issues (e.g., a nonverbal or aphasic patient, a classroom observation of behavior, a client who is a native English speaker). However, the need to communicate test results and interpretations with family members or caregivers may arise. In situations where direct communication with the patient is required, language becomes an even more salient consideration. If the patient speaks only limited English, then the clinician must decide whether to refer the case to an available practitioner who speaks the patient's native language, to use an interpreter during the examination, or to proceed with the assessment while hoping that the patient's limited English will allow him or her to understand the test instructions and interview questions.

If simple evaluation of cognitive functioning is required, then one may consider nonverbal measures of domains such as visual attention, visuospatial functioning, or visual memory. However, this approach will not be helpful if a wider range of verbal and complex cognitive abilities must be tested, or if the evaluation is to include personality or emotional functioning measures. In such situations, the clinician may decide to employ translated instruments or conduct the assessment in the client's native language. The use of an interpreter may be helpful if detailed information about the patient's background or presenting problem must be obtained. In addition, an interpreter could ensure that test instructions are communicated clearly to the patient, which will increase the validity of test performances. It is generally recommended to use a trained interpreter who, in addition to translating information, can also interpret cultural and social cues between the examiner and client (Lynch & Hanson, 1999). An interpreter trained in medical or social services translation would be ideal, as opposed to a family member or other layperson who happens to speak the client's language. Although interpreters can be a great help during the interview process and in explaining test instructions, only a mental health professional with the requisite psychometric training should actually administer psychodiagnostic instruments.

With regard to bilingual patients who speak English, it may be perfectly suitable to test the patient using English-language assessment tools. However, fluency in English does not necessarily correspond to having the cultural and historical knowledge that may be inherently assumed in tests developed in the Western world. In addition, clinicians must be wary of the fact that, for some bilingual clients, their non-English language dominates their verbal abilities, while other bilingual clients demonstrate differential strengths within each language. Depending on the type of assessment being administered, there may be cause to test in different languages within a single evaluation (e.g., clients may be strong in their native language for verbal working memory tasks, but strong on English academic achievement tests because all of their schooling was in English-language settings). It is widely established that perfect bilingualism may not exist, and that every bilingual individual tends to have a dominant language (Lyons, 1981).

The Presenting Problem

The description of a client's presenting problems is what guides the assessment and informs the clinician's interpretation of test results. When asking about symptoms, complaints, and other relevant history, it is important that the information is gathered in a collaborative effort between clinician and client (and family members, if applicable). There may be some details of the presenting problem that the client or family members wish to convey that is not typically asked for in clinical intake interviews. For example, a religious client (or family member) may wish to report a detailed spiritual experience as the precipitating event for a psychological symptom. Similarly, the examiner may ask clinically relevant questions that could be perceived as nonessential or inappropriate to clients' conceptualization of their complaints. For instance, disclosing information about family history may be viewed as intrusive and irrelevant to an individual who is unfamiliar with how diagnostic interviews are conducted. Furthermore, some clients may have difficulty answering questions about substance use behavior or sexual activity due to feelings of guilt or the social stigma such topics can carry within the Muslim community. The potential divergence between clinical significance and cultural significance underscores the fact that each individual's schemas and constructs of psychological well-being will influence his or her idea of what "normal" behavior is. Evidence has shown that cultural differences in how one construes the self can lead to differing expectations for how to process information cognitively and emotionally (Markus & Kitayama, 1991).

Clinicians will be more effective in treating the presenting problem if they can gain an understanding of the client's religious and cultural beliefs pertaining to psychological health. Research indicates that a significant barrier for minority groups who seek mental health services is the incongruence between clients and service providers in their beliefs of the causes of psychological conditions (Hoberman, 1992; Leong & Lau, 2001). When seeking services for their children, ethnic minority parents are less likely than white Americans to endorse a biopsychosocial cause for their children's conditions (Yeh, Hough, McCabe, Lau, & Garland, 2004). Muslims have been shown to be more likely than other minority groups to cite religion or spiritual causes for mental health problems (Cinnirella & Loewenthal, 1999). Thus, clinicians should be mindful when probing the clients' beliefs about the disease course or symptom history that preceded their appointment for a psychological assessment.

In some Asian cultures, there is a tendency for clients to focus primarily on physical symptoms instead of affective complaints, even when the underlying problem is psychiatric in nature (Lin & Cheung, 1999). This trend has also been noted in Middle Eastern cultures (Al-Krenawi & Graham, 2000). However, clinicians should also beware of overlooking the client's somatic complaints by assuming that they are just manifestations of a psychiatric disorder when in fact there may also be concomitant medical issues that need to be addressed.

Expectations and Goals of the Assessment

Muslim clients coming from cultural groups that are unfamiliar with Western psychology may require psychoeducation regarding the purpose and benefits of an assessment. For example, a family bringing their child in for cognitive or aptitude testing may assume that the evaluation itself will "treat" the client, in which case the clinician may need to clarify that a more appropriate expectation of the assessment is to characterize the child's current level of functioning in order to make treatment recommendations. If the client was referred by another treatment provider or medical professional, he or she may come to the assessment without any expectations at all, or perhaps wonder what value there is in seeing a mental health professional. A clear understanding of the purpose of the assessment will facilitate the client's cooperation and motivation, which in turn will help to ensure valid responses on psychometric tests and questionnaires.

During the Assessment

There are a number of logistical factors that clinicians must consider when it comes to conducting a psychological testing session with a Muslim client. These factors could potentially affect the manner in which the evaluation is administered, requiring clinicians to be flexible with their assessment procedures. Although making accommodations for a client by altering the testing environment may compromise the standardization of test administration or may affect the client's performance, the overall benefit of the assessment to the client's condition should be prioritized. To determine whether any modification to standard procedures should be used, the clinician must estimate the contribution such a change would make in answering the referral question and in producing useful recommendations. Importantly, it is possible (and sometimes quite likely) that no major adjustment in testing protocol would be required with a Muslim client, and this matter should be judged on a case-by-case basis.

The Testing Environment

The first practical issue to consider is simply the physical space in which the assessment will take place. If the clinician and client are of opposite gender, this can pose an initial challenge. In some Muslim communities, interaction between opposite genders may be limited and closely controlled. Assessment procedures involving direct contact with the client (e.g., neurological exam, tests of tactile abilities, etc.) may have to be delegated to another clinician of the same gender. Occasionally, a client may refuse to be tested alone with an examiner of the opposite gender unless a family member can view the assessment in plain sight (either through a large window or from inside the testing room). Given that some clients may feel embarrassed or remain silent due to cultural etiquettes of showing respect, the simplest approach is for clinicians to directly ask clients if they would prefer such accommodations.

Another issue to negotiate is the participation of family members in the assessment. Generally speaking, Muslim families tend to be quite involved in the health care decisions of their family members, with possibly several members of immediate and extended family discussing treatment with health care providers (Lawrence & Rozmus, 2001; Dwairy, 2006). It may not occur to family members that a psychological testing session typically does not include anyone other than the clinician and client, with the rare exception of additional individuals whose presence is necessary for medical or communication purposes (e.g., a nurse or an interpreter). In the case where the client is a child, the guardian(s) may not realize that their presence could affect the child's test performance and willingness to respond to questions. After hearing an explanation of the standard protocol, most families will likely comply. In the few instances when there is a strong objection to leaving the client alone with the clinician, judgment should be used in deciding which family members can sit in during the testing session, bearing in mind the potential distraction that may occur. Whatever is decided regarding the presence of others during the session should also be affirmed by the client's (or the client's guardian's) consent.

Timing and Scheduling

Clinicians should also be mindful of additional issues that may arise with regard to the timing and scheduling of assessment sessions. When scheduling a lengthy assessment session, breaks should be given to allow for religious clients to offer prayers at the appropriate times. If the assessment takes place during the month of Ramadan, then care should be exercised in making sure that the session does not interfere with the time for breaking fast. Clinicians should also be aware that there are some religious holidays based on the lunar calendar that clients may observe throughout the year and thus appointments may have to be moved in rare instances.

Selection of Assessment Tools

Tests and questionnaires used in a psychological assessment will only be useful if they can contribute meaningful information about the client's underlying cognitive, emotional, or behavioral condition. However, selecting tests that are inappropriate for a particular individual because of inherent cultural biases in the way the tests are developed, administered, and scored could end up causing more harm than good if the results are interpreted as true representations of the client's condition. Challenges in selecting an appropriate measure of a psychological construct for Muslim clients may arise whether the domain being assessed is cognition, personality, or emotion.

Cognitive Functioning When utilizing cognitive tests to characterize intellectual or neuropsychological ability, clinicians must consider whether cultural factors may be altering the cognitive process that each test was originally designed to assess. For example, using visual attention or verbal processing tests containing printed words that were standardized in Western societies where left to right is the dominant direction of written language may result in performances by native speakers of Arabic, Urdu, or Farsi (which are languages written and read from right to left) that underestimate the client's true ability. In the case of bilingual clients, a suboptimal performance on a verbal learning and memory task (e.g., a word list learning test or a story memory test) may be attributable to language difficulties and not necessarily indicate a deficit in memory or recall. In such a situation, measures of visual memory (e.g., complex figure copy and recall) may be one way of circumventing this problem. In general, nonverbal measures of cognitive abilities can be used to characterize strengths and weaknesses in intellectual functioning when verbal communication is complicated by language differences. Table 5.1 summarizes various nonverbal tests of general intellectual functioning that have been used in non-English-speaking populations from a variety of different cultures. It is important to note that an over-reliance on nonverbal measures will fail to capture some clients' cognitive symptoms, particularly those with left-hemisphere deficits involving verbally mediated processing.

Caution should be exercised when using translated versions of cognitive tests. A simple exchange of written stimuli into a translated version could potentially alter the psychometric properties of the test, rendering it invalid as a measure of neuropsychological function. For example, an Arabic version of a letter-sequencing (Trail Making) test was shown to have a high false-positive rate, resulting in performances by healthy Arabic-speaking individuals that appeared similar to those of brain-injured clients in the American normative sample (Stanczak, Stanczak, & Awadalla, 2001).

Beyond the issue of translation, clinicians may need to examine whether clients have difficulty with the content of a cognitive test due to a lack of cultural context. Without knowledge of American history or familiarity with the nuances of Western proverbs, even an examinee with excellent

Table 5.1 Summary of Nonverbal Tests of Intellectual Functioning

Test Name	Author(s)	Clinical Characteristics
Comprehensive Tests of Nonverbal Intelligence, 2nd Edition (CTONI-2)	Hammill, Pearson, & Wiederholt (2009)	• For age range 6–90 years • Multiple-choice format, examinee can point to response • Provides a Pictoral IQ score, Geometric IQ score, and Nonverbal IQ score
Kaufman Assessment Battery for Children, 2nd Edition (KABC-II)	Kaufman & Kaufman (2004)	• For age range 3–18 years • Contains nonverbal subtests that can be administered using standardized pantomimed instructions • Provides age-based standard scores, age-ranks, and percentile scores
Leiter International Performance Scale–Revised (Leiter-R)	Roid & Miller (1997)	• For age range 2–20 years • Useful for children and adolescents with limited language ability, poor motor coordination, or cognitive delay • Contains two standardized batteries assessing: Visualization/Reasoning and Attention/Memory
Raven's Progressive Matrices (RPM)	Raven, Raven, & Court (1998)	• For age range 6–80 years • Standard form tests visual problem solving and is based on Spearman's measurement of "g" • Does not assess multiple domains of cognition but is widely used in many cultures across the world
Universal Nonverbal Intelligence Test (UNIT)	Bracken & McCallum (1998)	• For age range 5–18 years • Uses multiple response modes including manipulated stimuli, paper and pencil, and multiple choice • Provides index scores for memory, reasoning, and Full Scale IQ
Wechsler Nonverbal Scale of Ability (WNV)	Wechsler & Naglieri (2006)	• For age range 4–21 years • Uses pictorial directions that aid administration without the need for pantomiming • Provides a Full-Scale IQ based on subtests that are well established and common to other Wechsler batteries

English could easily lose points on some intelligence tests (e.g., the different Wechsler scales of intelligence). For some Muslim immigrants and their children, there may be animals or objects on a confrontation-naming task that they are unfamiliar with or have no reference to in their everyday life. The inability to identify a picture of a pretzel or a beaver on a naming test could simply reflect how foreign the item is to the client, and would not suggest a word-retrieval deficit. In some cases, it may be useful to substitute culturally relevant alternatives to items on cognitive tests that would otherwise unfairly penalize clients. While testing Arabic-speaking Muslim patients, Escandell (2002) found that inserting culturally appropriate words on a confrontation-naming test as well as replacing passages in a story memory test with culturally relevant content yielded useful results in differentiating patients with cognitive disorders from those with normal cognitive functioning.

Personality Functioning With regard to personality measures, it is possible that a Muslim's worldview could influence his or her approach to the test and result in seemingly non-normative responses when compared to Western norms. For example, Muslim clients responding to the Minnesota Multiphasic Personality Inventory-2 (MMPI-2) may produce elevations on various scales that would falsely suggest psychopathology. Pondering one's mortality, being fatalistic about the future, and showing little interest in the material world are all considered praiseworthy exercises in Islamic spiritual discipline. However, endorsing these perspectives could result in a significant elevation on the depression scale that is not clinically meaningful. Similarly, strong beliefs in an unseen world (e.g., angels or life after death) and endorsing spiritual experiences outside the realm of the body's physical senses could be mistaken for a thought disorder, when in fact they are considered acceptable in some Muslim communities and do not have any correlation with the ability to function in daily life. Studies have shown that although religious people in general tend to produce elevations on the "lie" scales of personality inventories, their responses are a consequence of their worldview and do not necessarily indicate a desire to hide the truth (Francis, Pearson, & Kay, 1988; Pearson & Francis, 1989).

The use of projective measures could also be problematic if Muslim clients are unable to relate to the stimuli or tasks with the same frame of reference that was originally intended by the test-makers. The Draw a Person Test could raise objections from a client who follows a strict interpretation of Islamic practice that forbids the drawing of human figures. Asking a child to draw a picture of their family could result in a drawing containing every member of the child's extended family because of how the concept of a family is perceived in some Muslim cultures. When asked to describe ambiguous images or scenes, a failure to insert innuendo or symbolic meanings that are similar to responses by Western examinees does not mean that the client is naive or lacking in emotional depth. Rather, differences in worldview and the cultural narrative used to decode particular images or situations could explain the response. De Vos and Miner (1989) found that North African Muslims who had more formal French education exhibited responses on the Rorschach test that showed greater similarity to Western norms compared to individuals who were primarily exposed to only Islamic educational environments. Given that the stimuli on some projective tests (such as the Thematic Apperception Test or TAT) depict Western people and settings that may be viewed as alien to a Muslim client, responses to the tests may tell more about the client's stereotyped image of Westerners than his or her own personal experience (Dwairy, 2006).

Emotional Functioning   One of the most relied upon sources that inform a clinician's understanding of the client's emotional state is the client's own report. Fortunately, a number of self-report measures of mood and psychosocial functioning have been used and validated in various Muslim populations, including the Beck Depression Inventory (BDI-II; Alansari, 2005; Kapci, Uslu, Turkcapar, & Karaoglan, 2008), the Hamilton Depression Rating Scale (HDRS; Hamdi, Amin, & Abou-Saleh, 1997), the Center for Epidemiologic Study Depression Scale (CES-D; Ghubash, Daradkeh, Al Naseri, Al Bloushi, & Daheri, 2000), the Hospital Anxiety and Depression Scale (HADS; Malasi, Mirza, & El-Islam, 1991), the Beck Anxiety Inventory (BAI; Al-Issa, Al-Zubaidi, Bakal, & Fung, 2000), and the State Trait Anxiety Inventory (STAI; Abdel-Khalek, 1989). These studies indicate that while the constructs of mood and psychological distress are present in different Muslim cultures, the expression and reporting of the associated symptoms on self-report measures tend to produce patterns of responses that differ from the original normative samples. For example, many Muslim clients' emphasis on the somatic nature of their emotional complaints results in the greater endorsement of physical symptoms in the areas of energy/fatigue, psychomotor speed/slowing, appetite, and sleep (Al-Krenawi & Graham, 2000).

Despite simplifying the testing experience by eliminating the need for direct interaction between client and clinician, the use of self-report questionnaires or inventories can present some unique challenges when assessing Muslim clients. Some individuals may find it difficult to respond in a completely open and revealing manner because of the religious conviction that disclosing intimate details of potentially shameful feelings or experiences is improper. They may question the wisdom in exposing their faults and sins that God has mercifully veiled from others. If the measure is assessing self-esteem, it may inaccurately characterize some Muslim clients as having low self-worth when in fact their desire to minimize their accomplishments or downplay their abilities is considered a praiseworthy expression of humility before God. Whatever data is gathered from self-report measures, it should be corroborated with a diagnostic interview, clinical impressions, and any other sources of background information.

After the Assessment

Following the assessment, the clinician must integrate all the information gathered from the interview, behavioral observations, and test results in order to formulate a coherent profile of the client's psychological condition. There is little difference in this process when working with a Muslim client versus a client of another faith. However, it may be prudent for the clinician to seek additional input from the family members to understand the unique factors that contribute to the client's religious and cultural identity as an individual. In addition, seeking consultation from an Islamic scholar or an imam may be helpful to the clinician in understanding the broader religious and cultural framework from which the client originates.

Reporting and Interpretation of Findings

If the psychological assessment was conducted in a way to accommodate cultural factors, then any conclusions drawn from the test results should be interpreted in that context. The influence of language difficulties, nonstandardized test procedures, or responses that are culturally acceptable from the client's point of view but potentially non-normative from a Western standpoint should be diligently discussed and accounted for by the clinician. For example, if a family member was present during the evaluation, then the clinician must consider whether the client's performance on tests or willingness to respond openly to questions was in any way affected by the presence of the additional person. It is only the clinician who can provide a qualitative description of what transpired during the testing session. This becomes of utmost importance when writing a report that other medical or mental health professionals may read, particularly if the reported scaled scores alone could mislead another clinician. If there are no adequate norms to properly illustrate the client's performances, then one might consider reporting only the raw scores as a way to describe the client's strengths and weaknesses within the assessment.

Providing Feedback

Just as psychoeducation may have been required to initially orient the Muslim client and his or her family to the purpose of the assessment at the beginning of the session, additional background and context may be required before providing feedback after the evaluation has concluded. Clinicians should be sensitive to the worldview of the client and family when explaining diagnostic impressions that may not completely fit with their beliefs about the causes of illness or deficits. In many cases, feedback will receive wider acceptance if the clinician's recommendations can incorporate the positive role of the larger family system in the client's treatment and care. If applicable, clinicians should encourage religious clients to also incorporate their spiritual traditions during treatment and intervention, particularly if they reported having spiritual beliefs about their mental health.

CASE EXAMPLE

> Nayif is a 14-year-old boy who is brought in for a psychological evaluation by his parents who are immigrants from an Arabic-speaking country with a predominantly Muslim population. His parents speak limited English and describe the presenting problem as their son's "laziness" and his academic struggles in keeping up with classmates. His parents state that they know he has no intellectual problems because he excels in the video games he plays. Nayif is bilingually fluent in Arabic and English, with Arabic his primary language at home and English used outside of the home. He reports that the subject matter taught in school is very difficult for him and he would rather play sports because it is his goal to be a professional athlete when he grows up. His parents are requesting an evaluation to seek recommendations that will "cure" him of his lack of motivation.

Given that the family may not be familiar with Western mental health practice, it would be prudent to gather information regarding their knowledge and expectations of a psychological assessment. It is likely that they would require some psychoeducation about what role the evaluation can play in providing recommendations and treatment options. In addition, it may be useful to review the protocol for the assessment, including who will be present during the testing and how long the sessions will take.

Language will be an important consideration during this assessment. For example, the clinician should probe the parents' statement that Nayif is "lazy" and try to determine what was meant by that description. Initial hypotheses about the case could guide this process. If the underlying cause of Nayif's problems is psychiatric in nature (such as a mood disturbance), then what the parents call "lazy" could refer to apathy or general slowing. If Nayif is having trouble in school due to a possible learning disability, then "lazy" in that situation may refer to a general adverse attitude toward schoolwork that is actually fueled by feelings of discouragement. Nayif's own language abilities should be assessed given that his bilingual status may be contributing to his presenting problem. Will the clinician be able to obtain a valid reflection of Nayif's intellectual and academic abilities if the assessment is conducted in English using standard cognitive tests? Should some of his abilities be tested in his native Arabic? If the examiner does not have the ability to test bilingually, then perhaps an interpreter could be used to aid in the evaluation.

It is likely that assessment measures and questionnaires used during the evaluation may not be normed for Nayif's ethno-linguistic group. This must be taken into consideration when interpreting results. It is possible that raw scores may be more informative than standardized scores when describing his strengths and weaknesses. What qualitative information about Nayif's performances on tests and responses to questions should be included in the report?

As the clinician prepares to give feedback, the family's beliefs about the causes of Nayif's psychological condition must be considered. The potential for a cultural gap between an acculturated youth and his immigrant parents may mean that Nayif and his parents disagree about the underlying problem and what the solutions should be. Given that Nayif's parents believe he has no cognitive problems and simply lacks motivation, how should the clinician present the interpretation of the test results if there seems to be evidence for neuropsychological deficits?

Conclusions

When evaluating Muslim clients, the use of assessment tools common to the practice of psychology in the West poses many difficult but not insurmountable challenges. Although there is no such thing as a completely culture-neutral test that is applicable to all peoples, research in cross-cultural testing indicates that clinicians who are sensitive to the backgrounds of their clients, the cultural biases of the tests in their battery, and their own cultural self in relation to others can tailor the process of assessment in ways that still inform psychological interventions (Lonner, 1985; Hwang & Wood, 2007). Importantly, no single test should be used as the sole basis for making a diagnosis or conclusion about the client's functioning. Clinicians must be responsible in incorporating multiple converging sources of evidence before making definitive statements about a client's cognitive status, personality, or emotional state. As Muslims in the West continue to become more familiar with mental health services in general, the availability of culturally competent psychological assessment must increase because Muslims will begin to seek out such evaluations to aid in decisions pertaining to academic placement, mental health treatment, and overall psychological well-being.

References

Abdel-Khalek, A. M. (1989). The development and validation of an Arabic form of the STAI: Egyptian results. *Personality and Individual Differences, 10*(3), 277–285.

Alansari, B. (2005). Beck Depression Inventory (BDI-II) items characteristic among undergraduate students of nineteen Islamic countries. *Social Behavior and Personality, 33*(7), 675–684.

Al-Issa, I., Al-Zubaidi, A., Bakal, D., & Fung, T. S. (2000). Beck Anxiety Inventory symptoms in Arab college students. *The Arab Journal of Psychiatry, 11*(1), 41–47.

Al-Krenawi, A., & Graham, J. R. (2000). Culturally sensitive social work practice with Arab clients in mental health settings. *Health & Social Work, 25*(1), 9–22.

Bracken, B., & McCallum, S. (1998). *Universal Nonverbal Intelligence Test*. Chicago, IL: Riverside.

Butcher, J. N., Nezami, E., & Exner, J. (1998). Psychological assessment of people in diverse cultures. In S. Kazarian & D. R. Evans (Eds.), *Cross-cultural clinical psychology* (pp. 61–105). New York, NY: Oxford University Press.

Cinnirella, M., & Loewenthal, K. M. (1999). Religious and ethnic group influences on beliefs about mental illness: A qualitative interview study. *British Journal of Medical Psychology, 72*, 505–524.

De Vos, G. A., & Miner, H. (1989). Oasis and Casbah: Acculturative stress. In G. A. De Vos & L. B. Boyer (Eds.), *Symbolic analysis cross-culturally: The Rorschach Test* (pp. 201–245). Berkeley, CA: University of California Press.

Dwairy, M. (2006). *Counseling and psychotherapy with Arabs and Muslims: A culturally sensitive approach*. New York, NY: Teachers College Press.

Escandell, V. A. (2002). Cross-cultural neuropsychology in Saudi Arabia. In F. R. Ferraro (Ed.), *Minority and cross-cultural aspects of neuropsychological assessment* (pp. 299–325). Lisse, The Netherlands: Swets & Zeitlinger.

Francis, L., Pearson, P., & Kay, W. (1988). Religiosity and lie scores: A question of interpretation. *Social Behavior and Personality, 16*(1), 91–95.

Ghubash, R., Daradkeh, T., Al Naseri, K., Al Bloushi, N., & Daheri, A. (2000). The performance of the Center for Epidemiologic Study Depression Scale (CES-D) in an Arab female community. *International Journal of Social Psychiatry, 46*(4), 241–249.

Hamdi, E., Amin, Y., & Abou-Saleh, M. (1997). Performance of the Hamilton Depression Rating Scale in depressed patients in the United Arab Emirates. *Acta Psychiatrica Scandinavica, 96*, 416–423.

Hammill, D., Pearson, N., & Wiederholt, J. (2009). *Examiner's manual: Comprehensive Test of Nonverbal Intelligence* (2nd ed.). Austin, TX: Pro-ed.

Hoberman, H. M. (1992). Ethnic minority status and adolescent mental health services utilization. *Journal of Mental Health Administration, 19*, 246–267.

Hwang, W., & Wood, J. J. (2007). Being culturally sensitive is not the same as being culturally competent. *Pragmatic Case Studies in Psychotherapy, 3*(3), 44–50.

Kapci, E., Uslu, R., Turkcapar, H., & Karaoglan, M. (2008). Beck Depression Inventory II: Evaluation of the psychometric properties and cut-off points in a Turkish adult population. *Depression and Anxiety, 25*, E104–E110.

Kaufman, A. S., & Kaufman, N. L. (2004). *Kaufman Assessment Battery for Children: Technical manual* (2nd ed.). Circle Pines, MN: American Guidance Service.

Lawrence, P., & Rozmus, C. (2001). Culturally sensitive care of the Muslim patient. *Journal of Transcultural Nursing, 12*(3), 228–233.

Leong, F. T. L., & Lau, A. S. L. (2001). Barriers to providing effective mental health services to Asian Americans. *Mental Health Services Research, 3*(4), 201–214.

Lin, K., & Cheung, F. (1999). Mental health issues for Asian Americans. *Psychiatric Services, 50*, 774–780.

Lonner, W. J. (1985). Issues in testing and assessment in cross-cultural counseling. *The Counseling Psychologist, 13*(4), 599–614.

Lynch, E., & Hanson, M. (1999). Steps in the right direction. In E. Lynch & M. Hanson (Eds.), *Developing cross-cultural competence: A guide for working with children and their families*. Baltimore, MD: Paul H. Brookes Publishing Co.

Lyons, J. (1981). *Language and linguistics: An introduction*. Cambridge, UK: Cambridge University Press.

Malasi, T., Mirza, I., & El-Islam, M. (1991). Validation of the Hospital Anxiety and Depression Scale in Arab patients. *Acta Psychiatrica Scandinavica, 84*, 323–326.

Markus, H. R., & Kitayama, S. (1991). Culture and self: Implications for cognition, emotion, and motivation. *Psychological Review, 98*(2), 224–253.

Padilla, A. (2001). Issues in culturally appropriate assessment. In L. A. Suzuki, J. G. Ponterotto, & P. J. Meller (Eds.), *Handbook of multicultural assessment* (pp. 5–27). San Francisco, CA: Jossey-Bass.

Pearson, P., & Francis, L. (1989). The dual nature of the Eysenckian lie scales: Are religious adolescents more truthful? *Personality and Individual Differences, 10*(10), 1041–1048.

Raven, J., Raven, J. C., & Court, J. H. (1998). *Manual for Raven's Progressive Matrices and Vocabulary Scales*. San Antonio, TX: Harcourt Assessment.

Roid, G., & Miller, L. (1997). *Leiter International Peformance Scale–Revised: Examiner's manual*. Wood Dale, IL: Stoelting.

Stanczak, D. E., Stanczak, E. M., & Awadalla, A. W. (2001). Development and initial validation of an Arabic version of the Expanded Trail Making Test: Implications for cross-cultural assessment. *Archives of Clinical Neuropsychology, 16*(2), 141–149.

Wechsler, D., & Naglieri, J. A. (2006). *Wechsler Nonverbal Scale of Ability (WNV)*. San Antonio, TX: Harcourt Assessment.

Yeh, M., Hough, R., McCabe, K., Lau, A., & Garland, A. (2004). Parental beliefs about the causes of child problems: Exploring racial/ethnic patterns. *Journal of the American Academy of Child & Adolescent Psychiatry, 43*(5), 605–612.

CHAPTER 6

Individual Psychotherapy/Counseling
Psychodynamic, Cognitive-Behavioral, and Humanistic-Experiential Models

MONA M. AMER and BALAND JALAL

Islam represents the second largest religion in the United Kingdom after Christianity (Weatherhead & Daiches, 2010), and Muslims constitute the fastest-growing and soon to be largest religious minority in the United States (Haniff, 2003; Ali, Liu, & Humedian, 2004). Evidence suggests that Muslims living in these countries (and most likely other countries in Europe and North America) have experienced intensified psychological distress since 9/11 (Ahluwalia & Zaman, 2010; Ali, Milstein, & Marzuk, 2005; Amer & Hovey, in press; Rippy & Newman, 2006; Weatherhead & Daiches, 2010). This has yielded an increase in the demand for mental health services specifically targeting this population.

Notwithstanding an increased need for effective services, the substantial literature on culturally sensitive psychotherapy is deficient of material targeting Muslims (Hodge, Baughman, & Cummings, 2006; Sheridan & North, 2004). In order for mental health professionals to provide the most effective and culturally sensitive interventions it is essential that they are aware of fundamental aspects of Muslims' faith. That being said, evidence suggests that mental health professionals are generally very little, if at all, educated in the basic tenets of Islam and the practices of Muslims (Carlson, Kirkpatrick, Hecker, & Killmer, 2002; Furman, Benson, Grimwood, & Canda, 2004).

Moreover, it has been suggested that Muslims living in the West do not trust mental health professionals (Hodge, 2005; Kelly, Aridi, & Bakhtiar, 1996). There is a growing concern among Muslims that mental health professionals either do not respect their religious beliefs or simply are not aware of basic Islamic values, and thus offer a therapy that is incongruent with their belief system (Hodge & Nadir, 2008).

Western psychotherapeutic models may prove futile if used without proper consideration of the social and religious beliefs and values of Muslim clients (Shah, 2005). The theoretical frame in which Western psychology is embedded is largely secular and culturally dependent, and in many instances contradicts Islamic views on mankind. For example, many models regard humans as biological outputs, or focus on the observable and quantifiable, and thus they overlook a spiritual or transcendental dimension (Haque, 2004a). As such, psychotherapy approaches are value laden, and in some cases advocate principles that contradict the worldviews of Muslim clients (Shah, 2005).

The purpose of this chapter is to offer a critical examination of the applicability of well-known individual psychotherapy[1] models for Muslims living in regions such as North America and Europe. The chapter begins by presenting common conceptual and practical counseling considerations germane to all therapeutic orientations. Next, the psychodynamic, cognitive-behavioral, and humanistic-experiential paradigms are discussed, both in terms of theoretical congruence with Islam and the suitability of interventions to Muslims from diverse cultures. Each section integrates specific and practical recommendations for therapists and concludes with a case study[2] that illustrates both successful and unsuccessful therapeutic interventions. The chapter ends with references to other promising psychotherapy models as well as research evidence on the effectiveness of integrating religiosity into traditional psychotherapy.

Religio-Cultural Considerations for Individual Psychotherapy/Counseling

It is important for therapists to recognize that the Muslim community is quite heterogeneous. Muslims come from different ethnicities, national origins, sociopolitical histories, and cultural traditions, and they may endorse varying levels of adherence to Islam. As such, therapists should aspire to be culturally sensitive and consider the religio-cultural nuances of their clients. Notwithstanding this multicultural diversity, there are

---

[1] Throughout this chapter the terms "counseling" and "psychotherapy" and "therapy" are used interchangeably, as are terms such as "counselor" and "mental health practitioner."
[2] These case studies represent fictional amalgamations based on the first author's clinical experiences. All potentially identifying information has been modified to ensure anonymity.

several considerations that may arise in the individual treatment setting with Muslims from different backgrounds, regardless of the particular theoretical orientation used.

For example, Muslim clients, particularly those from Arab, South Asian, and Hispanic/Latino origins, may inquire about their therapists' backgrounds or personal experiences, and be confused or offended if the therapists decline to answer. Some clients, such as Arab Muslims, may expect the therapists to express their emotional reactions in session (Al-Abdul-Jabbar & Al-Issa, 2000), and clients coming from cultures that value family honor may ask therapists from that same culture about their family lineages. As such, a therapeutic stance of neutrality may be an obstacle in developing an effective therapeutic alliance. Therapists are advised to show greater flexibility in navigating the therapeutic boundaries, particularly if clients ask questions that are relatively innocuous such as, "Are you married?"

Paradoxical to Muslim clients' expectation for therapist candidness is the clients' own patterns of not disclosing personal or intimate details (Chaudhry & Li, 2010). Many Muslims come from cultures that use metaphors to symbolize emotional reactions (Dwairy, 2006) or display indirect communication styles. As such, explicitly acknowledging, labeling, and discussing intimate experiences may be seen as confusing or even offensive (Hodge, 2005). Clients may avoid revealing issues that are sensitive or taboo, such as substance abuse and premarital sex (Ahluwalia & Zaman, 2010; Hammoud & Siblani, 2003). Another barrier to self-disclosure is the post-9/11 context, in that many clients may conceal information (such as domestic violence) to prevent further tarnishing the reputation of their community. Additionally, as discussed by previous authors (Al-Abdul-Jabbar & Al-Issa, 2000; Ali et al., 2004), many Muslims come from cultural backgrounds in which people are taught not to divulge personal or familial secrets to strangers. It is important to note that because of the collectivistic family-oriented culture forming the backdrop to many Muslims' lives, revealing personal information will by default be associated with revealing family information.

Because the family is held in high esteem for Muslims, it is not uncommon for clients to bring family members to sessions for emotional or even linguistic support. For example, Muslim women may bring their children to session (Carter & Rashidi, 2004). Muslims often indicate that they cannot make decisions without the consultation of family members (Ali et al., 2004; Carter & Rashidi, 2004; Chaudhry & Li, 2010). It would be a mistake for counselors to respond with confusion or irritation at these events, or assume that the client is overly dependent or enmeshed. On the contrary, family members are a source of mental health support for Muslims in the West (Weatherhead & Daiches, 2010) and may serve as a valuable asset to the therapeutic process (Hodge, 2005). Family members can even support the therapist in the implementation of interventions such as in vivo exposure or behavioral modification (Takriti & Ahmad, 2000).

Even when meeting with clients without the presence of family members, family issues may factor prominently in the therapeutic process. For example, Dwairy (2006) argued that in light of the collectivistic Arab culture, therapists working with Arab Muslim clients are encouraged to focus on family issues during the assessment and treatment processes. On the other hand, more individualistic approaches aimed at enhancing individuation may be counterproductive when working with Muslims from patriarchal and collectivistic cultures. For Muslims of all ethnicities, faith, collaboration, and harmony with others typically take precedence over autonomy and self-determination. Therapists should aim at enhancing interdependence and developing behaviors and beliefs that are more smoothly aligned to religious and cultural norms (Al-Abdul-Jabbar & Al-Issa, 2000; Chaudhry & Li, 2010).

Religious and cultural factors can also influence gender interactions in the individual therapy setting. For example, the Qur'an instructs Muslims to lower their gaze when interacting with persons of the opposite sex (24:30–31). Additionally, avoiding direct eye contact with the opposite sex and with authority figures is a mark of humility and respect in many Asian and Middle Eastern cultures. Therapists should not misunderstand these behaviors to be signs of low self-esteem or dishonesty (Carter & Rashidi, 2004). Moreover, because it is religiously unacceptable for a man and woman to be enclosed alone in a private room (Carter & Rashidi, 2004), counselors should ask Muslims who are more adherent to their faith if they would prefer a same-sex counselor or if an alternative arrangement (e.g., leaving the door slightly ajar, inviting family members to session) would be preferable.

As shown by the previous examples, Islam is a holistic and comprehensive way of life that not only permeates the spiritual life of Muslims but also their familial, social, political, and economic lives. Due to the encompassing nature of Islam, it often constitutes an essential and central part of Muslims' identities. In this respect, it has been argued (e.g., Hamdan, 2008) that it would be useful to integrate relevant spiritual and religious components in the counseling process. Of course, such an approach would be more pertinent for clients who express higher levels of religious commitment. Previous research has shown that Muslims desire therapists who recognize and respect the role of God and religion in their lives, and prefer for the content of the therapeutic interventions and advice to be rooted in religion (Weatherhead & Daiches, 2010).

A first step toward religious competence for mental health practitioners is gaining accurate knowledge about Muslim clients' faith and cultures. Unfortunately, the popular media is riddled with biases and falsehoods regarding Islam and Muslims (Haque, 2004b). Consumers of such media may not be aware of their own prejudices and misconceptions, which can unknowingly negatively impact the way they interact with their clients. Practitioners should invest effort into becoming aware of and eliminating their own biases (Dwairy, 2006; Kobeisy, 2004). Greater trust and stronger therapeutic alliance can be established if they demonstrate to their Muslim clients their efforts used to obtain valid and accurate information (Ahluwalia & Zaman, 2010; Kobeisy, 2004). Part of this educational process is to gain information on the religio-cultural applicability of actual psychotherapeutic techniques used, as discussed in the following sections focused on psychodynamic, cognitive-behavioral, and humanistic models.

Psychoanalytic/Psychodynamic Model

Theory

Psychoanalytic theory has left a considerable mark on Western civilization, having influenced not only psychology, but also disciplines such as anthropology, sociology, political science, art, and literature. In fact, psychoanalysis has permeated mainstream Western culture inasmuch as an expression such as *Freudian slip* has crept into everyday language, and the name Sigmund Freud has become a household name similar to Einstein and Darwin (Carver & Scheier, 2008). Although it is difficult to pinpoint a single aspect of Western intellectual culture that has not been influenced in one way or another by Freudian theory, psychoanalysis has generally been ignored or explicitly scorned in the Muslim world.

Undoubtedly one of the principal explanations for lack of popularity of psychoanalysis among Muslims is the theoretical foundation upon which it rests. Classic Freudian theory posits that human beings—similar to primitive animals—are driven by unconscious sexual and destructive urges (Shah, 2005). Such ideas do not resonate well in the Muslim world, where mankind is viewed in high esteem as the vicegerents of God. The Qur'an states,[3] "Note that occasion, when your Rabb [i.e., Lord] said to the angels: 'I am going to place a vicegerent on earth . . .'" (2:30). Albeit influenced by sexual drives, human beings are chiefly seen as rational creatures, endowed with an intellect to influence their own course of behavior (e.g., Qur'an 2:269).

Moreover, Freud's notions on psychosexual development are not in accordance with Islamic thought. That is, while psychoanalytic

---

[3] Readers should recognize that English translations of the Qur'an do not necessarily capture the full meaning of the original Arabic Qur'an. The translation used for all verses in this chapter is the *Al-Qur'an: Guidance for Mankind* (6th ed.), translated by Muhammad Farooq-e-Azam Malik, and published by the Institute of Islamic Knowledge, Houston, Texas, USA (2006).

theory posits that children go through psychosexual stages associated with obtaining satisfaction of libidinal drives (e.g., through oral gratification, or desire to sexually possess the parent of the opposite gender; King, Viney, & Woody, 2009), such ideas are alien to the Islamic belief system. In contrast, Islam stresses that children are born innocent with a natural inclination (*fitrah*) toward goodness (Obeid, 1988). Although human drives including sexuality are not discounted, certainly Freud's conceptual dominance of the sexual drive even during infancy is not compatible with Islamic beliefs.

Despite the theoretical incongruence between psychoanalytic theory and Islamic principles, there have been attempts to reconcile the two. For example, it has been argued that the Freudian tripartite divisions of the psyche—the id, ego, and superego—parallel three types of "souls" or "selves" mentioned in the Qur'an: *Nafs Al-Ammara, Nafs,* and *Nafs Al-Lawwama* (for a review, see Aydin, 2010). The *Nafs Al-Ammara* (the Commanding Soul) has been likened to the id. It is the evil self that inclines to basic bodily desires and pleasures. For example, the Qur'an describes, "Man's soul [or self] is prone to evil, except the one to whom my Rabb [i.e., Lord] has shown mercy" (12:53). Analogous to Freudian theory, Sufi Islamic literature has suggested that this passionate self should be acknowledged and not completely stifled and eliminated, although it does not constitute a genuine source of energy (Ismail, 2008).

The *Nafs*, which simply means "soul" or "self" in Arabic, has been paralleled to the ego. In Islamic scholarship *Nafs* originally implied self-conscience and self-awareness (Aydin, 2010). According to Freudian theory, however, the ego is said to mediate the demands of reality and the conflicting forces of the id and superego. Although the ego, according to psychoanalytic theory, operates on both a conscious and an unconscious level, it is more conscious than both the superego and id (Segrist, 2009). On the other hand, the ego that Jung described, unlike the Freudian ego, is the center of the total psyche and awareness and is the "*I* or the *me* of the personality" (King et al., 2009, p. 398). In this respect, the *Nafs* as understood within Islamic scholarship may be more consonant with Jung's concept of the ego (Aydin, 2010).

Lastly, the *Nafs Al-Lawwama*, which means The Blaming Soul, has been equated with the superego. For example, the Qur'an describes how peoples' own consciousness can translate into feelings of burden: ". . . So despondent were they that the earth, with all its vastness, and their own souls, seemed to close upon them" (9:118). In Islamic scholarship *Nafs Al-Lawwama* has been defined as a part of the self that keeps warning about straying from the path of orthodoxy (Aydin, 2010), often by producing a sense of guilt. For Freud, the superego is a product of a childhood exposure to parental demands and discipline (George, 1999). However, Henry Murray expanded this concept to also entail the ongoing influences of culture, including other authority figures, peer groups, and religion

(Murray, 1959; 1940/2008). Thus, Murray's broader definition of the superego is more consistent with the Islamic concept of the *Nafs Al-Lawwama*, which according to Aydin (2010) is most profoundly influenced by religious and societal values.

In this respect, Ismail (2008) argued that contemporary Islamic scholars tend to stress the likelihood of internal conflicts that build up as a consequence of inner passions and desires on the one hand, and societal pressures and expectations on the other. Aside from the three souls/selves that have been likened to Freud's tripartite personality structure, Freud's pleasure-pain principle—that is, the idea that people are driven to seek pleasure and to avoid pain—is a widespread concept in the Sufi literature (Ismail, 2008).

Intervention

Despite any similarities that can be drawn between psychoanalytic and Islamic concepts, psychoanalysis is not a favored therapeutic intervention for most Muslims (Al-Abdul-Jabbar & Al-Issa, 2000; Azhar & Varma, 2000). For example, Hodge and Nadir (2008) argued that while the intrapsychic conflicts that form the hallmark of psychoanalytic theory tend to yield inward-pointing insights, Muslims in general tend to form their identity based on more external factors such as religion and family. Thus, Muslims are more outward looking, favoring a sense of communal actualization over self-actualization, which might lead Muslims to be less interested in the introspective psychoanalytic approach.

Classic long-term psychoanalysis in particular is not suitable for the majority of Muslim clients (Dwairy, 2006). Paying for a long-term therapeutic process may be financially unfeasible for those Muslims who are not wealthy, and the process of exploring past childhood experiences may be perceived by many Muslim clients as irrelevant or even impolite (Kobeisy, 2004). Al-Abdul-Jabbar and Al-Issa (2000) went as far as to describe Arab Muslims as "intolerant" toward insight-oriented exploratory therapy that in some cases can induce even more severe anxiety for clients (p. 281). However, Freudian psychoanalysis may perhaps be suitable for a minority of Muslim clients, particularly more individuated and acculturated individuals who come from higher educational backgrounds and are more psychologically minded. In such cases, these individuals may purposely seek more exploratory psychotherapy (Dwairy, 2006).

Shorter-term psychodynamic therapy can be modified to better suit the cultural experiences and needs of Muslim clients. For example, Dwairy (2006) recommended that when working with Arab Muslim clients, counselors should focus on the familial conflicts and relationships rather than the intrapsychic conflicts. He argued that the intrapsychic dynamics that developed from previous childhood experiences are difficult to distinguish from the salience of clients' present-day family experiences: "An encounter with a traditional Arab/Muslim individual is an encounter with a group of people that live inside her and still play a major role in directing her behavior" (p. 58). The id, ego, and superego are not viewed as autonomous structures but rather interconnected and constantly impacted by present-day cultural and familial factors. Furthermore, defense mechanisms may not be unconscious and intrapsychic, but rather social mechanisms used to cope with the external "oppressor" (p. 63). Based on these observations, it follows that object relations therapy may be more effective when working with Muslim clients because it focuses more on human interactions rather than aggressive and sexual drives.

Interpreting to clients their aggressive and sexual drives is an intervention that counselors should approach in a delicate and sensitive manner. Clients may receive such interpretations as threatening or guilt provoking, particularly among Muslims for whom such topics are considered taboo or sensitive (Dwairy, 2006). Acknowledging resentment toward a parental figure, which is common in Western psychotherapeutic dialogues, is culturally taboo in many Muslim cultures (Al-Abdul-Jabbar & Al-Issa, 2000). As such, therapists may be advised to give feedback or recommendations to clients without divulging the therapists' underlying interpretations of the inner conflicts (Dwairy, 2006).

Another important issue to consider is the role of religion and spirituality in the therapeutic process. Because the Freudian tradition has generally ignored or discounted religion, the integration of religiosity in treatment has not been characteristic of the psychodynamic tradition; this is not compatible for Muslims (Badri, 1979). Muslims report that prayer, meditation, and other religious practices provide them with peace and emotional comfort (Khan, 2006), and thus integrating such practices as part of the therapeutic process may be more effective than depending solely on insight-oriented techniques (Chaudhry & Li, 2010).

Despite modifications, therapists working from a psychodynamic approach may find it challenging to work with Muslim clients, particularly immigrants and those from Arab and South Asian backgrounds. These clients typically pursue therapy with the expectation of obtaining clear, practical advice from experts. Thus, therapy that is exploratory and less directive may be met with skepticism from the clients, who view their therapists as passive, incompetent, and ineffective. In fact, in the absence of receiving immediate, concrete feedback from the therapist, many Muslims may prematurely terminate treatment (Dwairy, 2006; Haque, 2004b).

Furthermore, it is important to note that Muslims often confide in and depend on strong support systems such as their families and religious communities. Accordingly, they may pursue therapy only to request assistance with a specific pressing matter that has not been solved through natural supports. For that reason they may not see the usefulness or need for exploring on a deeper level other aspects of their present or previous life experiences (Chaudhry & Li, 2010). Brief and structured psychodynamic models that focus more on present-day conflicts may therefore be more suitable.

CASE EXAMPLE: "SUMEYA'S NIGHTMARE"

Sumeya is a 24-year-old whose family emigrated from Pakistan to New York when she was 15 years old. She sought services from a private-practice psychologist to cope with anxiety and depression. Sumeya was recently divorced after having been married for three years to a Muslim convert of Caribbean origin. She met her ex-husband at university and married him despite her parents' objections to his ethnic background. After the divorce, Sumeya decided to live alone in her own apartment rather than move back into her parents' home, which was located in the same city. This decision led to frequent arguments with her parents, who were concerned about the potential stigma and shame their daughter would bring upon the family as a woman living alone. This, they said, would intensify the shame already produced by the divorce.

After the first few sessions of listening to Sumeya, the therapist began to feel irritated toward Sumeya's parents for what she perceived to be interference in Sumeya's life, and impatient with Sumeya's passiveness in the face of so much parental criticism. The therapist attributed this response to diagnostic countertransference. The therapist was not aware, however, that Sumeya experienced increased irritation toward the therapist for not offering her direct advice, and had begun to question the worth of paying so much money per session when the therapist was mostly silent. Sumeya believed that it was impolite to raise such concerns with the therapist, but made subtle hints of her frustration, which the therapist understood to be transference stemming from Sumeya's unexpressed frustration with her parents.

Nearly two months into the therapy Sumeya reported that her anxiety had increased and that she had begun to dread nighttime after having dreams of her mother dying in an airplane crash. The therapist offered the interpretation that these nightmares were symbolic of the anger and resentment Sumeya had toward her mother for smothering her with criticisms related to the failed marriage while having the "perfect" marriage with Sumeya's father. In response, Sumeya became visibly agitated and told the therapist with a shaky, tearful voice that this was a "horrible thing to say" and she was ashamed that the therapist could hold such a negative opinion of her and her kind parents. The therapist was so startled at this sudden display of negative emotionality that she apologized, but anticipated that Sumeya would not return for the following session.

Prior to the next session the therapist sought consultation from a local Muslim psychiatrist. He explained that in many Muslim cultures, and as documented in the Qur'an, parents are to be revered and respected. Thus, the suggestion that a child may hate or resent her parents was an unacceptable—and maybe even sacrilegious—notion. Because expressing anger toward the therapist (an authority figure) would have been culturally unacceptable, Sumeya had reacted by experiencing shame. The psychiatrist also normalized Sumeya's family dynamics. He argued that her insistence on living alone was in fact the "abnormal" behavior within her cultural context, and that her parents were unusual in their tolerance of Sumeya's repeated behaviors in defiance of their culture. He hypothesized that Sumeya's parents were therefore probably very supportive and caring, and she may not have mentioned acts of kindness in session because reporting positive experiences was not part of the traditional psychotherapy discourse. He also highlighted the complexity of Sumeya's multiple identities and urged the therapist not to assume that because Sumeya appeared acculturated in one aspect of her life (biracial marriage) that she did not adhere to other aspects of her traditional culture and religion.

Sumeya did return for the following session. At the advice of the Muslim psychiatrist, the therapist did not explicitly discuss the interaction from the previous session out of concern that it may intensify Sumeya's anxiety. However, over the coming sessions the therapist made a concerted effort to provide more feedback and direction in session, and to also become more aware of how her own cultural and familial histories shaped her countertransference. The coming sessions saw an increased focus on exploring Sumeya's process of differentiation from her parents. Also explored was her identity development, particularly as a child immigrant to the United States who (Sumeya later revealed) had frequently been on the receiving end of prejudice and hostility. Sumeya eventually came to the realization that her nightmares may have been triggered by all the news reports she had been watching regarding potential terrorist threats, as well as a collective guilt over sharing the religion of the 9/11 hijackers.

Cognitive-Behavioral Model

Theory

Cognitive-behavioral therapy (CBT) has been found to be effective for a wide variety of psychological disorders such as anxiety and depression, and is among the most evidence-based therapies (Chambless & Ollendick, 2001). It has been argued that cognitive-based therapies are more congruent with the religious beliefs of Muslims than, for example, psychoanalysis (Al-Abdul-Jabbar & Al-Issa, 2000; Hodge & Nadir, 2008).

According to Hodge and Nadir (2008), CBT emphasizes reason, logical discussion, education, and consultation—notions that are well known and commonly stressed within Islamic-religious discourse. For instance, the values of education and consultation date back to the time of Prophet Muhammad (PBUH[4]). He taught his followers that whoever ". . . treads the path in search of knowledge, Allah would make that path easy, leading to paradise for him . . ." (Sahih Muslim, Book no. 35, Hadith no. 6518). As far as consultation, the Prophet's companions would eagerly consult him for advice when afflicted with calamity and distress (Al-Munajjid, 1999).

Muslims may easily understand behavioral theories. For one thing, the Qur'an makes numerous references to rewards and punishments both during life as well as in the Hereafter[5] (e.g., Heaven and Hell). These rewards and punishments serve as consequences to behaviors. Much like behavioral theories, the Islamic literature emphasizes the importance of behaviors when it comes to coping with life events. In this respect the Qur'an advises the following: ". . . Seek Allah's help with patience and Salah [the prayer] . . ." (2:45). *Salah* refers to the ritualistic prayer involving movements of the entire body (e.g., bowing and prostrating) while reciting soothing verses, and it is preceded by ablution in which certain body parts are washed. Much like meditation, prayer is meant to promote relaxation and alleviate psychological distress.

Modeling, or observational learning as described by Albert Bandura, is another concept that is easily recognized by Muslims (Dwairy, 2006). The Islamic faith places emphasis on the importance of parents and authority figures modeling positive behaviors, and it encourages Muslims to look to Prophet Muhammad (PBUH) as a model to emulate. For example, the Qur'an reminds Muslims, "You have indeed, in the life of Allah's Rasool [i.e., the Prophet Muhammad], the 'Best Model' for him whose hope is in Allah and the Day of the Hereafter" (33:21).

Another principal feature of present-day CBT is the cognitive therapy that was promoted by therapists like Aaron Beck. Cognitive therapy focuses on identifying maladaptive and distorted thoughts that produce psychological disturbance and unproductive behavior. These irrational cognitions and automatic thoughts are modified during the therapy

---

[4] PBUH is an abbreviation of the phrase "peace be upon him." The expression is commonly used in Islamic discourse when referring to the Prophet, a tradition rooted in the Qur'anic verse: "Allah and His angels send blessings on the Prophet: O ye that believe! Send ye blessings on him, and salute him with all respect" (33:56).
[5] According to Islamic teachings the Hereafter or Afterlife refers to the events that unfold subsequent to death (e.g., being resurrected on the Day of Judgment, and residing evermore in either Heaven or Hell).

process, and are replaced with more productive cognitions that foster psychological well-being and more adaptive patterns of behavior (Beck, 1976). Islamic discourse likewise highlights the role of intellect, reflection, and seeking knowledge in maintaining positive mental health (Haque, 2004b). Logical analysis is particularly emphasized (Obeid, 1988). There are numerous verses in the Qur'an that stress this rational aspect of humans, for instance, "Surely, in the creation of the heavens and the earth and the alternation of the night and the day, there are signs for men of understanding" (3:190), and "This Book (Al-Quran) which We have sent down to you (O Muhammad) is highly blessed, so that they may ponder upon its verses and the men of understanding may learn a lesson from it" (38:29). In light of this emphasis on rationality, cognitive therapies may be especially congruous with the Islamic faith (Carter & Rashidi, 2004).

However, it is important to note that what is considered "rational" and "irrational" may itself be embedded in cultural values. For example, many of the common irrational beliefs identified by Albert Ellis (1962) may be normative within Muslim cultures. To illustrate, many Muslims believe that there is indeed a correct way to implement everyday matters in their lives (Chaudhry & Li, 2010) and that they should strive toward perfection using Prophet Muhammad (PBUH) as an example. Muslims are encouraged to feel upset over other peoples' problems because humans are one *Ummah* or community. Islamic literature includes examples of people who are evil and villainous who should be punished for their deeds. These concepts all relate to (albeit somewhat less extreme) versions of Ellis's core irrational beliefs.

Intervention

Muslim clients who are pursuing therapy that is active, directive, goal-oriented, and focused on practical tasks generally look favorably upon cognitive-behavioral techniques (Dwairy, 2006). For Arab Muslim clients in particular, the therapist's persona as an empathic and directive coach or advisor is easily aligned to the patriarchal culture, and therapists are often perceived in a parental role (Al-Abdul-Jabbar & Al-Issa, 2000). Moreover, parallel to other Islamic relationships of healing and learning, Muslims may view the roles of therapists and their clients to be akin to teachers and their disciples (Haque, 2004b).

Behavioral techniques, including behavior modification, systematic desensitization, and flooding, may be successfully implemented with Muslim clients. Muslims who already spend significant portions of their days involved in prayer and meditation may find techniques like guided imagery and relaxation to be congruent with their faith (Carter & Rashidi, 2003).

Furthermore, the Qur'an and Sunnah[6] offer numerous behavioral suggestions for addressing emotional and behavioral ailments that can easily be integrated in the therapy process. For example, Prophet Muhammad (PBUH) advised, "When one of you becomes angry while standing, he should sit down. If the anger leaves him, well and good; otherwise he should lie down" (Sunan Abudawud, Book no. 41, Hadith no. 4764). This is a simple and effective strategy for anger management that reduces the risk that the angry person will engage in behaviors that he or she would subsequently regret. Other examples of behavioral techniques to reduce anger as prescribed by Prophetic traditions include performing ablution, taking sips of water, and changing location (i.e., leaving the place in which a person was angered) (Haque, 2004b).

Moreover, ablution and prayer can be assigned to relieve tension, and activity scheduling can include events at the local Islamic community center. Clients can be reminded of out-of-session target behaviors (such as behavioral monitoring, practicing progressive muscle relaxation, or following through with contingency management plans) by scheduling them to coincide with the five daily prayers.

Previous authors have advised that effective behavioral therapy should be implemented in a warm and empathic therapist–client relationship, and that effective psychoeducation about behavioral principles can prevent clients from feeling as though they are nothing more than animals or robots (Goldfried & Davison, 1994). This advice applies well to practitioners working with Muslims. When working with Muslim children in particular, care must be made to not emphasize the mechanistic aspects of the therapy and consider their applications within the cultural contexts. For example, many Muslims may perceive techniques like "time out" as cruel and inhumane, and parents may be hesitant to offer positive reinforcement for behaviors that are expected to be followed and respected within the religious or cultural framework.

For the most part, cognitive techniques may also be effective for Muslim clients (Carter & Rashidi, 2004). Many clients benefit from strategies aimed at identifying and challenging maladaptive and irrational cognitions and enhancing awareness of how their thoughts relate to feelings and behaviors. Moreover, taking inventory of and claiming responsibility for one's thoughts is a part of many Muslims' daily routine.

As mentioned previously, however, the perceived rationality of certain beliefs may be culturally embedded. As such, Muslim clients may be wary

---

[6] Although the Arabic expression Sunnah is often translated as practice or habit, in traditional Islamic discourse it specifically refers to the sayings or actions (i.e., the practice) of Prophet Muhammad (PBUH). The Prophet's Sunna is documented in books that compile these sayings, known as ahadith (hadith in the singular).

of counselors who attempt to challenge beliefs; in fact, some clients may be concerned that their valued beliefs may be discounted, particularly beliefs regarding the supernatural (Carter & Rashidi, 2004). Western discourse emphasizes rationality and examination of the evidence, as well as a more internal locus of control (Carter & Rashidi, 2003). This may not be congruent with many Muslims' belief in the power of external forces like God and the supernatural (e.g., angels, *jinn*[7]) in influencing their lives. Therefore, it is recommended that therapists be cognizant of their own belief systems and respectful of the fact that they may differ from those of their clients' (Carter & Rashidi, 2004).

One way to enhance the success of cognitive interventions with more religious clients is to integrate religious cognitions as part of the therapeutic process. Hamdan (2008) proposed a series of cognitions from the Islamic literature that may be used during the religiously informed CBT, such as the Islamic emphasis on the temporality of the worldly life. This is the concept that the life of this world with all its trials and tribulations is not eternal, but rather a temporary journey toward the Hereafter. For example, the Qur'an states the following: "The things which you have been given are but the provisions and adornments of this worldly life; and that which is with Allah is better and more lasting..." (28:60). As Hamdan elucidated, Muslim clients may overcome irrational beliefs related to despair and hopelessness when reminded of the temporality of this life.

Another Islamic cognition highlighted by Hamdan (2008) is trusting and relying on Allah, a concept known as *tawakkul*. *Tawakkul* implies that the individual is cognizant that God single-handedly has authority and control over all domains in the universe, and as such people should rely solely on Him to facilitate their needs. Such a mental framework alleviates worries and anxiety as people submit their affairs to God, well aware that He has promised to help those who put their trust in Him. In this regard the Qur'an says, "And when you make a decision to do something, then put your trust in Allah ... Allah loves those who put their trust in him" (3:159).

Hamdan (2008) also recommended that Muslim clients focus on Allah's blessings instead of the misfortunes afflicting them, which can yield a sense of thankfulness. The Qur'an emphasizes in this regard that "... if you want to count the favors of Allah, you will never be able to count them" (14:34), which reminds Muslims that the blessings bestowed upon them by Allah outweigh the hardships and trials. A related Islamic concept is comparing misfortunes with those who are less fortunate, in order to appreciate God's blessings. Prophet Muhammad (PBUH) said, "Look at those who are less

---

[7] The *Jinn* or genies in Islamic tradition refer to supernatural creatures that exist in parallel with humans as a part of God's creation. Unlike angels, but similar to human beings, they are held accountable for their actions by God.

fortunate than yourselves, not at those who are better off than yourselves, so that you will not belittle the blessings that Allah has bestowed upon you" (Al-Mundhiri, 2000, n.d., Book no. 68, Chapter 13, p. 11115, as cited in Hamdan, 2008).

Despite the consensus among scholars regarding the general effectiveness of CBT over other techniques when working with Muslims, there are some practical challenges that may arise during the therapeutic process. One relates to asking clients to conduct tasks between sessions (sometimes called "homework"). Many clients, particularly those who present as passive recipients waiting for a magical cure (Al-Abdul-Jabbar & Al-Issa, 2000) and those unfamiliar with the psychotherapy process, may not follow through with these target behaviors. This may come as a surprise to the therapist who is aware of how the daily Islamic rituals promote self-discipline (Carter & Rashidi, 2003) and who knows that following through with promises or plans is a valued Islamic principle. However, it is important to note that many Muslim immigrants come from countries in which educational systems do not incorporate the use of frequent assignments (grades are determined based on a final examination) and thus the concept of homework per se may not be as familiar. Additionally, therapists should remember that many Muslim clients already have numerous religious "tasks" to accomplish on a daily basis and thus adding to these tasks may be overwhelming. Therefore, integrating into therapy tasks that are already being performed (such as ritual prayers, supplications, reading the Qur'an, etc.) may be a better strategy.

There are also interventions that may be counterproductive when working with Muslim clients. For example, assertiveness and social skills training often coach clients in communicating leadership, maintaining eye contact, hand-shaking, and presenting firm requests. However, for Muslims coming from collectivistic cultures in which modesty, humility, and interdependence are emphasized, such behaviors may be perceived as impolite (Dwairy, 2006). In the case of direct eye contact and hand-shaking with the opposite sex, such behaviors may be viewed as violations of religiously mandated modesty. Moreover, many CBT interventions require clients to monitor and document specific details of their behavioral or cognitive patterns. This process may be experienced as intrusive or anxiety provoking if the behaviors or thoughts are associated with issues that are taboo or culturally sensitive.

CASE EXAMPLE: "RAYYAN THE LITTLE MAN"

Rayyan is a 12-year-old boy of Palestinian-Jordanian origin who was referred by his school to a mental health clinic due to worsening grades and disruptive behaviors such as making loud jokes during the teacher's lessons and releasing the class's pet rabbit from its cage. The referral from the school stated that as a private Islamic academy they had zero tolerance for unruly behaviors and did not have a psychologist on staff who could counsel the boy.

After missing the first scheduled appointment, Rayyan and his mother arrived late for the second. This was not surprising to the counselor who had worked with many Arab clients who were often tardy. At first glance, the mother seemed anxious and the boy depressed. The mother, an immigrant physician, spoke in a loud, rapid, high-pitched voice and repeatedly straightened her *hijab* (headscarf). Rayyan, on the other hand, stared silently at the ground and grunted short answers to questions. However, the counselor remembered that rapid speech was not uncommon among people from the Levant, and that the mother's anxiety could be a consequence of the shame of being referred for counseling. The counselor asked the mother about Rayyan's eye contact and was told that Rayyan recently began lowering his gaze in imitation of how his father interacted with women.

Although typically the counselor meets separately with a child during the child's first session, she knew Rayyan's mother might perceive this arrangement as offensive or it would raise her suspicions that the counselor was not trustworthy. Additionally, the mother refused to sign the forms consenting to exchanging information with Rayyan's pediatrician and teacher due to fear of stigma—a decision that the counselor respected but cautiously revisited in later sessions. To enhance confidentiality the counselor scheduled Rayyan's appointments at times that did not intersect with those of other Muslim clients from the same community. Despite such efforts, invitations to the father to attend were declined; he stated that it was a child-rearing issue that the mother should take care of and he could not risk his reputation as a medical school professor should someone see him at the clinic.

The counselor provided greater ongoing psychoeducation regarding the conceptualizations and interventions than she typically would have with other clients. One challenge arose when she asked the mother and son to identify the antecedents, behaviors, and consequences of Rayyan's classroom conduct. Both were quite silent, and the mother admitted that she did not wish to say anything that would entail backbiting against the teacher and principal, who were both sisters in Islam. From this, the counselor suspected that the family was unhappy with the management of the school and classroom but she was not able to obtain further information on these issues.

Focusing on the reinforcements for Rayyan's behavior—primarily the laughter and admiration of his classmates—was a more effective strategy. It was discovered that his unruly school behaviors coincided with increased pressure in the home environment for Rayyan to "act like a man," obtain high scores that would enable him to pursue a medical career, and "stop wasting time" with video games. When Rayyan had become more withdrawn and "careless" in his schoolwork, the parents had responded with heightened criticisms and urgency in their demands. Rayyan, on the other hand, admitted that he did not care much for his school work but was unhappy that he did not have any friends because his parents "kept [him] locked in a prison at home" where video games were his only escape.

The counselor worked with the mother (who agreed to share the information with the father) to instead focus parental attention and praise on Rayyan's prosocial behaviors. She also helped the mother identify some of her irrational cognitions that were contributing to the family stressors, such as

- Because Rayyan is on the cusp of manhood this is the most critical year in which everything must go perfectly.
- Rayyan's careless school behaviors show that he is doomed to academic and career failure.
- Rayyan is a rude and heartless boy for throwing away all that we have invested in trying to give him a good education.
- I have been a failure as a mother to pursue my medical career at the expense of my son.
- If Rayyan goes to the mall or cinema he will be corrupted by Western practices and end up a drug addict.

Within the context of systematically evaluating the evidence in order to modify some of these cognitions, the counselor asked the mother to produce examples and metaphors from the Qur'an and Sunnah that could challenge the beliefs. Additionally, she provided psychoeducation on normal developmental expectations and typical childhood behaviors seen among acculturating second-generation youth. The parents agreed to give Rayyan greater opportunities to socialize with friends outside of the home, and video games were instead used as a reward for completing homework. Over the 10 weeks of counseling, Rayyan became more verbally expressive and his grades began to improve. During the final session the father accompanied the mother in order to thank the counselor.

Humanistic-Experiential Model

Theory

Humanistic psychologists have criticized other schools of psychology for providing a diminished and reductionist view of humans. An example of this criticism came from two prominent figures of the humanistic tradition, Abraham Maslow and Rollo May, who castigated the schools of psychoanalysis and behaviorism for trying to explain the complexity of the human experience by drawing from their research on neurotic patients and laboratory animals. A main challenge of the humanistic movement has thus been to provide a new epistemology in the study of human psychology that, in contrast to other established schools, emphasized the higher forms of human behavior. In this regard, the main themes that have emerged from the humanistic movement are the importance of human achievement and potential (Moss, 2001).

Perhaps one of Maslow's most profound contributions to the field of humanistic psychology is the theory of the self, or self-actualization. Maslow came to formulate a psychology that focused on the study of healthy human beings, and in particular he turned his attention to those individuals who were self-actualized and hence had reached their full human potential. He concluded that the highest form of self-actualization centered on a type of self-transcending altruism (Dhiman, 2007; Moss, 2001).

This aspect of humanistic psychology in many respects dovetails nicely with the Islamic belief system. For instance, unlike the psychodynamic theoretical framework in which psychic conflict is often tied to childhood events, both humanistic psychology and the Islamic faith stress the prospects of self-transformation and human potential at any given moment without shackling the individual to past experiences. For example, the Qur'an emphasizes that whoever follows up sin with "good deeds ... Allah will change his evil [i.e., sins] into good, and Allah is Most Forgiving, Most Merciful" (25:70). This aspect goes to show how the Islamic faith, similar to humanistic psychology, does not promote the idea of dwelling in the past, but instead encourages self-actualization (i.e., in this case by resorting to virtuous and righteous deeds).

The Qur'an contains countless narrations of self-actualized individuals, particularly prophets, who reached their full potential, displaying self-transcending and altruistic attributes. An outstanding example of this is Prophet Muhammad (PBUH), whose sense of altruism was so profound that although he was rejected, scorned, and persecuted, he never abdicated his mission to serve God. In this regard, Maslow argued that the self-actualized person is characterized by a devotion to a cause that he or she understands as his or her life mission (Dhiman, 2007).

In Islamic psychology, self-actualization can be seen as the *Nafs Al-Mutma'inna*, which literally means the soul (or self) of serenity and tranquility (Aydin, 2010). The Qur'an says about this type of soul, " ... O fully satisfied [or serene] soul! Return to your Rabb [i.e., Lord] well pleased with him and well-pleasing to Him. Join My servants, and enter My paradise" (89:27–30). According to Islamic scholarship, a serene soul inhabits the God-fearing and spiritually enriched individual. This idea is somewhat similar to Maslow's concept of the self-actualized person, who likewise reaches a certain spiritual dimension or mode of being, called peak experience (Dhiman, 2007). Of course, peak experience according to mainstream humanistic theory is devoid of any theological connotations per se (Aydin, 2010).

Another pioneer of humanistic psychology is Carl Rogers, whose view of human beings was optimistic. For instance, he regarded infants as having an intrinsic inclination to self-actualize. This view of human nature is likewise shared by the Islamic faith. As touched upon briefly in the previous section on psychoanalytic theory, Muslims believe that human beings are born pure with a natural inclination (*fitrah*) toward good (Obeid, 1988). People who follow their *fitrah* would automatically seek to self-actualize. On the other hand, deviation from this natural inclination can be a source for psychological distress. Akin to humanistic theory, Islamic thought holds that people are lured into partially renouncing their *fitrah* due to external factors ranging from parental pressures to whispers of the devil (Philips, 1989), in which case self-actualization may be stifled (Haque, 2004b). In this regard, it is commonly held in Islamic tradition that prophets were guided solely by their *fitrah*, and with God's divine aid they were able to subdue any societal pressures that could have potentially blocked them from reaching their full human potential.

Rogers believed that the path to full human potential starts during childhood. He postulated that when children become self-aware, they yearn for nurturance and protection from significant others, or *positive regard*. Privileged and fortunate children are exposed to ample positive regard, or *unconditional positive regard*, which consequently has a positive impact on how they come to perceive themselves. Rogers called this self-perception *self-regard*. On the other hand, Rogers argued that individuals who constantly experience selective or conditional positive regard by significant others were more likely to develop anxiety or other psychopathology (Thorne, 2003). In Rogers' client-centered therapy, a main aim is therefore to offer clients unconditional positive regard in order to awaken their will to self-actualize.

The idea of unconditional positive regard is in some respects not in accordance with Islamic beliefs. For instance, the Qur'an and Sunnah clearly elucidate how there are certain facets of human behavior Allah detests, such as mischief (Qur'an 2:205) and arrogance (16:22). Prophet Muhammad (PBUH) said, "A slave (of Allah) may utter a word which pleases Allah without giving it much importance, and because of that Allah will raise him to degrees (of reward): a slave (of Allah) may utter a word (carelessly) which displeases Allah without thinking of its gravity and because of that he will be thrown into the Hell-Fire" (Sahih Bukhari,

Book no. 76, Hadith no. 485). Put differently, Islam as a belief system does not offer unconditional positive regard when peoples' actions or behaviors explicitly contradict Islamic codes of conduct.

On the other hand, the Islamic faith also embraces certain principles that may bear resemblance to the concept of unconditional positive regard. For example, Islam encourages people to be forgiving and to avoid judging others. The Qur'an says that God forgives all sins irrespective of magnitude and quantity as long as the person sincerely repents, for example, "Say: 'O My servants who have transgressed against their souls, do not despair of Allah's mercy, for Allah forgives all sins. It is He Who is the Forgiving, the Merciful'" (39:53).

As opposed to other theories of psychology that largely advocated a deterministic view, Rogers emphasized the free will of the client, including during the therapeutic process (Rogers, 1995). According to the Islamic belief system, humans are endowed with free will with which they can pursue knowledge and truth that can bring them closer to their divine purpose on earth (Haque, 2004b). Because of this endowment of both free will and intellect, people will be judged and held accountable for their actions (Achoui, 1998). However, unlike some humanistic psychologies (particularly from the past) that emphasized absolute free will, Islam assumes a middle path in which Muslims believe that although they have the immediate choice between good and evil, Allah has ultimately decreed everything that is going to befall them (Philips, 1989). The intersections between free will and fate/predestination represent a complex theological dialogue for Islamic scholars that is beyond the scope of this chapter.

Although some humanistic psychologies also take a moderate approach in acknowledging environmental forces that form limitations to free will, the role of God is generally overlooked (Achoui, 1998). A more extreme paradigm that negates the presence of God is the existential school. Unlike traditional humanistic psychologies, existential psychology as formulated by prominent thinkers such as Rollo May and Victor Frankl is less congruent with Islamic thought. For example, existential psychology views the world as a meaningless existential vacuum in which people shape their own phenomenological experience and reality (Frankl, 1984). In other words, the individual is responsible for providing meaning to his or her otherwise meaningless existence (May, 1983). In a similar fashion Frankl states, "People have enough to live by but nothing to live for; they have the means but no meaning" (Frankl, 1984, p. 142).

According to Islamic thought there is instead an unambiguous and objective meaning to life that transcends one's phenomenological and subjective experience of the world. For instance, the Qur'an says, "I (Allah) have not created ... mankind except to worship[8] Me (alone)" (51:56) and that Allah "created death and life, so that He may put you to test, to find out which of you is best in deeds" (67:2). Thus, the Qur'an formulates what the objective purpose of life is, that is, to worship God, and always strive to engage in acts that are pleasing to Him. However, one aspect of existential theory that may be acceptable to Muslims is the emphasis on accepting responsibility for one's decisions and actions in life. For example, the Qur'an states "... Allah never changes the condition of a people until they change what is in themselves ..." (13:11).

Because of the importance of worship to Muslims' everyday lives, a more spiritual approach to counseling may be more conceptually palatable. One of the relevant branches of therapy endorsed by Abraham Maslow is transpersonal psychotherapy, in which developing the spiritual dimension of humans is at the core of psychological healing. However, therapists should consider that Muslims view their relationship with God to be the essence of their spiritual development, and appreciate the influence of God's will even on the therapeutic process. Transpersonal therapy per se does not acknowledge this divine guidance. Thus, spirituality for Muslims is not only an energy and life force, but rather it is merged with the divine faith of the formal religion (Hamzah & Maitafsir, 1999).

Intervention

From the outset, it would seem that client-centered therapies like Rogerian therapy would be particularly suitable for Muslim clients. In the post-9/11 sociopolitical context, Muslims face prejudice, discrimination, and religious profiling, in other words, a cultural environment that is hostile and judgmental (Ahluwalia & Zaman, 2010). Many Muslims feel like they have to shed or hide significant aspects of their identities (or they experience confusion about their identities) as a result of being constantly bombarded with information maligning the core of their religion and cultures. As such, Muslims may be relieved to meet with a counselor who offers unconditional acceptance, empathy, and warmth. Such an environment can promote trust and provide a space for clients to take risks (Carter & Rashidi, 2004), explore their sense of self, strive for a more genuine lifestyle, and increase their self-acceptance. Counseling can even offer an opportunity for Muslims to examine their belief systems with more clarity and freedom without being judged or pressured by their own cultural and religious communities.

---

[8] According to the Islamic faith, worship (*'ibaadah* in Arabic) is a comprehensive term that encompasses all words and actions that are pleasing to Allah. Thus, worship can range from tasks such as praying and fasting in Ramadan to treating other people with respect and dignity.

Although nondirective approaches like Rogerian therapy may be suitable for some Muslims who were born and raised in the West, immigrants and those from Arab, Asian, and Central/South-American backgrounds may seek therapists who are more directive. Such clients may become frustrated with a therapeutic approach that places the responsibility on the client to guide and direct the session. For example, as described by Dwairy (2006), Muslim Arab clients may become disappointed and confused with nondirective humanistic approaches, and will likely prematurely terminate therapy. For that reason, more structured and directive therapies are preferred. One example of a potentially useful approach may be process-experiential therapy, which is an empirically supported emotion-focused treatment that incorporates directive, action-oriented tasks, some of which are experiential (Elliott, Watson, Goldman, & Greenberg, 2004; Greenberg, Rice, & Elliott, 1993).

Process-experiential is one of the neo-humanistic approaches that are less concerned with man's ultimate purpose on earth and rather focus on clients' immediate phenomenological experience and creation of meaning within session. Many of these therapies, such as Fritz Perls' Gestalt therapy, incorporate experiential tasks aimed at enhancing awareness of emotion, thought, and bodily sensation. For emotion-focused therapies (e.g., Greenberg, 2002), emotions are seen as the focal point of clients' experience (not cognitions or behaviors as in the CBT tradition). Thus, therapy works to, for example, recognize, reflect upon, unblock, and regulate emotions, and emotional insights open pathways to more adaptive and genuine ways of living.

Emotion-focused techniques can be particularly effective for Muslim clients who come from cultures in which emotions are openly acknowledged and expressed. Clients from European descent, for example, may be open to such techniques. Also, in some Middle Eastern cultures it is not uncommon to see individuals engaged in passionate, emotive discussions and even to see adult men cry openly. The Arabic language is replete with vivid expressions to describe refined variances in emotional experiences. Thus, emotion-focused techniques may be congruent for such individuals and offer the benefit of exploring reactions to sensitive issues without necessarily having to self-disclose specific behavioral details about the issues themselves.

On the other hand, many immigrant clients experience frustration when trying to express themselves in the European languages, which are perceived as stale and constricting in contrast to the richness of their languages of origin. When the facility with language is a barrier, therapists can give license to clients to verbalize emotions in their own language (even if the therapist does not understand it) or use focusing techniques (Gendlin, 1981) in which emotional experiences are instead represented in metaphoric terms or by visual imagery.

It is important to remember, on the other hand, that many other Muslims come from cultures in which expression of negative affect is looked down upon, and discussion of emotions may be viewed as a sign of weakness. Moreover, many Muslims from immigrant backgrounds are likely to experience their emotions through somatic complaints (Hodge, 2005) and thus emotional reflection may be minimal. In such cases, emotion-focused techniques may be challenging to implement, and may be experienced by clients as irritating.

Many of the techniques for enhancing emotional awareness are experiential, such as focusing and empty chair and two-chair work. For Muslims who are new to the process of psychotherapy or have a belief that treatment lies in purely verbal exchange, such interventions may be met with confusion. Additionally, these techniques can be powerful in evoking strong emotional reactions, which some Muslims may not feel comfortable sharing with the therapist, particularly if they are already anxious or ashamed about receiving treatment. Therefore, greater psychoeducation than is typical may be essential when introducing such techniques, or the techniques can be implemented in later sessions after a stronger therapeutic alliance has been established. Furthermore, chair work should be implemented in a manner that is culturally sensitive. For example, it is not uncommon for therapists to guide clients to engage in dialogue expressing anger, resentment, or despair toward an imagined parent or God. Such a technique can intensify anxiety and guilt for Muslim clients (especially those who are more religious); in the case of the parent it may be religio-culturally taboo, and in the case of God it can be seen as blasphemous.

Finally, humanistic therapies tend to appreciate therapists' genuineness and their own moment-by-moment experiencing during sessions. Therapist self-disclosure may be more common in the humanistic traditions when it is conducive to the therapeutic process (Carter & Rashidi, 2004); this may increase comfort for Muslims. Therapists who are accustomed to revealing their reactions should gain greater knowledge of the religion and culture of their clients to anticipate session content that may inevitably evoke negative reactions. For example, Muslims often say "*inshallah*" (if God wills it) to future planning, or appear submissive to the realities of their lives. For therapists who are entrenched in a cultural and theoretical worldview that emphasizes free will and self-determination, this may involuntarily induce a reaction of irritation or impatience that the client may sense, potentially compromising the therapeutic alliance.

CASE EXAMPLE: "TAMER'S PATH OF TRUTH"

Tamer, a 40-year-old immigrant Egyptian, visited the outpatient public mental health center at the urging of his wife and teenage children who were concerned about his depression. Tamer was fired from his job as a company accountant nearly six months ago and since then had been sleeping most days and complaining of headaches, fatigue, and low motivation. He also frequently smoked marijuana. During the intake session Tamer stated that he did not want to "get into that childhood nonsense" and preferred to "focus on here and now." He was assigned to the next therapist on the rotation list.

During the first few therapy sessions Tamer became annoyed with what he perceived as the mechanistic and heartless process of identifying measurable objectives, completing depression inventories, and dissecting his thinking patterns. He asked the outpatient services director to transfer him to the male Lebanese clinical social worker that he heard worked there, but the director refused, stating it was against agency policy and Tamer should discuss his dissatisfaction with his therapist. Considering Tamer's drug use, exaggerated expressions of speech, and resistance to the services, the therapist added to the diagnostic impressions, "Personality Disorder Not Otherwise Specified." Tamer stopped coming to sessions and was eventually hospitalized for a suicide attempt.

Tamer was referred back to the mental health center after his release from the inpatient ward. The clinician of Lebanese heritage who was aware of Tamer's case believed that it had been handled in a prejudiced and culturally insensitive manner. He advocated for Tamer to be reassigned to his caseload. The director finally agreed. In their first meeting the clinician told Tamer that he was Christian and did not speak very good Arabic because he was raised in the United States. Tamer stated that he did not care about these factors but rather simply wanted a therapist who would have some familiarity with the Arabic culture. He said he had been upset because once after lamenting to the first therapist, "Why did God take my job away from me?" the therapist had enthusiastically replied that she would be happy to explore with him the factors that led to the unemployment. He said that since then he felt like he was restrained in his inability to make references to God or religion.

The next few sessions focused on exploring how Tamer's unemployment had shattered his sense of self, particularly as a Middle Eastern male who should be responsible for his family. He also felt confused about his religious and cultural identities, and realized that he had been acting so many different personas with his children, wife, friends, ex-boss, people on the street, and even the previous therapist, that he had lost connection with his true identity. He was fearful that with his drug use and suicide attempt he had fallen from God's grace and would be destined to misery in this life and the Afterlife. He yearned to return to the "more truthful and faithful" person he was before he uprooted his family from a city in the Northern Egyptian delta area and let himself become enveloped by the fast-paced Western society.

The clinician showed warmth and genuinely expressed his emotional reactions and thoughts to Tamer during the sessions, which enhanced Tamer's comfort and trust. Tamer was articulate in describing his emotional experiences, although many times he spontaneously produced descriptions and metaphors that were in Arabic; the clinician only understood the gist. Tamer was increasingly able to acknowledge and experience primary emotions, such as the shame he felt after being fired. He moreover disclosed—albeit with visible discomfort—that other areas of his life had suffered as a result of his depression, such as sexual relations with his wife. The therapist guided him in exploring his emotional reactions and thoughts to these issues without explicitly referring to the details.

Much of the sessions concentrated on encouraging Tamer to explore the person that he wanted to become rather than the person he used to be and make efforts to reach that ideal self with the help of God. This meant exploring the importance of religiosity in his life and his relationship with God. Tamer began to gain deeper meaning from his experiences and refocus what he believed his purpose in life to be. He also gained the realization that he had never fully committed to living permanently in the United States, and this had prevented him from truly engaging in the present moments of his life. In later sessions the therapist engaged Tamer in two-chair work, for example, to process the opposition between the part of him that believed he had failed his religious duties and the part that was hopeful for God's mercy. Eventually, Tamer reported feeling more motivated and confident enough to apply for jobs. The therapist removed the personality disorder diagnosis from his chart and replaced it with "Acculturation Problem" and "Religious or Spiritual Problem."

Additional and Alternative Psychotherapy/Counseling Models

Three main psychotherapy orientations were reviewed in this chapter. However, there are countless therapeutic approaches available to practitioners, many of which may be congruent for Muslims. As discussed by Chaudhry and Li (2010), one of the most overlooked therapies that promise to be effective for Muslims is the solution-focused model. This therapeutic orientation is strengths based, goal oriented, short term, and focuses on finding practical solutions to problems rather than gaining deeper self-insights. The therapist collaborates with the client in a structured manner, and self-disclosure by the client can be minimal. Such characteristics are consistent with the needs and expectations of Muslim clients. Moreover, a previous interview study found that British Muslim participants referred to using positive thinking and searching for inner strength and solutions when coping with problems (Weatherhead & Daiches, 2010). As with other therapies, solution-focused therapists are encouraged to integrate religious concepts when working with more religious clients. For example, the miracle question can be framed as a scenario in which God suddenly solves the problems overnight.

Another potentially suitable therapeutic intervention mentioned in the literature is metaphor therapy. Dwairy (2006) discussed how metaphor therapy could be an effective and religio-culturally sensitive approach because it allows for the integration of Qur'anic metaphors as a healing approach. As reviewed by Ahammed (2010), therapeutic metaphors can help bypass clients' resistances or defenses and stimulate greater imagination in the problem-solving process. Moreover, Muslims from diverse cultural backgrounds are exposed to the frequent use of metaphors, similes, and parables in the Qur'an (Obeid, 1988), and thus integrating examples in therapy can be a natural and effective intervention.

Beyond the European-American techniques, healing approaches originating from other parts of the world may also hold promise for treating Muslims. Carter and Rashidi (2004) discussed the potential usefulness of Asian psychotherapies when working with Muslim clients, because such holistic approaches tend to emphasize spirituality, communal relationships, benevolence, and clarity of consciousness. Treatment can incorporate prayer, meditation, and belief in a higher power (Carter & Rashidi, 2003). This may be a more suitable fit for Muslim clients in contrast to Western therapies that are secular and emphasize individualism and independence.

Research Evidence for Religiously Informed Psychotherapy/Counseling

Several studies conducted in Malaysia have shown the advantages of incorporating religious themes into psychotherapy for Muslim clients. For example, a double-blind experimental study evaluated the use of religious CBT for patients suffering from generalized anxiety disorder or depression (Razali, Hasanah, Aminah, & Subramaniam, 1998). Participants were randomly assigned to standard CBT or CBT plus religio-cultural interventions. In the latter condition, maladaptive cognitions were subsequently replaced with cognitions from the Islamic faith, and religious and cultural issues were discussed. More rapid symptom reduction (using standardized symptom rating scales rated by psychiatrists blind to the patients' condition) was seen for the religious condition, but at the six-month follow-up these differences had diminished.

A similarly designed study with patients with generalized anxiety disorder further classified participants as religious or nonreligious (Razali, Aminah, & Khan, 2002). Religious patients in the experimental religious condition improved more rapidly compared to religious patients in the standard CBT condition (nonreligious patients did not differ between the experimental and control conditions). The differences in symptom status diminished at the six-month follow-up. Other controlled studies likewise showed that religious psychotherapy in addition to standard treatment (i.e., supportive psychotherapy and in some cases medication) was superior in enhancing faster symptom reduction for religious patients. This was found for those with generalized anxiety disorder (Azhar, Varma, & Dharap, 1994), depression (Azhar & Varma, 1995b), and depression with bereavement (Azhar & Varma, 1995a).

Taken together, these studies show that the integration of religious components in treatment is effective for Muslim clients, especially when religious psychotherapy is congruent with their faith values. Religious treatments were associated with accelerated symptom reduction in the early months of treatment. As patients continued to maintain this improvement, the other patients from nonreligious treatments eventually improved to the same levels. Although these studies were conducted in Malaysia, it is likely that the findings may also apply to Muslims living in Muslim-minority nations, particularly as it is consistent with the observations of previous scholars as discussed in the Religio-Cultural Considerations section in this chapter.

Conclusion

Muslims may have varying preferences with regard to the religion of their counselors, and research has indicated that what is more essential to clients is their counselors' demonstration of cultural and religious respect and competence (Ahluwalia & Zaman, 2010; Kelly et al., 1996; Weatherhead & Daiches, 2010). This chapter aimed to support mental health practitioners in this process of becoming religio-culturally sensitive by providing practical information on the theoretical and technical applications of different therapeutic orientations.

As discussed previously, there has been general consensus among scholars that the psychoanalytical/psychodynamic approach is not suitable for most Muslims. However, it is important to appreciate the diversity not only within the Muslim community, but also within the psychodynamic model that can generate points of congruence for successful client-therapy pairings. On the other hand, cognitive-behavioral techniques have been generally touted as the most effective modality when working with Muslims, although there are numerous conceptual and technical concerns that should be considered. It is unfortunate that the more structured and directive humanistic approaches have been ignored from the previous literature despite their potential for many Muslims.

Regardless of therapeutic orientation, mental health practitioners working with Muslims should be flexible and may need to accommodate modifications to their theories or interventions to better suit their clients. In order to be successful at doing this, practitioners should conduct an assessment of their clients' religiosity (Ahluwalia & Zaman, 2010) and develop a grounded understanding of their clients' multicultural backgrounds. Constant self-reflection, reading educational materials, and consultation with an imam or cultural/religious expert can be helpful (Ahluwalia & Zaman, 2010; Hodge, 2005).

Notwithstanding these sources of education, mental health practitioners are encouraged to avoid making assumptions and rather directly ask their clients about their values and preferences. For example, practitioners can ask, "What do I need to know about your religion or culture that would allow me to help you better?" or they can instruct the client to "please let me know if I say something or ask you to do something that contradicts your faith." Asking the client is a simple way to foster a strong therapeutic alliance and develop an intervention plan that is religio-culturally tailored with more positive outcomes.

Acknowledgments

We would like to extend our appreciation to Robert Elliott for the time he took to offer feedback on the writings in this chapter, particularly related to the humanistic-experiential models. We would also like to thank Shamala Shaukat and Mohamed Elsamra for offering their valuable insights.

References

Achoui, M. (1998). Human nature from a comparative psychological perspective. *The American Journal of Islamic Social Sciences, 15*(4), 71–95.

Ahammed, S. (2010). Applying Qur'anic metaphors in counseling. *International Journal for the Advancement of Counseling, 32*, 248–255.

Ahluwalia, M. K., & Zaman, N. K. (2010). Counseling Muslims and Sikhs in a post-9/11 world. In J. G. Ponterotto, J. M. Casas, L.A. Suzuki, & C. M. Alexander (Eds.), *Handbook of multicultural counseling* (pp. 467–478). Thousand Oaks, CA: Sage.

Al-Abdul-Jabbar, J., & Al-Issa, I. (2000). Psychotherapy in Islamic society. In I. Al-Issa (Ed.), *Al-Junūn: Mental illness in the Islamic world* (pp. 277–293). Madison, CT: International Universities Press.

Ali, O. M., Milstein, G., & Marzuk, P. M. (2005). The imam's role in meeting the counseling needs of Muslim communities in the United States. *Psychiatric Services, 56*, 202–205.

Ali, S. R., Liu, W. M., & Humedian, M. (2004). Islam 101: Understanding the religion and therapy implications. *Professional Psychology: Research and Practice, 35*, 635–642.

Al-Munajjid, M. S. (1999). *Islam's treatment for anxiety and stress.* Riyadh, Saudi Arabia: International Islamic Publishing House.

Amer, M. M., & Hovey, J. D. (in press). Anxiety and depression in a post–September 11 sample of Arabs in the United States. *Social Psychiatry and Psychiatric Epidemiology.* 1–10. Pre-publication electronic version is available at http://www.springerlink.com/content/g4r10x02118x1417/

Aydin, H., (2010). Concepts of the self in Islamic tradition and Western psychology: A comparative analysis. *Studies in Islam and the Middle East, 7*, 1–30.

Azhar, M. Z., & Varma, S. L. (1995a). Religious psychotherapy as management of bereavement. *Acta Psychiatrica Scandinavica, 91*, 233–235.

Azhar, M. Z., & Varma, S. L. (1995b). Religious psychotherapy in depressive patients. *Psychotherapy and Psychosomatics, 63*, 165–168.

Azhar, M. Z., & Varma, S. L. (2000). Mental illness and its treatment in Malaysia. In I. Al-Issa (Ed.), *Al-Junūn: Mental illness in the Islamic World* (pp. 163–185). Madison, CT: International Universities Press.

Azhar, M. Z., Varma, S. L., & Dharap, A. S. (1994). Religious psychotherapy in anxiety disorder patients. *Acta Psychiatrica Scandinavica, 90*, 1–3.

Badri, M. B. (1979). *The dilemma of Muslim psychologists.* London, UK: MWH London Publishers.

Beck, A. T. (1976). *Cognitive therapy and the emotional disorders.* New York, NY: Meridian Books.

Carlson, T. D., Kirkpatrick, D., Hecker, L., & Killmer, M. (2002). Religion, spirituality, and marriage and family therapy: A study on family therapists' beliefs about the appropriateness of addressing religious and spiritual issues in therapy. *American Journal of Family Therapy, 30*, 157–171.

Carter, D. J., & Rashidi, A. (2003). Theoretical model of psychotherapy: Eastern Asian-Islamic women with mental illness. *Healthcare for Women International, 24*, 399–413.

Carter, D. J., & Rashidi, A. (2004). East meets West: Integrating psychotherapy approaches for Muslim women. *Holistic Nursing Practice, 18*(3), 152–159.

Carver C. S., & Scheier M. F. (2008). *Perspectives on personality* (6th ed.). Boston, MA: Pearson.

Chambless, D. L., & Ollendick, T. H. (2001). Empirically supported psychological interventions: Controversies and evidence. *Annual Review of Psychology, 52*, 685–716.

Chaudhry, S., & Li, C. (2010). Is solution-focused brief therapy culturally appropriate for Muslim American counselees? *Journal of Contemporary Psychotherapy* [electronic version], 1–5. DOI 10.1007/s10879-010-9153-1.

Dhiman, S. (2007). Personal mastery: Our quest for self-actualization, meaning, and highest purpose. *Interbeing, 1*, 25–35.

Dwairy, M. (2006). *Counseling and psychotherapy with Arabs and Muslims: A culturally sensitive approach.* New York, NY: Teachers College Press.

Elliott, R., Watson, J., Goldman, R., & Greenberg, L. S. (2004). *Learning emotional-focused therapy: The process-experiential approach to change.* Washington, DC: American Psychological Association.

Ellis, A. (1962). *Reason and emotion in psychotherapy.* New York, NY: Lyle Stuart.
Furman, L. D., Benson, P. W., Grimwood, C., & Canda, E. (2004). Religion and spirituality in social work education and direct practice at the millennium: A survey of UK social workers. *British Journal of Social Work, 34,* 767–792.
Frankl, V. (1984). *Man's search for meaning: An introduction to logotherapy* (3rd ed.). New York, NY: A Touchstone Book.
Gendlin, E. T. (1981). *Focusing.* New York, NY: Bantam Books.
George, F. (1999). Freud's concept of the superego: Review and assessment. *Psychoanalytic Psychology, 16,* 448–463.
Goldfried, M. R., & Davison, G. C. (1994). *Clinical behavior therapy.* New York, NY: John Wiley.
Greenberg, L. S. (2002). *Emotion-focused therapy: Coaching clients to work through their feelings.* Washington, DC: American Psychological Association.
Greenberg, L. S., Rice, L. N., & Elliott, R. (1993). *Facilitating emotional change: The moment-by-moment process.* New York, NY: Guilford.
Hamdan, A. (2008). Cognitive restructuring: An Islamic perspective. *Journal of Muslim Mental Health, 3,* 99–116.
Hammoud, M. M., & Siblani, M. K. (2003). Care of Arab Americans and American Muslims. In J. Bigby (Ed.), *Cross-cultural medicine* (pp. 161–194). Philadelphia, PA: American College of Physicians.
Hamzah, M. D., & Maitafsir, M. G. (1999). Transpersonal psychotherapy: The Islamic perspective. *Insight, 14*(38). Retrieved from http://www.ifew.com/insight/14038rch/transpsy.htm.
Haniff, G. M. (2003). The Muslim community in America: A brief profile. *Journal of Muslim Minority Affairs, 23,* 303–311.
Haque, A. (2004a). Psychology from the Islamic perspective: Contributions of early Muslim scholars and challenges to contemporary Muslim psychologists. *Journal of Religion and Health, 43,* 357–377.
Haque, A. (2004b). Religion and mental health: The case of American Muslims. *Journal of Religion and Health, 43,* 45–58.
Hodge, D. (2005). Social work and the House of Islam: Orienting practitioners to the beliefs and values of Muslims in the United States. *Social Work, 50,* 162–173.
Hodge, D. R., Baughman, L. M., & Cummings, J. A. (2006). Moving toward spiritual competency: Deconstructing religious stereotypes and spiritual prejudices in social work literature. *Journal of Social Service Research, 32,* 211–232.
Hodge, D., & Nadir, A. (2008). Moving towards culturally competent practice with Muslims: Modifying cognitive therapy with Islamic tenants. *Social Work, 53,* 31–41.
Ismail, G. A. (2008). *Islam, Sufism & psychotherapy: In search of unifying values and epistemologies.* James Madison University, Harrisonburg, VA. Unpublished doctoral dissertation.
Kelly, E. W., Aridi, A., & Bakhtiar, L. (1996). Muslims in the United States: An exploratory study of universal and mental health values. *Counseling and Values, 40,* 206–218.
Khan, Z. (2006). Attitudes toward counseling and alternative support among Muslims in Toledo, Ohio. *Journal of Muslim Mental Health, 1,* 21–42.
King, D. B., Viney, W., and Woody, W. D. (2009). *A history of psychology: ideas and context* (4th ed.). Boston, MA: Pearson.

Kobeisy, A. N. (2004). *Counseling American Muslims: Understanding the faith and helping the people.* Westport, Connecticut: Praeger.

May, R. (1983). *The discovery of being: Writings in existential psychology.* New York, NY: W. W. Norton & Company.

Moss, D. (2001). The roots and genealogy of humanistic psychology. In K. J. Schneider, J. F. T Bugental, & J. F. Pierson (Eds.). *The handbook of humanistic psychology: Leading edges in theory, research, and practice.* Thousand Oaks, CA: Sage Publications.

Murray, H. A. (1959). Preparations for the scaffold of a comprehensive system. In S. Koch (Ed.), *Psychology: A study of science* (vol. 3). New York, NY: McGraw-Hill.

Murray, H. A. (1940/2008). *Explorations in personality* (70th Anniv. Ed.). New York, NY: Oxford University Press.

Obeid, R. A. (1988). An Islamic theory of human development. In M. R. Thomas (Ed.), *Oriental theories of human development: Scriptural and popular beliefs from Hinduism, Buddhism, Confucianism, Shinto, and Islam* pp. 155–174. New York, NY: Peter Long Publishers.

Philips, A. A. B. (1989). *The fundamentals of tawheed: Islamic monotheism.* Birmingham, UK: Al-Hidaayah Publishing and Distribution.

Razali, S. M., Aminah, K., & Khan, U. A. (2002). Religious-cultural psychotherapy in the management of anxiety patients. *Transcultural Psychiatry, 39,* 130–136.

Razali, S. M., Hasanah, C. I., Aminah, K., & Subramaniam, M. (1998). Religious-sociocultural psychotherapy in patients with anxiety and depression. *Australian and New Zealand Journal of Psychiatry, 32,* 867–872.

Rippy, A. E., & Newman, E. (2006). Perceived religious discrimination and its relationship to anxiety and paranoia among Muslim Americans. *Journal of Muslim Mental Health, 1,* 5–20.

Rogers, C. R. (1995). *On becoming a person: A therapist's view of psychotherapy.* New York, NY: Houghton Mifflin Harcourt.

Segrist, D. J. (2009). What's going on in your professor's head? Demonstrating the id, ego, and superego. *Teaching of Psychology, 36,* 51–54.

Shah, A. (2005). Psychotherapy in vacuum or reality: Secular or Islamic psychotherapy with Muslim clients. *Pakistan Journal of Social and Clinical Psychology, 3,* 3–20.

Sheridan, L. P., & North, A. C. (2004). Representations of Islam and Muslims in psychological publications. *International Journal for the Psychology of Religion, 14,* 149–159.

Takriti, A., & Ahmad, T. (2000). Anxiety disorders and treatment in Arab-Muslim culture. In I. Al-Issa (Ed.), *Al-Junūn: Mental illness in the Islamic world* (pp. 235–250). Madison, CT: International Universities Press.

Thorne, B. (2003). *Carl Rogers* (2nd ed.). London, UK: Sage Publications.

Weatherhead, S., & Daiches, A. (2010). Muslim views on mental health and psychotherapy. *Psychology and Psychotherapy: Theory, Research, and Practice, 83,* 75–89.

CHAPTER 7

Family Systems Therapy and Postmodern Approaches

MANIJEH DANESHPOUR

Over the past century, due to war, political unrests, and dictatorships, Muslim families from diverse countries with distinct cultural backgrounds have immigrated to a variety of nations across the globe. Therefore, it is difficult to make universal statements about the relationship of Muslim men and women, and their attitudes about family life. Local ethnic, social, and historical factors affect the ways in which the Islamic faith is interpreted and applied. These influences determine how strict and traditional or how flexible and open the interpretation of Islam is in any given place. Most importantly, the attitudes of the family members toward their own ethnicity and its values, and their own perceptions of their position in the dominant culture influence every Muslim family differently. This is sometimes to the point that even family members have difficulty separating cultural issues from Islamic perspectives. Furthermore, in many Western countries, there has often been confusion regarding what characteristics come from being raised as a Muslim.

Nevertheless, Islamic ideology creates a fundamental link between cultures and establishes a common framework for understanding Muslim family life. Family structure, which derives from these belief systems, is predominantly patriarchal and values the extended family. Traditions and rituals celebrating important events in both individual and family life cycles often have religious underpinnings. These religious influences foster important similarities in individual and family developmental tasks through the life cycle (Daneshpour, 1998).

There seems to be an increasing interest among family scholars, researchers, and therapists in understanding cultural diversity, couple and family systems, and the impact of Islam as a religious ideology on family life (Daneshpour, 1998, 2009a, 2009b; Hedayat-Diba, 2000; Springer, Abbott, & Reisbug, 2009). Of this growing literature many consider clinical work with Arab Muslim families (Abudabbeh & Aseel, 1999; Al-Krenawi & Graham, 1997, 2000, 2005; Abu Baker, 2003; Nasser-McMillan & Hakim-Larson, 2003; Sayed, 2003), but there are no integrated systemic and comprehensive clinical approaches in working with the diverse Muslim immigrant populations living in the West.

This chapter is an attempt to identify, discuss, and clarify some important issues for mental health professionals working with Muslim couples and families using systemic approaches and postmodernist perspectives. It is important to note that this chapter focuses on Muslims who live in Western countries who are either immigrants or their descendants. It does not deal with the other major groups such as the converts or Muslims living in their countries of origin. Also, even though there are numerous Shi'ii, Sunni, and Sufi groups living in the West, as a minority, the Muslim "sameness" is greater than that of their "differences," providing them with a sense of community, which in turn is an essential source of consolation and support (Hedayat-Diba, 2000).

This chapter has three major goals. The first goal is to familiarize readers with the basic premises of Islamic ideology as it relates to family. Islamic ideology provides guidance about creating and sustaining ideal couple and family relationships. These ideals may differ significantly from the actual dynamics of couple and family relationships, which are influenced by cultural beliefs, values, and practices. It is important for mental health professionals to be introduced to very general yet basic premises set forth in Islam for marriage and family life to prevent false stereotypes from interfering with clinician–client rapport (Daneshpour, 1998).

The second goal is to discuss the dynamics of Muslim couple and family relationships in terms of family systems theory and postmodernist perspectives. And, finally, the third goal is to provide guidance and insights that can assist mental health professionals in working with this population.

Dynamics of Family Relationships in Islam

Family in Islam

Muslims believe that the family is a divinely inspired and predestined institution. They believe that family was not evolved through human experimentation involving a process of trial and error spread over time. Instead, family was an institution that came into existence with the creation of human beings.

The family can be the source of comfort, pleasure, and happiness as well as the source of intimidation and pressure. The response of the family may bring satisfaction and happiness when the individual's conducts and attitudes fit the will of the family and add credit to the family reputation and coherence, and may cultivate shame feelings when the individual displays any deviance from the family consensus. For many Muslims, the self is not often differentiated from the family's identity, thus self-concept and self-esteem will have collective meanings, depending on the family's reputation and approval and reflections of the family's identity (Dwairy, 2006).

Institution of Marriage
Although marriage is a divinely ordained institution, each marriage is a contract. The word *nikah*, used for marriage in the Qur'an, means that the marriage as a social contract engenders a set of mutual rights and obligations. Divorce is permitted when partners have not been able to successfully work on their differences and manage their conflicts. The power to dissolve the marriage is the responsibility of both parties, and based on Islamic principles specified conditions should be laid down for it. Remarriage is allowed and even encouraged in Islam even though in some Muslim cultures there is stigma attached to remarriage or to marrying a divorced woman or a widower.

It is important to note that even though marriage is first and foremost a relationship between the spouses, it in fact builds relationships between families. For this reason, other members of the family, particularly the parents of the spouses, typically play an integral and affirmative role in the whole process. This may mean that parents may have both administrative and emotionally supportive roles. Based on the Islamic principles, consent of both the bride and the groom is crucial and indispensable, and even though free mixing of the sexes is not often allowed, it is mostly permitted for the intending partners in marriage to see each other before the marriage. The main point, however, is that marriage in Muslim society is not simply a private arrangement between the husband and the wife. The entire family is part of the whole process and contributes effectively toward its arrangements, manifestations, and fulfillments. This factor has played an important role in the stability of Muslim families, because when families are part of the selection process, they are more likely to provide support when the couples are later struggling with marital and family issues.

Family Systems Theory

Systems theory can be used as a foundation and integrating force for understanding Muslim family behaviors and dynamics. Similar to Islamic values about family relationship, family systems theory identifies the interactional milieu of the family as central to emotional development, behavioral patterns, values, and loyalties for individual members. In Islam, the family is a part of the greater social order. Families establish an ideological society, with a high level of moral awareness and purposive orientation of all human behaviors where a high degree of social and familial responsibility prevails. Therefore, every family member is responsible for healthy family functioning. In the same manner, family systems theory assumes that the appearance of symptoms is an expression of systemic dysfunction. Such dysfunctions, or imbalances, may appear in an early generation and be passed across numerous generations, or be displayed as symptoms in individuals, marriages, or parent–child relationships.

Most traditional theories of individual psychopathology, like cognitive behavioral and person-centered models, focus on the individual or internal aspects in isolation from the emotional and interactional milieu of the individual. Clearly, other individualistic theories such as psychodynamic, cognitive, and behavioral may contribute to an understanding of certain individual components within a Muslim family system, but they are inadequate to explain the broad patterns of family structure and process or the powerful influences of interactional and intergenerational loyalties (Boszormenyi-Nagy & Spark, 1973; Minuchin, 1974). Family systems theory is a practical model to use with Muslim families because it represents an organismic approach that considers the interaction and roles of each member across the generations as potentially influencing and affecting the emotional makeup and behaviors of all members and their relationship patterns within the entire system (Nichols, 2009).

Family system theory views the family as more than the sum of its parts (Figure 7.1). It also understands internal or external events for a family to have a circular causality. This means that any singular action by a family member will influence not only all other family members, but their responses will be reciprocal to that first action by influencing the initial actor and the nature of the family's overall response (Nichols, 2009).

Based on this broad view of circular and reciprocal interactions, and the recognition of presenting symptoms as part of a wider family system dysfunction, family systems therapists working with Muslim couples and families may respond to the symptoms, or they see the symptoms only as a method of entrance into the system to correct the broader dysfunction. The acting out of a young Muslim child at school, for example, may be an expression of an underlying marital dysfunction between the child's

> **The principal components of family system therapy with Muslim families:**
>
> - Family patterns are circular rather than linear.
> - All parts of family systems are interdependent.
> - Families try to maintain stability of their patterns even when it is not functional.
> - Family systems always have subsystems that can make family function well or become highly dysfunctional.
> - The subsystems within a large family system are separated by boundaries, and interactions across boundaries are governed by implicit rules and patterns.

Figure 7.1 The principal components of family system therapy with Muslim families.

parents. Thus, family systems therapists may work with individual, marital, parent–child, and sibling subsystems; nuclear family systems; family of origin and intergenerational systems; and social networks to understand what patterns affect the whole system and to develop strategies for change throughout the system. Because family system therapists use genograms to track intergenerational roles and events and to analyze triangular relationship patterns, it is a very helpful model given the extent of interdependence or heavy involvement in most Muslim families. Family system therapists can challenge rigid boundaries and shift the structural organization of a Muslim family or dramatize the symptoms themselves in order to further imbalance the system and cause internal change.

Postmodernist Perspectives

Postmodernism embraces the contradictions and complexities of postmodern life, envisions nondichotomous possibilities, challenges cultural constructions of sex and gender, and ultimately reclaims and redefines couple and family relationships by assuming that grand utopias are impossible (De Reus, Few, & Blume, 2004). Postmodernism rejects grand narratives and favors "mini-narratives"—stories that explain small interactions, rather than large-scale universal or global concepts. In this view, Islam and Muslim families can be examined from many different perspectives. Therefore, culture and cultural differences do not become transhistorical entities (Sandoval, 2000) or homogeneous (Grewal & Kaplan, 2002). Internal class, religious, ethnic, and regional divisions crisscross each culture. Therefore, even though Muslim "sameness" is greater than its "differences," sociopolitical changes impact each Muslim country in many different ways, and systemic issues such as gender relations, power dynamics, extended family support, education, class, and age impact each Muslim couple and family relationship.

Thus, the guidelines proposed in this chapter are an attempt to create some sense of "sameness" for Muslim couples and families so therapists can gain understanding regarding the Muslim populations living in the West. In any specific situation, however, the postmodernist's perspective should be used to understand Muslim couples' and families' own "mini-narratives" to help them repair their relationships (Figure 7.2).

The principal components of postmodern therapy with Muslim families:

- *The therapist is the participant-manager of the conversation, not the "expert"*
- *Meaning and understanding are achievable through continued efforts*
- *Difficulties are constructed in language system and can be "dissolved" through language*
- *Families come to therapy with a 'problem-saturated narrative' that has become internalized as their primary self-description*
- *Problem stories/identities are created, lived and kept alive by their connection to important others*

Figure 7.2 The principal components of postmodern therapy with Muslim families.

Muslim Couple and Family Relational Issues

Immigrant Muslim families often come from collectivistic cultures that value the connectedness of the community, tribe, or family more than the individual. Harmony within the family, sensitivity to the needs of others, and support between family members are priorities. Therefore, the autonomy of the individual, which is of significant importance in European and White Western identity development, is not a priority and, in fact, may be sacrificed for the good of the family. Further, due to the influence of a mixture of culture and religion, Muslim families may have a strict patriarchal family system with a hierarchy of generations, and females may be subordinate to males. Parents may be authoritarian, giving direction to children, and collaborative discussion may not be expected. This section reviews some of the common clinical issues that the family therapist may encounter. Several case examples are presented to demonstrate the use of family systems and postmodern perspectives.

Gendered Relationships

The question of gender relationships and the equality or inequality of the sexes is a very controversial issue for Muslims. Muslim are very diverse in their interpretations and understandings of the issues related to gender relationships. The dynamics of gender relationships may be the product of certain cultural and legal contexts, and are not always consistent with the Islamic ideology where the equality of men and women as human beings has been divinely confirmed and legally protected. Ideally, based on the Islamic principles, there is a differentiation of roles and responsibilities, and certain arrangements are made to meet the demands of family institutions—not on the basis of superiority or inferiority of the sexes—but in the light of the basic facts of life and the needs of society. Their roles are considered to be not competitive but complementary. Muslims may believe that one of the main reasons men have been made the head of the family is that order and discipline will be maintained. However, both parties should work together to discharge their respective functions with justice and equity. Therefore, conflict may arise when justice and equity are interpreted by one gender differently than the other.

CASE EXAMPLE[1]

Iman and Tarik are from Egypt. They have been married for 12 years and have two children aged 10 and 8. They immigrated to the United States about 10 years ago, and both were raised in traditional Arab

---

[1] All the names, geographic locations, genders of children, and ages in the case examples have been altered to protect the identity of families that are mentioned in this chapter.

families. Tarik, a mechanical engineer, works long hours and spends most of his evenings and weekends socializing with his friends to "relax and unwind." Iman takes care of family life including all the major responsibilities for children and household chores. Tarik does not allow Iman to visit her friends, claiming that he is responsible for her well-being and women should not socialize with anyone other than family members after they are married. Iman feels isolated and is upset about this double standard in their relationship. A genogram of their family of origin revealed the same interactional patterns in his family. Tarik's mother never socialized with anyone other than family members, and his father spent most of his time with friends after work. Iman's family of origin had the same pattern with her mother never socializing outside of the family circle; however, her father was always home after work helping his children with homework and doing some household chores. Iman believes that Tarik is not attending to his duties as a good Muslim husband and father, and Tarik believes that he provides for the family and can choose what to do with his own time after a stressful day at work.

Based on the family systems theory there is a clear family of origin influence on how this couple views their problems. Tarik continues his father's pattern and expects Iman to behave like his mother, even though they live in another country and she does not have any close relatives with whom to socialize. Iman expects Tarik to behave like her father, even though Tarik's job demands more social interaction than her father's farm-based job. Both are stuck with their own expectations of a perfect relationship.

Through the process of couple therapy, Tarik and Iman realized that their relationship would not improve unless they redefined their expectations of each other based on justice and equity in their own relationship. They agreed that they were bringing the family of origin's pattern to justify their expectations without realizing that every relationship is different and has its own dynamics. They realized that they live in another social context that demands different interactions and social relationships. Couple therapy was successful in helping them reevaluate their own expectations and create their own subsystem while respecting their family of origin's systems of relating and functioning. They both realized that a relationship is unfair when a partner's fair expectations are not being met.

Child-Rearing Practices

Child-rearing practices of any group are influenced by its local culture and religion. There seem to be some differences between the child-rearing practices of the Europeans and White Westerners and Muslims from mostly

Asian and Middle-Eastern cultural backgrounds. For example, the process of separation–individuation that is an important focus of child rearing in European and White Western cultures is not considered important at an early age for Muslim families. As in all other cultures, the success of children is reflective of good mothering and solid family relationships (Daneshpour, 1998).

Discipline begins at an early age and there are usually clear expectations of children to obey their parents without questioning them (Abudabbeh, 2005). Physical punishment may not be considered problematic, and scolding with a light strike may be accepted. As children grow up, they are instructed that they should not do certain things because God has said so, whether or not they understand the reasons behind it. Parents' expectations for compliance increase as children grow older and their cognitive abilities increase (Abudabbeh, 2005).

Many parents are rightfully concerned about the difficulty of raising their children in Western culture without being heavily influenced by it (Smith, 2010). The culturally sanctioned parental strictness becomes problematic after migration to a culture where flexibility and collaborations are considered a sign of healthy families. Raising children, especially girls, becomes a major issue in such a pervasive culture; not uncommonly, families with teenaged girls may consider returning to their home countries to avoid conflict.

This time period also can be traumatic for the child (Nobles & Sciarra, 2000) because in many immigrant Muslim families, open discussion and expression of emotions are not encouraged, which can lead to poor communication. A child that has difficulty understanding sexual and hormonal changes, for example, may find it difficult to approach his or her parents for guidance. Immigrant Muslim parents living in the West may find these issues even more challenging, because at some level they blame themselves for bringing their children and families to these countries and feel that doing so has caused an imbalance leading to subsequent behavioral or emotional problems for their children. Both children and parents struggle to balance acculturation while maintaining their own ethnic identity (Nobles & Sciarra, 2000).

Concerns around a person's sexuality, dating, and dressing are all controversial issues because there are sharp differences between Muslims' beliefs and Western culture. Islam has very clear guidelines on the issue of sexual relationships. Premarital sex is forbidden. This is considered a preventive step against teenage pregnancies, sexually transmitted diseases, and emotional challenges associated with having difficult relationships at a very young age, even though there are instances of early marriages for young girls in many Muslim families. Some Muslim parents, in general, may feel more comfortable when these issues are discussed in school, preferring to avoid discussing these issues with their children at home (Athar,

2010), while some may not want any issues related to sexuality to be discussed at school. The Islamic perspective on sex education involves not only knowledge about anatomy, physiology, and contraception, but also about the morality of sexual issues.

CASE EXAMPLE

Ahmed and Janan came in for couple and family therapy. Ahmed is from Jordan and has lived in the United States for the past 25 years. He is a devout Muslim believing that his religion has given him "all the answers for life challenges." Ahmed's deceased mother was a very spiritual and kind woman and had a strong role in his upbringing and his sense of religious identity. His father, on the other hand, was a very abusive man. Ahmed has many disturbing memories of being physically and emotionally abused by him. At age 18, Ahmed immigrated to the United States to study and work. He met his wife, a Scandinavian American, a few years later and after she converted to Islam, they got married. They have four children: three girls (Sanam and Sarah, 16, and Samaneh, 14) and one boy (Sadedgh, 10). Ahmed claims that his plan has always been to move back to Jordan once his children are older so his children can be raised in a Muslim country with Islamic values.

Janan was raised in a very chaotic family and claims that a family friend raped her at a very young age. As a result, she has no contact with her family of origin and has many unresolved emotional and psychological issues. She is extremely overprotective of her children and assumes that any conversation with the opposite sex is extremely dangerous and can have sexually abusive consequences. She constantly talks to her children about her own sexual abuse and follows her daughter everywhere they go. She volunteers at their school so she can observe their behaviors and listen to their conversations with friends. Whenever she complains to her husband about the children's behaviors, Ahmed blames the "corrupted American society" and blames Janan for not agreeing to leave the United States to live in Jordan.

The conflictual relationship between the parents has resulted in many behavioral problems with their children. The children do not show respect to their parents and defy them all the time. They secretly have dates with boys and have bought cell phones to talk to their friends. They sneak out of the house at night and come back home before morning only to find that their mother has been sitting in their room waiting for them. Over the years, the children have become more and more accustomed to living in the United States, and they have become very comfortable with their lifestyles. On the other hand, Ahmed has become more bitter and resentful and sees their behaviors as a result of the lack of moral character of American teenagers. He strongly believes that if they move back to Jordan, his children will become devout Muslims, marry devout Muslim men, and then life will become perfect. Janan, on the other hand, blames her children for their own behaviors and is very resentful of Ahmed for criticizing the American way of life and not holding their children responsible. She is extremely overprotective of her country and children. As a result, Ahmed and Janan fight constantly, blaming each other for what is happening in their family while their children have become more disrespectful and defiant. No one wants to take responsibility, and the vicious cycle of blame and disconnection constantly continues.

Family systems theory and postmodern perspectives were extremely useful in working with this family. The therapy concentrated on the parents' subsystem first. It seemed clear that Ahmed and Janan had a complementary relationship that was no longer effective. None of them took responsibility for what was wrong in their relationship and both blamed each other. The first step was to get them to realize that this dysfunctional pattern had developed over time and both of them had contributed to it equally. Ahmed had been able to blame Janan without seeing his own role, and she had been defending herself and her children without acknowledging her children's behavioral problems. Ahmed accepted the fact that it was his decision to move to the United States and marry an American woman, and he could not expect his children to live in the United States without being influenced by the culture. Janan accepted responsibility for being overprotective of her children without realizing that her own issues related to the childhood sexual abuse had never been resolved or dealt with. She was challenged to see that controlling her children's interactions with men was a way for her to gain control over her own unresolved issues. Ahmed's fantasy that his children would become devout Muslims only in Jordan was challenged by giving him examples of many devout young Muslims in the United States. Janan's fantasy that controlling her children would make them obey her was challenged by giving her examples of their sneaky and out-of-control behaviors.

Once they both resolved some of their own personal and relational issues, the children were invited to be part of the sessions. Each child told her or his "mini-narrative" about family life while the parents listened. Their wishes and desires for a better relationship with both parents were discussed. The family's understanding of the generational gaps that always exist between two age groups helped both parental and children subsystems to come closer to recognize the source of their miscommunications and misconnections. Parents listed some of their parental expectations and their hopes and dreams for their children, while the children listed some of their own desires and ideas. The pros and cons of living in Jordan versus the United States were discussed first from the parents' and then from the children's perspective. They all discussed likes and dislikes about both cultures. The children requested to have some privileges as long as they respected the parents' roles, the parents asked for more respect and responsibilities in return, and both subsystems agreed to honor them. For the first few months, both generations had lots of difficulties honoring their new boundaries, but over time they realized that the old system did not function well and they needed to respond to their family needs differently.

Problem Solving and Communication

Muslim families, like many other Asian and Middle-Eastern families from collectivistic cultures, may have a style of communication that is more restrained and indirect than in European and White Western societies, with less confrontation and more inference (Daneshpour, 1998; Al-Krenawi & Graham, 2000). This communication style is in contrast to European and White Western culture in which the family is expected to be more flexible, with more egalitarian relationships and direct, explicit communication. For example, the father may want to communicate rules with his children but he may not directly have a conversation with them about it and may ask his wife to explain his viewpoints to his children. This in turn (in the Western perspective) triangulates the mother and creates distance between him and his children.

CASE EXAMPLE

Sarah and Hamed have two children: a 14-year-old daughter, Hannah, and a 12-year-old son, Ali. Both Hannah and Ali have some emotional and behavioral problems at school and at home. Although in many situations parents agree on the unacceptable behaviors and support the same action plan, Sarah feels closer to her children and tends to try to mitigate the punishment, expressing some degree of empathic affection for them or dissatisfaction with the punishment, while Hamed is more remote and strict, and displays less affection and often does not talk to his children.

During couple therapy, it became apparent that Sarah tends to be ambivalent about supporting the behavioral plan for Hannah and Ali due to her own conflictual relationship with Hamed. She claimed that Hamed was very controlling and she needed to protect Hannah and Ali even though she expressed weariness with the burden she carried in disciplining them and acted very helpless. She often played the role of the weak agent obliged to fulfill the will of the stronger patriarchal authority, but she also threatened Ali and Hannah with their father's authority when they disobeyed. She used sentences such as "I will tell your father when he returns home" on a daily basis. Family systems therapy was able to get Sarah to realize how her attitudes in fact maintained the patriarchal system that she did not like. Hamed was able to process his family of origin issues and understand the reason behind his lack of connection with his children, which was related to how his mother always "translated" his father for him and his siblings. Hamed agreed that his parents did not act as a unified system mostly due to the hierarchical nature of their relationships. Sarah agreed that her helplessness in dealing with Hamed perpetuated the cycle of patriarchy and kept all of them stuck in the same pattern.

Because Hannah and Ali's behavioral problems were mostly related to Hamed and Sarah's own relationship issues, couple therapy helped them to come to mutual agreements about some of their own conflictual patterns. Once Sarah felt better about her relationship with Hamed, she was able to stabilize her relationship with Hannah and Ali and become less enmeshed. Hamed felt better about making his wife happy, and both agreed on disciplining Hannah and Ali if they have behavioral problems without becoming trapped in the previous cycle.

Clinical Implications in Working with Muslim Couples and Families

After coming to a Western country, immigrant Muslim families lose the support of the extended family and become very isolated, but do not know where to go or how to look for help. Religious places such as mosques and Islamic cultural centers are now recognizing this need. As a result, there is more awareness in the Muslim community, although there is still a lack of an organized structure to provide help in a systematic way. Muslims may expect help to be practical, specific, and directed to problems in the "here and now." For example, the use of family systems theory may lend to increased success in short-term therapeutic relationships if helping professionals use a more explanatory and instructional nature, similar to treatments for physical illnesses (Al-Krenawi & Graham, 2005).

Further, there are several stages in recognizing and addressing the impact of cultural influences in cross-cultural couples and family therapy. These stages can also be used with Muslim families and include gathering a history of the family's ethnocultural heritage, understanding the reasons for migration, conducting an assessment of the family member's adjustment, and gaining an understanding of the therapist's ethnocultural background for countertransference issues (Jacobsen, 1988). As in working in other cross-cultural situations, the clinician must explore his or her own preconceived notions about this cultural group. The clinician must also consider to what extent the family fits into expectations of the cultural group (Nobles & Sciarra, 2000).

After the family is engaged in treatment, there are several issues that should be considered in individual and family therapy. The therapist must realize that open and direct expression of causes of stress may be difficult for many immigrant Muslim families. The therapist must focus on encouraging partners to listen to each other rather than working on open communication (such as the use of "I statements") and remember that assertive communication may not be valued. Open discussion of issues in a family session may not be a comfortable situation and often does not help immigrant Muslim families who may perceive that as disrespectful. It is helpful to have some individual sessions with children or adolescents and some separate sessions with parents to discuss some fundamental issues and then conduct family therapy. This practice allows the clinician to focus on family orientation and interdependency rather than self-identity and independence with teenagers at first, and then use family systems theory to reconnect all family members at a healthier level. A multigenerational genogram may help the practitioner recognize the impact of the extended family on day-to-day functioning of the family in treatment (Daneshpour, 1998). For Muslim and non-Muslim therapists, one goal is to recognize the differences between Islamic and ethnocultural values and not impose their own ideas about proper ways of living. Sometimes, even Muslim families have a hard time separating Islamic values from the cultural ones.

Conclusion

It is important for mental health professionals to apply approaches that are congruent with Muslim values and their family processes. Family systems theory is the most applicable model to work with Muslim immigrant families because of its emphasis on the connectedness of relationships and the importance of family interactions for healthier functioning. Mental health professionals also need to be mindful that this value orientation sets the pattern of family life in a way that may be quite different from the Western culture. Family system theory helps practitioners understand family relationship dynamics in Muslim families to assess what the "functional" family structure is within the Islamic culture. It is important to note that the way in which a family problem is understood and the desired directions for change are colored strongly by religious ideology and the cultural belief system. It is important to note that Muslim families place high value on the process of integration and pay less attention to the process of differentiation (Daneshpour, 1998). Further, basic rules about gender relationships, family life, marriage, and divorce within Islamic ideology need to be taken into consideration. The goal is to respect Muslim immigrant families' sense of religious identity and interactional patterns while challenging their dysfunctional family dynamics. For this purpose, family systems theory and postmodernist perspectives are likely appropriate models to help family therapists engage with Muslim families without making them feel misunderstood and oppressed by the misrepresentation of their values and belief systems.

References

Abu Baker, K. (2003). Marital problems among Arab families: Between cultural and family therapy interventions. *Arab Studies Quarterly*, 25, 53–74.

Abudabbeh N. (2005). Arab families. In M. McGoldrick J. Giordano, & J. K. Pearce (Eds.), *Ethnicity and family therapy* (3rd ed., pp. 333–346). New York, NY: Guilford Press.

Abudabbeh, N., & Aseel, H. A. (1999). Transcultural counseling and Arab Americans. In J. McFadden (Ed.), *Transcultural counseling* (2nd ed., pp. 283–296). Alexandria, VA: American Counseling Association.

Al-Krenawi, A., & Graham, J. R. (1997). Spirit possession and exorcism in the treatment of a Beddouin psychiatric patient. *Clinical Social Work Journal*, 25, 211–222.

Al-Krenawi, A., & Graham, J. R. (2000). Culturally sensitive social work practice with Arab clients in mental health settings. *Health and Social Work*, 25, 9–22.

Al-Krenawi, A., & Graham, J. R. (2005). Marital therapy for Arab Muslim Palestinian couples in the context of reacculturation. *The Family Journal: Counseling and Therapy for Couples and Families*, 13, 300–310.

Athar S. (2010). *Sex education, teenage pregnancy, sex and marriage: Islamic perspective.* Retrieved from http://www.islamfortoday.com/athar19.htm on March 10, 2010.

Boszormenyi-Nagy, I., & Spark, G. (1973). *Invisible loyalties: Reciprocity in intergenerational family therapy* (2nd ed.). New York, NY: Harper & Row.

Daneshpour, M. (1998). Muslim families and family therapy. *Journal of Marriage and Family Therapy*, 24(3), 287–300.

Daneshpour, M. (2009a). Couple therapy with Muslims: Challenges and opportunities. In M. Rastogi & V. Thomas (Eds.), *Multicultural couple therapy* (pp. 10–121). Los Angeles, Sage.

Daneshpour, M. (2009b). Bridges crossed, paths traveled: Muslim intercultural couples. In T. A. Karis & K. D. Killian (Eds.), *Intercultural couples: Exploring diversity in intimate relationships* (pp. 207–229). New York, NY: Routledge, Taylor & Francis.

De Reus, L., Few, A., & Blume, L. (2004). Theorizing identities and intersectionalities: Third-wave feminism, critical race theory, and families. In V. L. Bengtson, A. A. Acock, P. Dilworth-Anderson, & D. Klein (Eds.), *Sourcebook of family theory and research* (pp. 447–469). London, Sage.

Dwairy, M. A. (2006). *Counseling and psychotherapy with Arabs and Muslims: A culturally sensitive approach.* New York, NY: Teachers College Press.

Grewal, I., & Kaplan, C. (2002). *Scattered hegemonies: Postmodernity and transnational feminist practices.* Minneapolis, MN: University of Minnesota Press.

Hedayat-Diba, Z. (2000). Psychotherapy with Muslims. In P. S. Richards & A. E. Bergin (Eds.), *Handbook of psychotherapy and religious diversity* (pp. 289–314). Washington, DC: American Psychological Association.

Jacobsen, F. M. (1988). Ethnocultural assessment. In L. Comas-Diaz & E. E. H. Griffith (Eds.), *Clinical guidelines in cross-cultural mental health* (pp. 135–147). New York, NY: Wiley.

Minuchin, S. (1974). *Families and family therapy.* Cambridge, MA: Harvard University Press.

Nasser-McMillan, S. C., & Hakim-Larson, J. (2003). Counseling considerations among Arab Americans. *Journal of Counseling and Development, 81,* 150–159.

Nichols, M. P. (2009). *Family therapy: Concepts and methods* (9th ed.). Boston, MA: Allyn and Bacon.

Nobles, A. Y., & Sciarra, D. T. (2000). Cultural determinants in the treatment of Arab Americans: A primer for mainstream therapists. *American Journal of Orthopsychiatry, 70*(2), 182–191.

Sandoval, C. (2000). *Methodology of the oppressed.* Minneapolis, MN: University of Minnesota Press.

Sayed, M. A. (2003). Psychotherapy of Arab patients in the West. *American Journal of Psychotherapy, 57*(4), 445–459.

Smith, J. I. (2010). *Women's issues in American Islam.* The Duncan Black MacDonald Center for the study of Islam & Christian–Muslim relations. Retrieved from http://macdonald.hartsem.edu/smithart1.htm on March 10, 2010.

Springer, R. S., Abbott, D. A., & Reisbug, A. M. (2009). Therapy with Muslim couples and families: Basic guidelines for effective practice. *The Family Journal: Counseling and Therapy for Couples and Families, 17*(3), 229–235.

CHAPTER 8

Islamic-Based Interventions

SABNUM DHARAMSI and ABDULLAH MAYNARD

The relationship between spirituality and therapy has become increasingly important in considering mental health (Sims & Cook, 2009). Although spirituality and religion may be variously defined, the term spirituality has been used to suggest a more numinous, experiential, and mystical approach—a way of knowing in contrast both to the following of institutionalized religion and the reductionism of science. It is in this context that Islamic counseling has emerged. It is both a response to, and a reflection of, these diverse approaches to religion and spirituality. These discourses exist in broader society as well as within many Islamic communities.

That this discussion takes place is itself significant, as spirituality, religion, and science are currently often seen in opposition to one another. Yet there is a need to relate these three in order to respond to the inner world of the believer and his or her mental well-being. To put this in another way, can there be an authentic way of treating Muslims in relation to mental health that is conducive to the believer in all his or her complexity? In this context, Muslims, and those working with them, have raised the question of whether there is a model of counseling or psychotherapy that can be called "Islamic." From this there are further questions that can be explored:

- Is there a way of working therapeutically that derives from Islamic knowledge and concepts?
- Is Islamic counseling more about the way that Muslim counselors bring their faith and inner reality to the counseling relationship and process, rather than a defined theoretical model or approach?

- Is it sufficient to integrate Islamic knowledge or teachings into a preexisting model of counseling or psychotherapy for the result to be Islamic counseling?
- Or, can Islamic counseling be what happens when a counselor, irrespective of his or her faith, is truly empathic and engages with a Muslim client at a spiritual as well as a psychological level?
- Or, is Islamic counseling and psychotherapy defined by the practical needs of Muslims at this time?

In this chapter we offer a discussion of these questions from the context of work in the United Kingdom. We propose that Islamic counseling and psychotherapy is not one approach, but an evolving paradigm. This paradigm is based on the spiritual teachings of Islam, contemporary expertise within psychotherapy, and the needs of the community. Further, we argue that combining these aspects in the evolution of Islamic counseling and psychotherapy is a process that is itself intrinsically Islamic.

Nafsiyyat—Islamic Science of the Self

So what is Islamic counseling/psychotherapy? In order to look at what Islamic counseling means, it is important to look at *nafsiyyat*—the Islamic Science of the Self. The Qur'an and *Sunna* (customs of the Prophet PBUH[1]) are full of detailed references to the nature of the human being.[2] These include descriptions of how to be in a successful relationship with oneself, with others, with the universe, and with God. These verses and sayings often touch on the development of insight, the need to pay attention to one's inner world, and how to live joyfully. It is this body of Qur'anic verses and the Prophet's utterances and practices that form the basis of the study of *nafsiyyat*.

It is *nafsiyyat* that provides much of the theoretical basis and terminology used in most models of Islamic counseling. For example, *nafsiyyat* provides the understanding that the human being consists of both *nafs* (self) and *ruh* (soul, spirit). The *ruh* is what brings each individual into existence. The Qur'an 17:85 (trans. by Shakir) describes it as follows: "And they ask you about the soul. Say: The Soul is one of the commands of my Lord, and you are not given aught of knowledge but a little." Emanating from the Absolute Divine, the *ruh* is perfect and limitless, whereas the *nafs*, reflecting relative reality, is imperfect and confined, having no existence at all

---

[1] The letters stand for "peace and blessings be upon him," commonly invoked by Muslims whenever the name of the Prophet Muhammad is mentioned.
[2] There are over 140 references to the *nafs* (self) in the Qur'an; see, for example, verses 74:38, 75:14–15, 6:164.

without the *ruh*. The *nafs* is the persona, or self. It is that limited sentience, that part of us that we normally identify with—the "I."

It is in the very imperfection of the *nafs*, and the constraints that it faces, that the ability to grow and develop toward perfection resides. The relationship between the divine *ruh* and the flawed *nafs*—two different paradigms of consciousness—is at the center of the nature of the human being and our relationship with both God and the universe. To grow and develop, the *nafs* needs to acknowledge the *ruh*, the divine within. This relationship is implicit in the following verse from the Qur'an, which shows how the human being is created with inner knowledge. When reflected and acted upon, there is purity and growth.

> And the self and Him Who made it perfect, Then He inspired it to understand what is right and wrong for it; he will indeed be successful who purifies it, And he will indeed fail who corrupts it. (Qur'an 91:7–10)

The interface of the soul and self is in the heart, and that is why the heart (*qalb* in Arabic) is of greatest importance in Islamic understandings of the human being:

> ... two different domains meet within the human heart. It is this convergence that can generate confusion as well as reliable guidance. ... These two worlds meet within every human being; they need to be acknowledged and their consciousness unified. (Haeri, 2008, p. xv)

When viewed from this perspective, Islamic counseling can be seen as rooted within the tradition of *nafsiyyat*, a model of the self and its place within the universe. It is also a way of working with spiritual, psychological, and emotional well-being. In Islamic terminology, we might describe this way of working as one that relates to both the seen (tangible, knowable) and the unseen (that which is unknown and empirically unknowable; believing in the unseen is an essential aspect of faith for Muslims).

The Historic Place of Islamic Counseling and Psychotherapy

In order to understand the development of Islamic counseling today, it will be useful to briefly consider a historical perspective on mental health in Islam, and how Islamic scholars responded to the challenges of their time. This is important for two reasons: first, to show how Islamic teachings have fostered a relationship between reason and religion, and second, to demonstrate something of Islam's breadth of understanding in relation to mental health.

The teaching of the Qur'an and the Prophet (PBUH), with their encouragement to seek understanding and knowledge of the human being and the natural universe, gave rise to numerous scholars and practitioners. Indeed,

Islam's "Golden Age" (c. 8th–13th century) refers to the burgeoning of knowledge across many fields including medicine, psychology, and mental health.

Revealed knowledge (meaning knowledge that comes from God through a variety of means such as prophesy and holy books) *combined with* rational inquiry has been the source of a long tradition of mental and spiritual health in Islam. These included Ibn Sirin (seventh century), who realized the importance of dream interpretation, and Abu al-Hasan Ali ibn Sahl Rabban al-Tabari (ninth century), who actively combined psychology with medicine and advocated wise counseling in working with patients (Haque, 2004). Similarly, in the same century, Al Razi (Razes) discovered that mental health and self-esteem helped patients recover faster (Al Ghazal, 2003), and he also developed medical ethics. Al-Farabi (9th–10th century) discovered the therapeutic effect of music and the importance of companionship (relevant to social psychology) (Haque, 2004), and Ibn-Sina, known also as Avicenna (10th–11th century), wrote the seminal books, *Kitab al Nafs* (*Book of the Self*) and *Kitab al Shifa* (*Book of Healing*). Ibn Sina's numerous contributions to the field included addressing conditions such as hallucinations, melancholia, and mania (Safavi-Abbasi, Brasilience, & Workman 2007). The legacy of Islamic scholars has been acknowledged for its significant contribution to modern understandings of health and treatment; it was in the Islamic world that people with mental illness were first recognized as those who deserved and needed treatment as evidenced by the building of hospitals with dedicated wings for the mentally ill.

In our view, what marks these contributions to medical progress and psychological understanding is that they successfully embodied both reasoning and revelation. In Islamic tradition, as exemplified by these scholars, there was no inherent conflict between the pursuits of scientific and spiritual knowledge as found in the Western world after the enlightenment. Islamic teachings emphasize seeking knowledge of the universe and its signs:

> And He it is Who spread the earth and made in it firm mountains and rivers, and of all fruits He has made in it two kinds; He makes the night cover the day; most surely there are signs in this for a people who reflect. (Qur'an 13:4)

Seeking to understand the universe includes reflecting upon—and being aware of—oneself (Qur'an 41:53). The historical perspective reminds us that Islam allows and indeed encourages the use of rationality and expertise, including from "non-Islamic" sources. We see Islamic counseling as being of this tradition, of having the capacity to bring together knowledge that crosses different paradigms to harmonize one's inner self with the outer world. As the Qur'an says, "Those who believe and whose hearts are set at rest by the remembrance of Allah; now surely by Allah's remembrance are the hearts set at rest" (13:28). This is what signifies contentment: "O contented self! Return to your Lord well-pleased with yourself and pleasing to Him. So enter among My servants. And enter into My Garden" (89:27–30).

Islamic Counseling and Psychotherapy in the Contemporary Context

So what is Islamic counseling/psychotherapy today? We have seen how Islamic counseling has a rich and authentic historical and spiritual basis, but how does it address the needs of Muslims today? Certainly, Muslims are a diverse population that requires help that is culturally sensitive. This help needs to take into account the diverse understandings of the values, beliefs, practices, and customs of the Muslim communities.

However, we believe that Islamic counseling not only incorporates cultural sensitivity, but also means recognizing the importance of working in a deeper continuum. Not only does Islamic counseling work with psychological, emotional, social, and subconscious material, but beyond—in relation to the spiritual. So what does that spiritual connection mean in a contemporary context? Human growth and change is more than self-actualization, but about reconnecting with a reality *beyond the self*. In contemporary *nafsiyyat*, the Islamic Science of the Self, all of these different facets of ourselves could be described as levels of consciousness (Academy of Self Knowledge, 2003; Wilber, 1993). At the root of all levels of consciousness is this reality, a supreme consciousness that is beyond the self, but also within it. In other words, consciousness—be it physical or metaphysical, individual or in relationship, immanent or transcendent—comes from God. The Qur'an states the following: "And Allah's is the East and the West, therefore, whither you turn, thither is Allah's purpose; surely Allah is Ample-giving, Knowing" (2:115).

A key theme uniting a number of approaches to Islamic counseling and psychotherapy is a foundation of openness to revealed knowledge and spirituality. Believing in revealed knowledge is a vital aspect of what makes a believer. In our experience, the significance of revealed knowledge for the believer is that it is authentic, immutable, and pure. To say "Islamic counseling" signifies that it is based on a relationship with revealed knowledge. It is this relationship that draws many Muslims to Islamic counseling and gives Islamic counseling its significance and credibility. This is an approach that means more to Muslims than sensitivity to the shared experiences of Muslim identity (although such work is also of great value).

Of course, not all those who identify as Muslims are practicing or religious. Furthermore, people have changing and varied relationships with their beliefs. The therapeutic offer, therefore, is not about Islamic advice, but the "psychological and spiritual space" that counseling of this form allows clients. This is the possibility of discovering "answers" for themselves within the context of their own lives—of working through issues such as relationships, depression, loss, as well as spiritual or religious dilemmas without being judged or swamped by the advice of others.

Indeed, counseling is an important resource for those who are not "religious." In many parts of the world, a decline in institutional religion has corresponded with a proliferation of counseling, which in many ways appears to take on the role of religion but also reflects the benefits of a mostly secular and scientific paradigm (Lines, 2006; West, 2000). There have been advantages to the greater emphasis that has been placed on evidence-based practice, and indeed, the support of behaviorist therapy by government institutions reflects the importance of attention to measurable and deliverable outcomes.

However, evidence-based therapy research literature has questioned the generalizability of evidence-based techniques, even finding that they are not empirically supported for minority ethnic groups.[3] There are mounting challenges, too, with the emphasis on behaviorist therapies, by studies that present a more nuanced consideration of what is effective therapy; for example, more important than techniques are qualities in the client themselves, and the relationship between client and counselor (Norcross, 2002). So where does Islamic counseling fit within this discussion? In many models of Islamic counseling (discussed later in the chapter) there are "both and" rather than "either or" approaches. In other words, Islamic counseling has a spiritual or transpersonal dimension but often includes behavioral techniques. This reflects both the Islamic teaching that the human being is both earthly and divine, and its historical tradition of combining reason with revelation.

Yet beyond this discourse is another consideration. We believe that the emergence of Islamic counseling can also be a response to a contemporary angst; a framework for healing some of the profound spiritual emptiness that marks the lives of many clients, both Muslim and non-Muslim. Within the milieu of postmodern, pluralistic societies, one observes more and more evidence of a yearning for a life beyond the confines of reason (Cottingham, 2005).[4] We are looking for ways of living with one's own self that draws upon a reliable unchanging source—a spiritual and/or moral framework that provides an anchor in what is otherwise a "flatland"

---

[3] Although not all Muslims are from minority ethnic groups, and being "Muslim" and/or "religious" and/or "spiritual" is a different category from ethnicity, one may infer from this research that those groups whose way of life, modes of thinking, and beliefs are dissimilar to the majority may not be as well served by behaviorist techniques.

[4] See, for example, Cottingham (2005, p. 146): "But for all that, to uphold the life of practical reason, as, so to speak, the last word on the good life for humankind seems in the end both a naively optimistic position, and at the same time an ultimately pessimistic one."

(Wilber, 2000) in which everything becomes relative and therefore eventually meaningless and directionless. This angst derives from a postmodernist worldview in which there are no absolute facts, only interpretations. In our view, Islamic counseling can and does provide an anchor in rudderless times, but also allows the flexibility of "spiritual and psychological space." In contrast to secular models, Islamic counseling implicitly acknowledges that human beings have within them something that calls them beyond what is rational and purely behavioral.

An Overview of Islamic Counseling and Psychotherapy Models

So far we have discussed how Islamic counseling and psychotherapy stem from Islamic teachings, practices, and history. This section explores different approaches to Islamic counseling and psychotherapy. We suggest that Islamic counseling and psychotherapy is not a single model, but may more properly be described as different models within an evolving approach to counseling and psychotherapy.

We have already implied that Islamic counseling or psychotherapy can be said to exist as an authentic way of working, based on a coherent body of work derived from Islamic sciences and practices that are therapeutic in nature. We have also suggested that Islamic counseling or psychotherapy embodies a relationship to revealed knowledge. In other words, there is a relationship between the spiritual and the psychological or psychotherapeutic, in which the spiritual contextualizes the psychotherapeutic. However, this is not necessarily the way that all practitioners see Islamic counseling. It is these different perspectives that indicate that, even though Islamic counseling is in its infancy, there are a number of distinct approaches to Islamic counseling. We hope to explore these perspectives through the work of their main proponents in the United Kingdom.

So what distinguishes these approaches to Islamic counseling? We propose three factors, which we believe are key to understanding each of these models:

1. Their conceptual basis
2. The way in which they relate to other models of counseling and psychotherapy
3. The impact of faith on the role of the practitioner

In the United Kingdom, the majority of approaches to Islamic counseling and psychotherapy have been developed from two distinct sources: the Islamic teachings of *tibb* medicine and/or the Islamic science of self-knowledge or *tasawwuf*. *Tibb an-nabawi* means "medicine of the Prophet" and relates to the words or actions of the Prophet Muhammad (PBUH) that have a bearing on sickness and disease. *Tasawwuf* is one of the classical Islamic sciences. Often translated as mysticism, Gnosticism, or Sufism, it combines esoteric, inward, and direct experiencing of God with the discipline of exoteric knowledge or the law. Another factor that we see as important to understanding the differences among models is the way in which they relate to and integrate contemporary models of counseling and psychotherapy.

So far, in framing the work in relation to the theoretical models, we have not explored the therapeutic relationship or the process of therapy within Islamic counseling. This denotes another key theme, where the counselor or therapist, in engaging with his or her own spirituality and faith, brings a different quality to the therapeutic relationship.

On this basis we will explore the adaptation of a mainstream model (cognitive therapy) to incorporate Islamic beliefs. We will then consider a *tibb*-based model of Islamic counseling. Following this we will consider a *tasawwuf*-based psychotherapeutic model. With this example we will explore how Islamic and Jungian theory are brought together. We will also briefly consider an Islamic psychotherapeutic relationship or process-based approach. This process-based approach combines Islamic and family therapeutic concepts. In the last example (our own), we explore how *tasawwuf*-based concepts and Islamic therapeutic process are combined.

An Adaptation of Mainstream Counseling Theory: Cognitive Therapy Incorporating Islamic Teachings

First, we would like to explore the way that Islamic teachings can be integrated into current counseling models and consider if this is also a form of Islamic counseling. There are therapeutic approaches to Muslim mental health that incorporate Islamic knowledge and understanding within a theoretical framework that predominantly derives from a modern (Western) psychotherapeutic tradition. This can be done effectively, as demonstrated by the work of Rameez Ali (2007), a United Kingdom-based practitioner and lecturer in Rational Emotive Behavioral Therapy (REBT) at the University of London. Ali's approach follows a classical application of REBT. When applied to Muslims Ali sees that what REBT brings to Muslim mental health is the flexibility of its approach to identity, cultural difference, and language. Further, he values REBT as a tool for Muslims, because rather than focusing on purely behavioral change, it acknowledges the significance of philosophical change (Ali, personal communication, April 2009). Philosophical change, with the acknowledgment of cultural difference and the development of a shared language between the Muslim REBT therapist and the client, enables the development of a therapeutic process. So, for example, in working with clients' irrational beliefs (a key technique in REBT and cognitive-behavioral therapy [CBT]), Ali is able to encourage the client to maintain his or her religious values and provide specific religious references to illustrate those irrational beliefs as well as rational beliefs. Hence, the client is enabled to work on personal goals within the context of Islamic beliefs. Ali finds that this shared language means that the work is collaborative and owned by the client, who is therefore more able to carry out REBT tasks between sessions (Ali, personal communication, April 2009). In other words, his practice is very traditional, in regard to its REBT history, and adaptive to encompass the religious identity of the client.

Ali argues that many modern therapeutic approaches do not acknowledge religious difference or religious significance in the development of mental health (Ali, personal communication, April 2009). For him, REBT allows not only the acceptance of the significance of faith in relation to thought processes, but can also be used in the context of a shared language to facilitate change through interventions such as metaphors, affirmation, mindfulness, and acceptance-based interventions.

The work of Ali is indicative of an approach to Muslim mental health through interventions based in current counseling and psychotherapeutic practice. Such work may or may not connect with the spiritual reality of the client, but it is indicative of good practice in the way it engages with the client's experience, and is accommodative of religion. It is our belief that such interventions are of great value. Certainly there are many examples of CBT-based models that have been adapted in relation to Christianity or Islam (e.g., Badri, 2000; Hawkins, Tan, & Turk, 1999).

However, it is our opinion that Ali's way of working remains REBT rather than Islamic counseling in that it is based on a theoretical framework of cognitive therapy. In our subsequent examples, we will be looking at approaches that attempt to integrate the psychological and emotional within a spiritual understanding of reality. This suggests that the client is "met" in a therapeutic space that is both psychological and spiritual. We consider this to be central to a counseling or psychotherapeutic process that is Islamic.

A *Tibb*-Based Model of Islamic Counseling

While *tibb an-nabawi* (prophetic medicine) is a specific method of treating illnesses, central to the approach of *tibb* medicine is a holistic approach to health that combines an understanding of the physical with the spiritual, psychological, and emotional. Our second practice example relates to The Mohsin Institute in the United Kingdom, founded by Dr. Salim Khan in 1978. In addition to client work, the Mohsin Institute provides Foundation and Diploma Courses in counseling and psychotherapy (*nafsiyyat*) alongside its Diploma in Herbal Medicine (*tibb*). Here, the treatment of illnesses with a range of techniques including nutrition and herbalism has been combined with the provision of support and counseling as a natural and holistic response to clients' health needs. Khan sees counseling as a specialism within *tibb*, wherein imbalance can manifest on a number of different levels including the physical and emotional. This holistic approach means that clients can receive a range of services catering to physical or emotional health needs through to the spiritual paradigm (Maynard, 2008). These ideas can challenge narrow and normative definitions of what illness and treatment are. Such a comprehensive approach to healing and counseling is not unique to work within the Muslim community (Skinner, 2010).

Looking at this from a user's perspective, clients conceptualize their concerns in different ways. For example, Muslim clients may choose to go to a doctor or a *hakim* (practitioner of *tibb*) if they see their issue as a physical one, or to a Sufi *Shaykh* for spiritual guidance. When Muslim clients come to a comprehensive service like the Mohsin Institute, even if they don't recognize the emotional and psychological, or somatize their problems, or are looking for spiritual guidance, the practitioner is able to respond. This is especially important in relation to Muslims because there may simply be no appropriate words in the clients' language for mental illnesses, as defined within Western constructs of mental health.

Khan's approach in terms of counseling is to combine Islamic guidance with mainstream integrative therapeutic practice, varying his way of working depending on his assessment of the client's needs. In part the rationale for this is the diversity of Muslims and the complexity of the situations they experience. Hence, when the patient is not clearly identifying with their *deen* (religion; literally, life-transaction), Khan advocates the use of culturally sensitive counseling (similar to a transcultural approach) before embarking on Islamic guidance based on faith. Here the model of Islamic counseling is about moving between mainstream counseling methods to Islamic guidance, with faith-sensitive work in the middle (Maynard, 2008).

To summarize, Muslims will approach different practitioners according to how they see the illness, imbalance, or sickness. Further, this will reflect how they see themselves and their understanding and implementation of their *deen* (religion). They may also approach the same practitioner with different articulations of their imbalance. *Tibb*, as practiced by Khan, facilitates this holistic and comprehensive approach. To us, this work suggests quite a different relationship between mainstream models and Islam to Ali's work, highlighted in the previous section. While the counseling techniques Khan uses are mainstream, his work is conceptually based on the Islamic science of *tibb*, is holistic, and incorporates Islamic guidance (Maynard, 2008).

A *Tasawwuf*-Based Psychotherapeutic Model

The concepts and practice of *tibb*-based Islamic counseling have a different basis and emphasis than approaches based on *tasawwuf*. We propose that these are distinct models within the field of Islamic counseling, with overlapping but different theories and practices. Exploring this using Islamic terminology, there is a spectrum within the self and therefore within *nafsiyyat*. This spectrum has been described in different ways, but we find Skinner's (2009) description useful. He states that imbalances/problems may be primarily biological, primarily emotional/psychological, or primarily spiritual. In this continuum, psychology (and by default psychiatry) sits in the middle ground.

As has been noted, *tasawwuf* forms the basis of a number of approaches to Islamic counseling and psychotherapy in the United Kingdom, including our own. *Tasawwuf*, with its emphasis on the process of growth and enlightenment, provides an approach that is developmental and that encompasses mental health and well-being in this wider frame. At its heart *tasawwuf* is "an arc of spiritual ascent during one's lifetime that human beings can partake (of) in the fullness of existence" (Allawi, 2009, p. 261).

Sitting in the middle of the biological–spiritual spectrum of the self is the work of both Skinner and Malik. Both work within the National Health Service, and in this capacity have developed Islamic psychotherapy using a combination of Islamic teachings and psychotherapeutic models (predominantly Jungian and family therapy). In this section we focus on the work of Professor Skinner.

Encompassing to a degree both the traditions of *tibb* and *tasawwuf*, Skinner incorporates a model of the self based on the work of both Salim Khan, and Haeri and Haeri (1990), to provide a wide vocabulary that the client will understand, combined with *fiqh* (Islamic jurisprudence). Predominantly a *tasawwuf*-based model, it is further supported by a Jungian approach.

Skinner's framework is based on a model of understanding the *qalb* (heart—that which connects the self to the divine through the soul), *nafs* (here defined as psycho-emotional drives), and the body, and how these interact within the person. Skinner has found that he is able to apply the same overall framework of understanding with both Muslims and non-Muslims (Maynard, 2008). In his work with non-Muslims, Jungian terms effectively substitute for Islamic terms. For Skinner, the Islamic psychotherapeutic process involves perceiving how the client understands shattering experiences in relation to the things that matter to him or her. Skinner finds that for Muslims, what matters to them most often is their Islamic understanding of the self and the world. In his experience it has been easier to work with Muslims and others of faith due to their holistic understanding of self and experiences in a greater spiritual context, so simple interventions have often been very effective. Where guidance is given to Muslims, it is in the framework of the *shari'ah*. "Shari'ah literally means road, drinking place, and the legal and social practice of a people based on the revelations of their prophet. Among present day Muslims, it has come to be understood as Islamic law or the Islamic code of conduct outlined by the Quran" (Ali, 1990, p. 1). Generally, Skinner finds that clients are not looking for advice that takes them out of shari'ah (Maynard, 2008).

So how does Skinner integrate the Jungian therapeutic model within Islamic psychotherapy? In Skinner's *tibb-* and *tasawwuf*-based model, Islamic psychotherapy takes account of the spiritual and experiential parts of the self, the cognitive processes, drives, and the soma (or body). Change is seen against a static model of balance. Stresses/problems create states of imbalance (consciously or unconsciously) that then optimally return to a state of balance when the stress is resolved. Within Skinner's model, symptoms can be located at different levels of self, mind, or body. Healing of symptoms involves a process by which the Self gains deeper understanding, and a reconciliation of these levels (Maynard, 2008). There are similarities to the Jungian concept of integration (the incorporation of the apparently negative into the whole personality). Skinner observes that this process of healing may be experienced as distressing and entails focusing on a particular aspect of the self. However, the process will always involve the *qalb* (the heart), as it is the connection between the self and the soul. According to Skinner, this concept is similar to Jung's theory of individuation. The outcome is that the self is more than balanced; the person has grown (Maynard, 2008).

In Skinner's model, Islamic and Jungian thinking combine in a way that can be seen as psychodynamic. However, Skinner also sees cognitive approaches, and reframing in particular, as useful tools to manage mental distress. These can work well within an Islamic framework, as the term *aql* indicates. This word, often translated from Arabic to English as "intellect," originates from a word meaning "to tether." The ability and purpose of the intellect is to tether the lower tendencies of the self (meaning "negative" emotions, such as jealousy, meanness, aggressiveness, etc.). However, key to an Islamic approach is the centrality of a spiritual dynamic in the counseling process, something Skinner feels is absent from many cognitive approaches to counseling and psychotherapy (Maynard, 2008).

Skinner argues that the strength of cognitive approaches rests on the client's ability to manage the lower self. However, the lower self, translated by Skinner as the psycho-emotive drives, can affect both the intellect and the heart, causing imbalance. Skinner also feels that ideally therapy should not simply respond to the anxieties of imbalance. Bringing one back to balance is only the beginning—it is simply clearing the way so that divine insights can flow from the heart. Skinner also categorizes this in another way. He terms the immediate cause of a psychological condition or personal state, as addressed through most therapeutic frameworks, as secondary causation. Primary causation, however, is always Allah. What this means is that reality exists by God's will, including the choices we make. This means that in Skinner's model, the therapeutic process includes in it the acceptance that no experience is random and all experiences have divine purpose. Thus psychotherapy entails helping the client explore both the spiritual and psychological meaning of the situation, with the objective being positive change and growth. The emphasis of the therapeutic process moves to primary causation (God) away from secondary causation. Skinner, in common with many transpersonal and Islamic counselors, finds that the combination of psychological intervention and spiritual development can have a profound impact on clients (Maynard, 2008).

An Islamic Approach to the Therapeutic Relationship

The model described previously shows how Islamic concepts can be combined with mainstream concepts. In addition to Skinner's combined Islamic/Jungian perspective, it will be important to consider Dr. Rabia Malik's work. This blends Islamic knowledge, primarily from *tibb*, with family therapy. Her work is influenced by the Islamic concept that the self is holistic—comprising an interconnection between mind, body, and spirit. (Dr. Malik has trained under Dr. Khan.) In her experience, Muslims often talk about their emotional distress in relation to both their physical and spiritual life experience. In addition, she has found that Muslim clients edit out spiritual and cultural aspects of their experience in general from the counseling relationship in the expectation of not being understood (Maynard, 2008). In her work, clients often talk about their internal world in connection to what Allah has decreed or wants from them. She notes that this has a direct impact on the individual's sense of autonomy. To understand a human being or a particular family unit she works from an understanding of the other relationships around it including social, cultural, and religious. Much of this is common with the systemic practice of family therapy. However, to share understanding of meaning with clients at a spiritual or religious level, Malik believes that practitioners themselves must spiritually engage to the same extent as the clients (Maynard, 2008). Aware that relationships are born out of religious and cultural assumptions, she brings to her work an engagement with Islam as a system of beliefs and meaning as well as her own cultural understanding of self and mental health. This enables Malik to work within the metaphors commonly used by her clients. Her faith perspective in her work is her relationship with Allah and clarity about her purpose. Her growth as a practicing believer facilitates her state of heart and acceptance in the counseling relationship, enabling greater understanding/sharing of the spiritual in the therapeutic relationship. In the relationship this starts with acknowledging the role of faith in people's lives. This provides opportunities to bring into the process clients' beliefs or faith by helping them to think about their lives in ways that draw on faith. It provides a therapeutic space in which clients may reflect on the meaning and significance of their experience or actions in relation to their understanding of Islam (Maynard, 2008).

Malik presents to her clients as a family therapist and a Muslim rather than an Islamic counselor. In part this is due to concerns (shared by the authors) regarding therapeutic competence. As the term Islamic counseling becomes popularly used, practitioners have raised questions regarding standards of practice, and the meaning of what it is to be an "Islamic counselor." This is made complicated by individuals who have neither counseling qualifications nor *idhn* (literally, permission—granted by an Islamic teacher following apprenticeship[5]). Currently, there is no clear delineation of who can call themselves counselors in the United Kingdom. Although it had been proposed that counseling in the United Kingdom would be regulated by statute, changes in policy now indicate a move away from regulation to an enhanced voluntary register.

In our opinion, this current lack of clarity regarding who can call themselves Islamic counselors has implications for the safety of clients. We believe counselors should have qualifications in Islamic counseling and/or *idhn* in order to practice as Islamic counselors. This would give some measure of safety to clients, but also allow clients to differentiate Islamic counselors from those who are counselors and Muslims, those who offer Islamic guidance but not therapy, and those who offer counseling that is faith sensitive or culturally competent, but not spiritual. We will explore what qualifying as an Islamic counselor means in talking about our model in the following, particularly in the latter section where we discuss implications for training. We are working with other practitioners, academics, and theologians to develop national standards for this nascent field.

Our *Tasawwuf*-Based Model of Islamic Counseling

We would now like to present our model (Stephen Maynard and Associates), which is based on *tasawwuf*. We work as an independent organization, involved in developing service provision as well as accredited practitioner training up to diploma level, with an emphasis on community and diversity. We begin by summarizing how our model relates to other Islamic counseling approaches.

---

[5] This authorization (*idhn*) relates to the transmission of spiritual education (*tarbiyah*); its use is most common among the Sufis. More well known is the term *ijaza*, which is permission or authority to teach or transmit legal jurisdictions or *hadith* (sayings of the Prophet, PBUH).

Like Skinner, the theoretical framework we use is based on a model of the self, devised by Haeri and Haeri (1990) and hence based in *tasawwuf.* The Haeri and Haeri model of the self combines the work of a number of previous scholars of *tasawwuf.* Another key aspect of our practice is a specific counseling process developed by Dharamsi (1998) that combines the therapeutic and theological or spiritual. (Aspects of this process model are discussed in the following.) Malik and Khan's approaches relate less directly to *tasawwuf*, being based more on *tibb*. However, all of these ways of working are related through a basis in Islam.

Different perhaps from the models mentioned previously, we see our work as a therapeutic model based wholly within Islamic teachings. To us, the fact that a number of different ways of working have been developed from integrating Islamic theory and contemporary models of counseling indicates the breadth and inclusivity of the Islamic perspective. So, in our model, at a level of technique, some practices are directly from the Qur'an and *sunna*, but a number of practices are derived from other counseling theories. What makes this integration different to those described previously is that these practices (from a number of other models) are all understood within an Islamic theoretical framework. This takes on the wider principle of inclusiveness and universality of Islamic teaching that whatever learning and knowledge is good and true and in tune with Islam's teachings comes from God, and is "Islamic." This approach can also be seen as part of a broader movement within contemporary Islamic thinking (Kamrava et al., 2006), which moves away from earlier more rigid interpretations of Islam to a more holistic understanding.

Tarbiyah—A Critical Process

In our model of Islamic counseling, *tarbiyah* (the development of or bringing up to one's highest potential) is a critical process. Although *tarbiyah* is sometimes translated as education, it is more properly the entire process of development including spiritual growth. In our work, *tarbiyah* sets the context for the *process* of therapeutic change within the counseling relationship, as well as the very nature of the Islamic *model* of the self. This process is about connecting to divine truth. In Islam, every event, both inwardly and outwardly, resonates with that truth. As the Qur'an says,

> We will soon show them Our signs in the Universe and in their own souls, until it will become quite clear to them that it is the truth. Is it not sufficient as regards your Lord that He is a witness over all things? (41:53)

Connecting to divine truth means recognizing the attributes of God that manifest in every life event. The attributes of God are also known as the names of God. These names offer invitations to worship and adore that resonate deep within our souls. Hence, every experience of one's life is an opportunity to acknowledge the ineffable, which can be called Allah, God, The One, or countless other names. As the Qur'an says, "Say: Call upon Allah, or call upon the Beneficent God; whichever you call upon, He has the Most Beautiful Names" (17:110).

One of the key aspects of our model is how the divine truth (that there is nothing but God, and everything reflects Him) is reflected in the therapeutic process and relationship. We call the method by which the counselor brings his or her faith and inner reality to the counseling relationship and process "orientation." Orientation means a deep understanding and internalization of this God-given truth by the practitioner that informs and transforms the process. We have named the process of "orientation" after the Islamic practice of facing *qibla*—the direction or orientation of prayer.

Concepts and Processes in Islamic Counseling

We would like to share the following case study and discussion to demonstrate key aspects of our Islamic counseling in practice. In particular we would like to draw attention to concepts of **tarbiyyah** and **orientation**, and the interplay of **self** and **soul** in relation to both client and counselor. The case study has been simplified to facilitate understanding of these concepts.

CASE STUDY

Khalid is 32 and has been struggling with a number of issues around anger and guilt following the breakup of his marriage to his beloved wife. He was finding it hard to reconcile his relationship with his mother, with whom he had previously been close, because he felt that she had destroyed his marriage through bitterness and jealousy. He responded quickly to Islamic counseling, evidently trusting the process and working seriously within the sessions. As sessions progressed, the counselor sensed a tension in the counseling relationship. The client began consciously or unconsciously attempting to test counselor boundaries through presenting conflicting stories or ones that were clearly not true. Further work indicated that Khalid was getting increasingly angry as he began to remember times when he'd done nothing to prevent the deterioration of his marriage and his relationship with his mother.

So how might an Islamic counselor interpret this? Khalid's response indicates conflicting levels of consciousness, or *nafs*, as he goes through a difficult transition in regard to his understanding of his circumstances. At one level of consciousness, Khalid's anger derives from his sense of powerlessness; his expectations of his marriage and of his mother in relation to his marriage had not been met. In Islamic terminology, this can be interpreted as *nafs al-ammara*, or the "commanding" self. This is a self or level of consciousness that is primarily reactive, often driven by and at the mercy of unconscious motivations. But there is more here—another (and higher) level of consciousness is struggling to emerge in Khalid. This is marked by guilt and is known as *nafs al-lawwamma*, or the "blaming" self. Here Khalid starts to take account of his inaction in relation to his responsibilities to his wife and marriage. Yet as Khalid's safety in counseling grows, so does his conscious awareness of the inappropriateness of his actions in his marriage, resulting in him becoming "stuck." The pain of this inner struggle manifests in dishonesty and more anger to avoid the realization of his weakness and failure. In Box 8.1, these and other levels of the self are identified.

But why is this truth of Khalid's fallibility problematic for him? Why isn't it "OK" to be limited or flawed? In Islamic teachings, fallibility and limitation are seen as not only a part of human nature, but as challenging by design, because of the fragility of the self's identity in relation to that which is absolute. The (relative) self (or *nafs*) cannot help but be confronted by its limitations because it aspires to the absolute. God created us to discover through life's experiences that anything less than Him will never be enough. This marks a paradox at the heart of our nature, to be dissatisfied with what is relative, including ourselves, *because* of its comparison to the light of the divine or absolute. Human nature is restless, unhappy with limitation because our deepest longing is to be absorbed by, and submitted to, divine perfection. This is worship, whether it is conscious or not. Khalid intended to have a long, happy marriage; he failed to realize this. Khalid's response is profoundly human, but its significance is divine. The guilt, the impossibility of the situation, and his failure are all part of the paradox of his existence, the relationship between the relative and the absolute.

So what difference does this paradox make to the practice of the Islamic counselor according to our model? Khalid's counselor begins by orientation. This means that the counselor sees all facets of Khalid's reality—his powerlessness, his love for his wife, his anger, his limitations and struggle to transcend them—as reflections of Allah's mercy. This is not necessarily shared with the client, but it is important that the counselor knows that Khalid's situation reflects the Islamic teaching that within our hearts is the soul or *ruh*, or God's "agent" (Haeri, 2008, p. 191). The soul is intangible and compelling, because it continually reflects God's attributes (as discussed previously). In *tasawwuf*, the soul is seen as reflecting the qualities of the absolute—perfect love, perfect absolute power, perfect justice, true

BOX 8.1 LEVELS OF THE SELF IN THE QUR'AN, IN ASCENDING ORDER

The Qur'an describes various "stations" of the self, which may also be understood in terms of levels of self-development or awareness or consciousness. These have been variously classified and expounded upon by Classical Islamic scholars, including Ibn Sina and al-Ghazzali, as well as more recently by Haeri (1991) and Frager (1999).

Nafs Al-Ammara   The Commanding Self   see the Qur'an 12:53
The lowest level of the self; childish, base, egotistical; wants instant gratification. Lacks introspection.

Nafs Al-Lawamma   The Blaming Self   see the Qur'an 75:2
Uncontrolled behavior but pricked by conscience, often characterized by self-questioning, defensiveness, guilt.

Nafs Al-Mulhamah   The Inspired Self   see the Qur'an 91:7
No longer ruled by conscientiousness or false sense of duty, this is a creative, artistic, liberal, loving self. This self often struggles with authority, rules, and discipline.

Nafs Al-Mutma'innah[1]   The Certain Self   see the Qur'an 89:27
Contained and remembering God. Confident and trusting, the self has become loyal to the path of worship and self-purification. Islamic counseling is not indicated at this level and beyond, although individuals may choose to explore particular areas for growth and development.

Nafs Al-Radiyah   The Content Self   see the Qur'an 89:28
Contented with whatever situation he or she is placed in, whether difficulty or ease. Seeing God in every circumstance.

Nafs Al-Mardiyah   The Self That Everything Is Pleased With   see the Qur'an 89:28
Contentment guides their choices and actions reliably so that individuals are in harmony with their environment.

Nafs Al Kamila   The Completed Self   see the Qur'an 4:55 and 5:54
The level of the Prophet. Living by Divine Love.

---

[1] This level of the self is also sometimes translated as the contented self and relates closely to the *nafs al-radiyah*.

and pure compassion, and so on. The self—our humanness—desires these qualities for itself, and is captivated and driven by them, but can never enduringly achieve them in this world. Well-being, therefore, depends on transcendence (going beyond the self, submitting to the soul) without being disassociated from reality (being in the self). In *tasawwuf*, this is known as "being in the world, but not of it"—operating and functioning and not denying the reality of life, but learning to let go of attachments and going beyond them. The paradox cannot be resolved utterly, but one can acknowledge and submit to it. Submitting is an active and dynamic process, not a fatalistic one. In the context of Islamic counseling, training (and similarly supervision) therefore centers on developing an understanding of this paradox, of the interplay of self and soul in the context of client work.

As practitioners gain deeper and deeper understanding of this interplay, they come to a greater acceptance of human frailty, not just of the client, *but their own*. This acceptance liberates practitioners, because they can see how, for example, wanting to rescue clients from their pain is an indication of the therapists' *own* desire for the absolute. God is the All Healer, not them. Therapists accept the discordance of witnessing another's pain and so, instead of trying to rescue the person, come to terms with the limitations of their own paradoxical nature. In acknowledging their own frailty as practitioners, they are enabled to truly let go of wanting to rescue the person in the knowledge that this process occurs not through them but by divine grace. Practitioners, in being released from their own projections, and by applying their own faith to the process, are perhaps more empowered, more peaceful, and more hopeful. They also are alert and open to the greatest possibilities of change in the client because they know that God is in charge. Thus, practitioners' belief or framing of the client's situation is a part and parcel of the healing, even if unspoken. Practitioners communicate safety and acceptance through a quality of heart that is a palpable experience for the client because of the practitioner's belief; Islamic counseling accepts the frailty of the practitioner *and* client and works with both.

This is not to say that the client and the counselor do not work to resolve practical difficulties experienced by the client. What is crucial, however, is that action rests upon a foundation of acceptance. With this inner knowledge, the practitioner can "face" the client without fear of what the client may bring, and genuinely hold a space for the client. The counselor both allows the client to safely express fears while also being actively supportive without foisting clichés (including therapeutic, religious, or spiritual ones) upon the client. In Islamic counseling, perhaps what we hope for and emphasize is that practitioners convey in the stillness of their heart their dynamic equanimity, a loving concern; this forms a context in which the client can discover his or her own healing. In this context, inspirations or insight of the client or counselor emerge. The classical scholar al-Ghazzali

(2008) refers to this process when he writes, "This opening of a window in the heart towards the unseen also takes place in conditions approaching those of prophetic inspiration, when intuitions spring up in the mind unconveyed through any sense-channel" (p. 22).

In other words, al-Ghazzali is saying that the heart can intuit things that are not accessed by our external senses, and moreover, that these intuitions can be from the unseen and of divine origin. Al-Ghazzali continues:

> The more a man purifies himself from fleshly lusts and concentrates his mind on God, the more conscious will he be of such intuitions. Those who are not conscious of them have no right to deny their reality. Nor are such intuitions confined only to those of prophetic rank. Just as iron, by sufficient polishing can be made into a mirror, so any mind by due discipline can be rendered receptive of such impressions. (p. 22)

In other words, the receptivity of the heart to high-quality insight can be increased by training the self and focusing on God. This inner discipline is a major component in our training of Islamic counseling practitioners.

Islamic Counseling Training

We would now like to give an applied example from Islamic counseling training of the inner discipline that we referred to previously. The training of practitioners is a key aspect of our work and focuses on the development of skills, but in the context of the spiritual development of the practitioner. This is because in Islamic teachings, the best actions are seen to proceed from good intentions and a pure heart. Box 8.2 contains an example of the kind of reflective exercises trainees are invited to use to develop and deepen their spiritual understanding.

In our Islamic understanding, every perception is relative to the observer and is seen as a fixation through which the clarity of the heart can become tarnished. However, although the world is illusory, it was also created with truth. Perceptions/illusions are still helpful in that through acknowledging and working through them, the self loses its attachment to these fixations and consciousness expands, and so the self comes closer to God. There is no outer reality independent of perception, apart from the absolute or God. So the counselor, in putting aside his or her agenda and letting go of desires (such as providing solutions, wanting to be liked and successful, or even to proselytize), is actually emptying out his or her own self. Through the discipline of "emptying out," the counselor hopes to be released from his or her own illusions and identification with them. This can be understood in the context of the following from Haeri (2008): "The awakened self hears the clear inner voice. Other selves battle with confusion and conflict before arriving at the safety of the knowing heart" (p. 223).

BOX 8.2 REFLECTIVE EXERCISE FOR PRACTITIONERS BASED ON ONE OF HIS BEAUTIFUL NAMES, AL-QAWI (THE MOST STRONG, THE ALL ABLE)

First, let us suggest that much of what we know is relative or in relation to something else—for example, we know heat only in relation to cold, or light in relation to dark.

Now, reflect upon an experience in your own life where you have felt weak.

Make an intention to see that weakness differently. This is not as opposed to a time when you felt strong, but see it as a shadow. The shadow is visible because of the light from your soul, as a longing for the divine attribute Al Qawi, the All-Able.

Suspend self-blame and see your wanting to overcome weakness as worship of Divine Power.

Momentarily let go of self, let go of identity, let go of effort and dive into soul; accept your weakness and melt in Divine Power.

In our courses, we teach students to acknowledge the client's feelings and context, to listen and to put aside their agenda and truly engage with the other person. The source of this practice in Islamic counseling is the Qur'an, which says, "By no means shall you attain to righteousness until you spend (benevolently) out of what you love . . ." (3:91). In the therapeutic context, giving of what one loves often means practitioners learning to let go of their ego, whether that is the desire to give advice, rescue others, or be liked.

This practice of putting aside one's agenda is exactly what many counseling models teach, and the skills are so far similar. Yet in Islamic teachings, putting aside one's agenda in service to another is a sacred and powerful act because it means disengaging with one's own illusions. With such disengagement comes the recognition of a universal truth that all of us are inevitably caught in perceptions that arise from our conditioning and experiences. The following quote from the Qur'an challenges the reader to see the perfection in God's creation, but also to recognize that any conception of imperfection relates to our own limitation.

Who created the seven heavens one above another: you see no incongruity in the Creation of the Beneficent God; then look again: can you see any disorder? Then turn back again and again; your vision shall come back to you confused while it is fatigued. (Qur'an 67:3–4)

To summarize, in our model of Islamic counseling, the process of putting aside one's agenda appears similar to humanistic counseling on the surface, but invites Islamic counselors to engage with a process of *returning to the One* root of all consciousness. They do this through an intense process of self-examination. This includes the discipline of examining their intentions, agendas, the quality of their empathy, their self-awareness, the techniques they use, and the results that come of them.

"Returning to the One" is an aspect of *tarbiyah*. As explained earlier, *tarbiyah* means development or refining to one's highest potential. Its etymology derives from Rabb, meaning Lord. Human potential is therefore based on the relationship of each self (as *abd*, or bondsperson) with his or her Creator through the divine Name of Al Rabb. Acknowledging the Rabb is conscious worship. In this context the growth process central to the practice of Islamic counseling rests very much upon the appropriate development of virtues within the person.

Inculcating Virtues

Counselors are encouraged in training and supervision to cultivate virtues. This makes the counseling relationship one in which clients feel not only very safe, but also trusting of their counselor as a reference point whose insights, tentatively and sensitively offered, they value. One of these virtues is humility. When working with a client, the counselor genuinely aspires and works with the concept and practice that it is a privilege to work with the client. This is because human beings are the highest aspect of creation—a paradox of both self and soul, seen and unseen, limited and yet drawn to perfection. In addition, after the session, both in supervision and through self-reflection, the counselor actively seeks out and acknowledges resonances with the client experience. This is because Islamic counseling presupposes that this interaction between counselor and client is also for the practitioner's own development. The client is a "gift" in that the therapeutic interaction enables the counselor to reflect and hence grow, knowing that in this transaction a mirror is being held both ways. Of course, one of the dangers of this kind of process is unintentionally "merging" or over-identifying with the client. Islamic counseling training also emphasizes checking perceptions through self-examination and feedback. Practitioners are therefore required to question their intentions in more and more depth as they develop greater understanding and skills.

Having made this caveat, the understanding of mutual benefit through the therapeutic process frames the counselor–client relationship and infuses the transaction with a deep and profound respect and parity. It is based on the understanding that therapeutic change is part of a greater therapeutic relationship in which both client and counselor are held. (This greater therapeutic relationship is with God.) Within this relationship it is important that counselors adhere to a clear code of ethics as well as *shari'ah* (revealed law and religious code of conduct). So, as we see Islamic counseling, it is not about dispensing Islamic legal jurisdictions, but about the counselor working within an ethical framework and allowing clients to discover truth for themselves.

In our understanding of Islamic counseling, discovering the truth for oneself is enabled through a number of practices. These include, for example, *huzoor* (presence), *tafakkur* (reflection), *tawbah* (returning to the One), *istighfar* (seeking forgiveness, acknowledging wrong), and *shukr* (gratitude). One of the key practices that we use in our model is "proactive listening." Here one listens with body, mind, and heart while seeking to hear the highest potential in one's client. It's important to distinguish hearing the highest potential from a "rosy spectacled approach" or simply seeing the positive in the person. The counselor acknowledges where the client is, not denying the client's pain, anger, doubt etc., but understanding that doubt and distress can often cloud the human heart from its true potential. Proactive listening involves being alert to the perfect soul that is guiding the imperfect *nafs*, and relating this to the specific context of the client. It is often "hidden in plain sight," that is, it may be obscured by apparently negative situations, "bad" actions, or problems. Part of this technique may involve highlighting this back to the client, but in proactive listening, the emphasis is on the counselor's conceptualization of the client and the client's situation. So in Khalid's case an example of proactive listening might be that the counselor focuses the insight of his or her heart on connecting with the love that Khalid has for his wife. The counselor recognizes how Khalid's love is a reflection of God's Attribute Al Wadud (the All-Loving). Connecting in this way is a skill enabled by Grace. The skill is developed and held in the orientation of the counselor and is part of the Islamic counseling process (mentioned previously).

In our Islamic counseling model, each of these skills can be seen to operate in a full spectrum, from the seen and tangible to the unseen. What this means in practice is that in the "seen world" counselor and client can interact at the level of concern for the client's circumstances. Yet, on an unseen level, we believe that sincere intentions on the part of the counselor and his or her client have a multiplier effect. God's grace elevates the quality of the healing to something that informs every skill and technique, but also can often go beyond the expectations of both client and counselor.

Conclusion

Islamic counseling and psychotherapy derive from an ancient tradition, not only of Islamic teachings, but perhaps more fundamentally, recognition and honoring of the primacy of spirituality in our lives. This spiritual truth is described in many faiths and some therapeutic models.

We discussed the way in which we believe Islamic counseling training supports practitioners in their spiritual development. We believe that this may be conducive to enhancing the therapeutic relationship. For Muslims today, we believe that providing accessible Islamic counseling is especially important because the therapeutic spiritual space it offers is one that enables growth and development that is in tune with *nafsiyyat*, but that does not impose religious teachings or advice.

We believe that when practitioners are able to connect with spiritual truth in a way that is appropriate to Muslim clients, the therapeutic relationship becomes transformed. This transformation enables the client to develop insight that is spiritual as well as psychological. Such work may not be seen as "Islamic counseling," but is indicative of the universality of the spiritual experience within us.

In this chapter, we hope we have presented aspects of our understanding of Islamic counseling in terms of its therapeutic application and techniques, but also in relation to that inner calling, which is also a universal call to look within one's own self—and to connect with one's Creator.

We have given an indication of how Islamic counseling relates to Muslim mental health across different models, highlighting key differences and similarities to mainstream models, but also from the perspective of the therapist and the client. We hope in this chapter that we have also shown how the application of these vast teachings to a contemporary counseling context has a universal offering in the majestic journey of self to soul, of reconnecting with and being in awe of the Divine, that Unifying Oneness that permeates our lives in a myriad of ways.

Acknowledgments

We would like to express our gratitude to our teachers, especially Shaykh Fadhlalla Haeri; to our editors for their kindness and painstaking comments; to colleagues and friends Jan Mojsa from CPCAB, Ruth Webster, and Muna Bilgrami for their support in the development of this chapter; to our colleagues Professor Skinner, Dr. Rabia Malik, Dr. Salim Khan, and Rameez Ali; and finally to our students and clients.

References

Academy of Self Knowledge. (2003). *Lesson seven evolving consciousness.* Retrieved from http://www.askonline.co.za/

Al Ghazal, S. (2003). The valuable contributions of Al Razi (Rhazes) in the History of Pharmacy During the Middle Ages. *Journal of the International Society for the History of Islamic Medicine, 2*(4), 9–11.

Al-Ghazzali. (2008). *The alchemy of happiness.* Charleston, SC: Forgotten Books.

Ali, L. (1990). *Introduction to Islamic law*. Retrieved from http://www.scribd.com/doc/19134789/Introduction-to-Islamic-Law-Luqman-Ali

Ali, R. (2007). Application of REBT with Muslim clients. *The Rational Emotive Behaviour Therapist Journal of The Association for Rational Emotive Behaviour Therapy, 12*(1), 3–8.

Allawi, A. A. (2009). *The Crisis of Islamic civilisation*. New Haven, CT: Yale University Press.

Badri, M. (2000). *Contemplation: An Islamic psychospiritual study*. Kuala Lumpur: Madeena Books.

Cottingham, J. (2005). *The spiritual dimension: Religion, philosophy and human value*. Cambridge, UK: Cambridge University Press.

Dharamsi, S. (1998). *Stephen Maynard & Associates Training Programme*. Unpublished.

Frager, R. (1999). *Heart, self and soul*. Wheaton, IL: Quest Books.

Haeri, F. (1991). *Journey of the self*. London: Harper Collins.

Haeri, F. (2008). *Witnessing perfection*. Alresford, Hampshire: O Books.

Haeri, F., & Haeri, A. (November 1990). *Islamic Counselling Training Programme*. London. Unpublished.

Haque, A. (2004). Psychology from Islamic perspective: Contributions of early Muslim scholars and challenges to contemporary Muslim psychologists, *Journal of Religion and Health, 43*(4): 357–377.

Hawkins, R. S., Tan, S. Y., & Turk, A. A. (1999). Secular versus Christian inpatient cognitive behavioral therapy programs: Impact on depression and spiritual well-being. *Journal of Psychology and Theology, 27*, 309–331.

Kamrava, M., et al. (2006). Reformist Islam in comparative perspective. In M. Kamrava (Ed.), *The new voices of Islam: Reforming politics and modernity—A reader*. (p. 1–28). London: I. B. Tauris.

Lines, D. (2006). *Spirituality in counselling and psychotherapy*. (p. 1–28) London: Sage.

Maynard, A. (2008). *Muslim mental health: A scoping paper on theoretical models practice and related mental health concerns in Muslim communities*. Retrieved from www.signposts.org.uk/.../Muslim%20Mental%20Health%20- %20Stephen%20Maynard.pdf

Norcross, J. C. (Ed.). (2002). *Psychotherapy relationships that work: Therapist contributions and responsiveness to patients*. New York, NY: Oxford University Press.

Qur'an (Shakir, M.H., Trans., 1982). New York, NY: Tahrike Tarsile Qur'an Inc.

Rumi Jalal al-Din. The Essential Rumi (C. Barks, Trans., 1995). San Francisco, CA: Harper.

Safavi-Abbasi, S., Brasiliense, L. B. C., & Workman, R. K. (2007). The fate of medical knowledge and the neurosciences during the time of Genghis Khan and the Mongolian Empire. *Neurosurgical Focus, 23*(1), E13, 3.

Sims, A. & Cook, C. (2009). Spirituality in psychiatry. In C. Cook, A. Powell, & A. Sims (Eds.), Spirituality and Psychiatry (p. 4). London: RCPsych Publications.

Skinner, A.-R. (2009). Paper delivered to the Academy of Self Knowledge UK Conference, Luton Hoo, July 25.

West, W. (2000). *Psychotherapy and spirituality*. London: Sage. Cited in Lines D. (2006). *Spirituality in counselling and psychotherapy*. London: Sage.

Wilber, K. (1993). *Spectrum of consciousness* (2nd ed.).Wheaton, IL: Quest Books.
Wilber, K. (2000). *Integral psychology consciousness: Spirit, psychology, therapy.* Boston, MA: Shambhala.

CHAPTER 9
Community-Based Prevention and Intervention

NADIA S. ANSARY and RAJA SALLOUM

Ummah, or community, is a vital part of the Islamic faith, and its significance is evidenced in many daily practices of Muslims. *Ahadith*, or important scriptures that serve as a guide for Muslims on how to live, state that the Prophet Muhammad (peace be upon him)[1] said, "Feed the hungry, visit the sick, and set free the captives" (Al-Bukhari, Vol. 7, no. 552). To illustrate the nature of this kinship further, Muslims are also expected to attend funeral services for community members with whom they may not be intimately acquainted (Abu-Ras & Abu-Bader, 2008).

This collectivistic nature, or an emphasis on family and community needs as opposed to one's individual needs, is simultaneously the Muslim community's greatest asset, as well as its greatest weakness, when considering the perception of mental illness and treatment. Given this emphasis on community, one would expect Muslims to turn to one another for support in times of crisis. However, many do not for fear of judgment from one's community as a result of disclosing familial problems, or worse, revealing a relative's mental illness. This unwillingness to share personal problems with others (Al-Krenawi & Graham, 2000; Khan, 2006; Khawaja, 2007), combined with the stigma associated with mental illness within the Muslim community, have created a formidable barrier to seeking mental health services.

---

[1] As a sign of reverence and respect, when Prophet Muhammad's name is mentioned, Muslims will say, "Peace be upon him."

In addition to the fear of shaming one's family by openly seeking mental health services, another obstacle for Muslims in need of mental health treatment is a deep-seated mistrust of Western treatment options (Abu-Ras & Abu-Bader, 2008; Abu-Ras, Gheith, & Cournos, 2008; Starkey et al., 2008). This is in large part due to cultural views on the etiology of mental illness that deviate from Western views.

Taken together, these two factors—namely, the fear of shaming one's family and the devaluing of Western mental health treatment—have resulted in an exceedingly low representation of Muslim consumers in all sectors of mental health services, and have minimized the exposure of non-Muslim mental health practitioners to Muslim clients. In effect, these factors have restricted the experience of non-Muslim mental health providers in treating these clients.

Research findings from other minority populations have documented that mental health services that are low on cultural competence are associated with poorer outcomes such as misdiagnosis (Delphin & Rowe, 2008; Rosenberg, 2000), as well as reduced levels of engagement and retention (Delphin & Rowe, 2008). Evidence suggests that many Muslims who have sought mental health services from non-Muslim providers have experienced this sort of disconnect and consequently inadequate treatment (Abu-Ras & Abu-Bader, 2008). This cycle is evidently self-reinforcing: Muslims fear treatment, and of the minority who do seek treatment, they often do so with non-Muslim mental health providers low on cultural competence, thereby fortifying the negative perception of Western treatment methods.

Given these very real obstacles to mental health treatment, our goal is to propose methods to de-stigmatize mental illness within the Muslim community, as well as to strengthen treatment options through community outreach. These prevention and intervention recommendations have three goals: (1) to strengthen the Muslim community through education about mental illness and available treatment options, (2) to provide support to non-Muslim mental health providers interested in working with and providing outreach to the Muslim community, and (3) to nurture a relationship based on mutual trust and respect between the Muslim community and non-Muslim mental health providers.

Challenges to Making Recommendations on Community Outreach with Muslims

There is no research to date that pertains to community outreach with Muslims. Therefore, some of the recommendations set forth in this chapter were garnered from existing community outreach research targeting other minority populations, while others were drawn from our own experiences working with several mosques and non-Muslim mental health organizations in the Northeastern United States.

Another challenge to creating useful recommendations is the large heterogeneity of this population. Muslims comprise approximately 1.2 billion of the world's population with 80% of these individuals living outside of Arabic-speaking countries (Council on American-Islamic Relations [CAIR], 2010). Muslim communities in the West are highly diverse in a multitude of characteristics ranging from levels of religious devotion to ethnic background (Khan, 2006). With respect to religiosity, Muslims vary a great deal in their level of adherence to the Qur'an (the Islamic holy book) and *Ahadith*, not to mention cultural practices that have their roots in Islam but have been modified over time so they may not be recognized by Muslims of other ethnic backgrounds (Kobeisy, 2006). Furthermore, as is the case in Australia (see Khawaja, 2007), there is great variability within Muslim communities in Western countries on characteristics such as immigration status and degree of acculturation.

Regarding mental well-being, Muslims who have emigrated to Western countries have unique experiences from their countries of origin—from cultural practices, ongoing racism, or in several cases, war and devastation—that have impacted their identity and potentially their mental well-being. This high level of diversity within the Muslim community constricts the range of useful recommendations that will apply to the majority of Muslims, and thus we have limited our suggestions for community outreach to those issues that are most fundamental to the overall community.

Theoretical Framework

In addition to making our recommendations sensitive to the heterogeneity of Muslims living in Western countries, our suggestions are also grounded in a theoretical approach. First, our recommendations are framed by our belief that mental health runs on a continuum, with mental illness at one extreme and mental well-being and happiness at the other—a belief that mental well-being is much more than simply the absence of illness or negative affect. This premise is perhaps one of the most critical ways to de-stigmatize mental illness and will be especially important in convincing the Muslim community to access mental health services.

Second, our suggestions are grounded in Bronfenbrenner's bioecological model of human development, which, in its most simplistic form, posits that all facets of day-to-day life—such as family, school, and community—interact with each other and with the individual's biological characteristics in informing the individual's development (Bronfenbrenner & Morris, 2006). We believe that this premise can be extended to inform and improve the treatment of individuals with mental illness, such that all environments in one's life contribute to psychosocial development and offer promise for the improvement of psychological well-being. Our views parallel the results of a focus group, conducted with an adolescent Muslim sample living in the United Kingdom, as many of these youth felt that treatment of children and families would be most successful when it involves parent, school, and practitioner (Randhawa & Stein, 2007). Consistent with these views, we adopted a holistic approach in developing our recommendations in that all aspects of the Muslim community—from schools to mosques— are targets of our prevention and intervention strategies.

Cultural Characteristics That Influence Help-Seeking

Beneficial Community Qualities

There are robust characteristics of the Muslim community that can be capitalized upon to develop community outreach. From the outset, it is important to note the strong faith inherent within this community. To illustrate, several studies document the fact that many Muslims turn to God—through prayer and reading of the Qur'an—to seek comfort and support during times of distress (Abu-Ras & Abu-Bader, 2008; Khan, 2006). Hence, strong faith is a quality that is entrenched in the Muslim community and certainly one that must be incorporated in successful community outreach efforts.

The role of family and the collectivistic nature of the faith are also central to the Muslim identity. In fact, several studies document that individuals in psychological distress often turn to their families and community as a primary source of comfort and support (Khan, 2006; Khawaja, 2007). Family and community can be sources of support protecting against the onset of mental illness; however, they can simultaneously serve to undermine treatment-seeking, with potentially grave consequences. Fear of shaming one's family is a very real dilemma for Muslims suffering from a mental illness experience (Kobeisy, 2006). Thus, although the emphasis on family and community can be viewed as a strength, they can also be seen as a major stumbling block for Muslims to overcome in seeking mental health treatment.

Additionally, the importance of community within Muslim networks has never been more important than it is today. Since 9/11, many Muslims have increasingly turned to their mosques and other community centers for support when they have experienced discrimination (Abu-Ras & Abu-Bader, 2008; Abu-Ras et al., 2008; Ali, Milstein, & Marzuk, 2005). This tight network often serves as an extended family, as is evidenced by the fact that elders are often referred to as "uncle" and "aunt" even when there is no biological relationship. Therefore, this support and sense of belonging is a key asset the community possesses and a major reason why community outreach efforts are a critical component of making mental health services accessible to Muslims.

Another feature of the Muslim community that is valuable is the belief that health is God given, and all Muslims have an obligation to safeguard their health (Rassool, 2000). For this reason, presenting mental wellness as a component of overall health is another key to drawing in Muslims in need of treatment.

In addition to valuing health, Muslims place a strong emphasis on education. In the first author's experience with giving lectures on family communication and adolescent mental health at a mosque in the United States, the attendance was surprisingly large. Moreover, it was the mothers who exhibited the most progressive views as many asked questions about mental illness and treatment, often on behalf of a loved one. Indeed, Muslim females have shown themselves to be powerfully motivated to support their families and willing to learn about mental health. They are likely to be one of the most vital components of a successful prevention and intervention strategy regarding Muslim mental health.

It is important to note that each Muslim community may have its own specific assets (i.e., advanced education, affluence, professional occupations, etc.). These may also be capitalized upon in order to promote mental wellness.

Qualities That Present Barriers to Treatment

For the most part, Muslims hold beliefs that deviate from—and are sometimes at odds with—Western views regarding the etiology of mental illness. For instance, within the Muslim community, psychopathology is often viewed as resulting from a weak character and lack of faith (Dwairy, 1998; Hedayat-Diba, 2000; Starkey et al., 2008). In particular, addiction disorders reinforce this notion because substance use and gambling are particularly *haram* (sinful) and shameful because these acts are explicitly forbidden in Islam. Another illustration of how Muslim views of mental illness diverge from Western beliefs is that sometimes mental illness is attributed to possession by an evil spirit (or *jinn*) and should be treated through the reading of certain verses of the Qur'an (Abu-Ras et al., 2008; McGraw Schuchman & McDonald, 2004).

Following from these perceived causes of mental illness is a profound doubt about the efficacy of Western treatment methods (Abu-Ras & Abu-Bader, 2008; Abu-Ras et al., 2008). This follows from three distinct premises. First, as noted earlier, the attributions Muslims typically make regarding the etiology of mental illness do not coincide with the Western treatment options available to them, and therefore there is little regard for their efficacy. In a similar vein, many Muslims residing in Western countries may not even be aware of the treatments that are available to address their mental health needs. Second, many fear that the disclosure of private information provided during therapy could, if leaked, cause shame to one's family and community (Al-Krenawi & Graham, 2000; Ali et al., 2005; Randhawa & Stein, 2007). Likewise, given the negative sociopolitical climate toward Muslims since 9/11, many fear that private information divulged during therapy could be passed on to their governments. Third, as noted earlier, many Muslims who have already sought formal mental health treatment have been met with services that lack cultural competence (Abu-Ras & Abu-Bader, 2008). Anecdotal evidence suggests that most Muslims who engaged in therapy in the West were often misunderstood or spent a good deal of therapy time educating the practitioner about their culture. The negative experiences of those who actually sought treatment solidify the general feelings of mistrust and futility held by the Muslim community regarding the Western treatment of mental illness.

In addition to these more direct barriers to treatment, there are cultural beliefs surrounding marriage that may indirectly prevent treatment-seeking. Marriage among Muslims typically involves the community, where families—not individuals—evaluate each other to select an appropriate union. In this context, mental illness within any family member (not just the bride- or groom-to-be) is oftentimes seen as shameful and a deterrent to marriage. In point of fact, Al-Krenawi, Graham, Dean, and Eltaiba's (2004) cross-national study reported that single Muslim females were significantly less likely to endorse help-seeking behaviors than their married counterparts. The authors concluded that this was attributed to the concern over getting married. Regarding married women, Abu-Ras and Abu-Bader (2008) reported that many wives feared their husbands' perception of them and even feared their children being taken away if they sought treatment.

Recommendations for Community Outreach

Prevention and Intervention Strategies Targeting the Muslim Community

Imams   One of the most fundamental steps in any prevention and intervention strategy and mental health is education. Given the centrality of community and religion within this population, this translates to targeting imams, or Islamic religious leaders, for education about mental wellness. Imams are often the first resource that Muslim families in crisis turn to after seeking support from family (Abu-Ras & Abu-Bader, 2008), and several studies have reported that many Muslims sampled sought help for a mental health issue from their imam (Abu-Ras et al., 2008; Khan, 2006). Additionally, imams have a wide audience during Friday prayer, a time equivalent to Christians' Sunday morning Mass, in which they can provide information in the *khutba* (sermon) that attempts to de-stigmatize mental illness and promote wellness. Hence, imams can be one of the key elements of a community outreach effort and are best positioned for education on mental health issues, from how to identify individuals and families in crisis to available and appropriate treatment options.

Mosques and Educating the Community The following are a few simple tasks that mosques can undertake to educate and support the mental well-being of its members: (1) invite mental health providers to lecture community members on topics of interest; (2) make reading materials on mental well-being and local appropriate treatment options freely accessible in several languages (in addition to pamphlets, the mosque's website could also provide this information to safeguard anonymity); and (3) circulate this information through existing support groups in the mosque such as women's groups, adolescent mentoring programs, weekend Islamic school education, etc. Potential seminar topics can range from specifics about mental illness (symptoms of postpartum depression, attention deficit hyperactivity disorder [ADHD], substance abuse, etc.) to themes related to daily life hassles (e.g., acculturative stresses, advocating for children in situations of school bullying, etc.).

Integrating Mental Health Treatment with Mosque Services Although imams are vital resources for educating the Muslim community about mental wellness and are key in assisting those in need, they cannot shoulder these burdens alone. Historically, imams are no strangers to supporting individuals in crisis through counseling; however, they often do not have the professional training required to identify and appropriately treat mental illness (Ali et al., 2005). In fact, imams reported this concern themselves in the focus groups conducted by Abu-Ras and Abu-Bader (2008). Interestingly, findings by Abu-Ras and colleagues (2008) suggest that many imams are supportive of clinical therapy, the use of psychotropic medication, and are interested in learning more about Western treatment methods.

The role of the imam encompasses many responsibilities—Western imams are charged with far more duties outside of religious guidance such as counseling and legal mediation than they are in their countries of origin (Kobeisy, 2006). Especially in larger mosques, imams can be overwhelmed by these expectations and, understandably so, their dedication to mental health issues may be less of a priority than their primary tasks.

Thus, integrating mental health services with the services mosques already provide is an essential step toward de-stigmatizing mental illness and making mental health services accessible to the Muslim community. Congregants could begin to trust the mental-health-related information dispensed through the mosque. Clearly, such a step would begin to legitimize the importance of mental wellness, de-stigmatize mental illness, and alleviate fears about treatment being antithetical to Islamic beliefs. We offer three suggestions for how mosques can begin to integrate mental health treatment with the services they already provide. From these suggestions, mosques can choose which option, or combination of options, best fits their needs.

First, at the most basic level, community outreach coordinators are vital in engaging the Muslim community. They possess the ability to perform community outreach, assess the ongoing problems of the population, supply members in need of assistance with the appropriate social service and mental health agency information, as well as make recommendations to the mosque in terms of needed services. Given their connection with congregants, community outreach coordinators could be important resources for providing the Muslim community with information on mental illness and treatment. Second, and another very practical solution, is for mosques to hire a nurse practitioner whose responsibility is to educate and promote physical and mental health, as well as to work with mosque members on the intersection of spirituality and health—supporting a holistic view of the individual (McGinnis & Zoske, 2008). Faith community nursing, also known as parish nursing, has its origins in the Christian faith, but has been effectively adopted by other religious groups (McGinnis & Zoske, 2008). Last, and most specifically addressing the mental health needs of the community, is the hiring of a masters level social worker or mental health clinician who can disseminate information, provide specific mental-health-related advice, and directly treat mentally ill members of the community.

Beyond assisting those in need of mental health services, integrating mental health services with the services already provided by mosques begins the greater task of de-stigmatizing mental illness. The integration of services unmistakably conveys the message that those suffering from mental illness should and will be helped. In terms of funding these positions, for smaller or financially challenged mosques, individuals can be sought to fulfill these roles on a volunteer or pro-bono basis. Alternatively, if feasible, outreach coordinators, nurse practitioners, or therapists could be paid employees shared by several centrally located mosques.

Islamic Schools   In addition to mosques, Islamic schools are also an essential component of prevention and intervention. The suggestions detailed previously are also appropriate for implementation in the education setting and may be even more critical in prevention because the information will be delivered to a younger audience. Research evidence suggests that the role of schools in circulating this information is vital within Muslim communities (Randhawa & Stein, 2007). Again, the emphasis here is not simply on raising awareness of mental illness, but also on shoring up mental well-being and supporting the Muslim family.

Internet The Internet is yet another tool for Muslim organizations to disseminate information on mental wellness. For instance, the Islamic Society of North America (ISNA; www.isna.net) has organized conferences, camps, and seminars directed toward Muslim youth and could potentially impact a wide audience of young Muslims with valuable information on mental well-being. Another example is the Council on American-Islamic Relations (CAIR, http://www.cair.com), which conducts an annual campaign called "Muslims Who Care" dedicated to myriad activities. During summer 2010, CAIR asked that Muslims volunteer in their local communities each month following a different theme such as "Health Awareness Month" and "For Our Youth" (CAIR; http://www.muslims-care.org/about-us.html).

Prevention and Intervention Strategies Targeting the Non-Muslim Community

Non-Muslim public schools, as well as mental health and professional organizations, represent critical areas in promoting awareness of mental wellness for the Muslim community. Detailed in the following are suggestions within each of these realms.

Schools Just as it is essential to educate the Muslim community about mental wellness, a viable prevention and intervention strategy requires addressing other facets of one's community. In areas densely populated with Muslims, school mental health providers should be conversant in the cultural practices and beliefs of Muslims as they relate to mental wellness. This would enhance their ability to relate to children and families of the Islamic faith, and would also help them to suggest appropriate treatment methods for them. In the following section, we discuss methods non-Muslim providers can employ to increase cultural competence. These same suggestions can be adapted to apply to teachers, guidance counselors, and, of course, school psychologists.

Mental Health Providers Many options exist for non-Muslim mental health providers to increase their exposure to, as well as to more effectively treat, Muslim clients. Primarily, these entail completing cultural competence training and initiating community outreach efforts to Muslims.

Cultural Competence Training The American Psychological Association (APA) has a long history spanning at least 20 years of emphasizing the importance of culture-specific training related to mental health service with minority clients (APA, 2003). In addition to encouraging mental health providers to reevaluate their assessment tools and typical modes of treatment when working with minority clients, the APA's guidelines on multicultural education and training also urge practitioners to seek out community leaders and traditional healers in order to most effectively treat their clients (APA, 2003). For additional resources, which are broadly applicable to minority populations, the reader is directed to the Office of Minority Health of the U.S. Department of Health and Human Services (http://minorityhealth.hhs.gov) and the Cultural Competency and Health Literacy Resources for Healthcare Providers produced by the U.S. Department of Health and Human Services (http://www.hrsa.gov/culturalcompetence/). A brief and general guide to cultural competence training of mental health providers in Europe is also very useful (Qureshi, Collazos, Ramos, & Casas, 2008).

The recommendations that follow are intended to assist non-Muslim mental health professionals interested in working with Muslims to increase their knowledge base about this community's perception of mental illness and barriers toward treatment.

First and foremost, non-Muslim providers must seek out cultural competence training in order to effectively treat Muslims. Outreach to mosques is the most fundamental step in this endeavor as imams and key community members can advise non-Muslim providers on their cultures, community views on the etiology and treatment of mental illness, and ways to engage Muslims in treatment.

A more formal cultural competence training should be designed with the input of community leaders, Muslim mental health providers, and published literature. This training should ultimately be approved or accredited by the appropriate continuing education governing body. As an incentive, those completing a Muslim cultural competence course can be given continuing education credits or a certificate of completion and ultimately be identified in a database of individuals who have knowledge and/or experience with providing mental health services to this population. Furthermore, non-Muslim mental health organizations should encourage cultural competence trainings by providing reprieve from work duties so that their staff are able to attend the training with ease.

In addition to the resources outlined previously, and in an effort to raise awareness of the beliefs and practices of the Muslim community that can affect mental health treatment, we have created an assessment tool. This Muslim Culture and Mental Health Service Scale (MCMHS) is presented in the Appendix. Intended for completion by non-Muslim mental health providers, the scale contains a series of statements pertaining to Muslim cultural norms and practices that could potentially impact treatment. The measure has not been piloted or validated as of this writing.

Conferences and Professional Training Professional conferences at the regional and national levels are also another avenue for the circulation of information on the Muslim community and mental illness. Ideally, Muslim mental health providers or practitioners with extensive experience working with the Muslim community can educate others about working appropriately and effectively with Muslim clients. Lectures and workshops in these venues can be powerful teaching tools and are open to a wide and diverse audience. Similarly, programs training students to become medical doctors, psychologists, social workers, clinicians and counselors, nurses, and school psychologists would be well served to have invited speakers discuss the cultural issues surrounding mental illness and help-seeking within the Muslim community.

Outreach to the Muslim Community Seminars, workshops, and brochures published in the most common languages of the community are imperative to raise awareness of mental health and treatment resources. These tools have proven effective in dispensing information on mental illness within Asian (Chen, Kramer, Chen, & Chung, 2005) and Latino (Rosenberg, 2000) populations and have also been efficacious in assisting the Asian American community to understand more about various forms of cancer (Chao et al., 2009; Grigg-Saito, Och, Liang, Toof, & Silka, 2008; Ngyuen, Tanjasiri, Kagawa-Singer, Tran, & Foo, 2008). These education aids should be created in close consultation with a Muslim advisory panel to identify topics of interest as well as the best strategies to engage the community.

Media campaigns, used to convey facts about an illness or to advertise for seminars and free screenings, have also proven effective with other minority populations. With respect to mental health and Asian Americans, an interactive radio program hosted by a clinician (Chen et al., 2005) and articles in a local newspaper commonly read within this community were modalities successfully used to circulate information (Chao et al., 2009; Grigg-Saito et al., 2008). Advertising in local grocery stores, businesses, and ESL classes have also been found to be effective tools (Grigg-Saito et al., 2008).

Mental Health Screenings Mobile and nonmobile mental health screenings, advertised in the media outlets noted previously, have also proven successful in raising awareness of mental illness and making treatment accessible to minority populations (Chao et al., 2009; Rosenberg, 2000).

Strengthening Ties between the Muslim Community and Non-Muslim Mental Health Providers

Now that we have delineated separate recommendations for both the Muslim community and non-Muslim mental health practitioners, it is critical to shift focus toward suggestions illustrating how both groups can work collaboratively to improve the mental well-being of Muslims.

Creation of a Community Advisory Panel   There is a clear benefit in the implementation of an advisory panel comprised of key Muslim community members as well as Muslim and non-Muslim mental health providers. In this way, the Muslim community can act as cultural informants on the mental-health-related beliefs of their people. This model has been successfully used with Asian populations and outreach aimed at reducing cancer rates (Chen et al., 2005; Grigg-Saito et al., 2008). In addition to providing knowledge about the internal workings of the community, an advisory panel can also serve as a model for the Muslim community to accept nontraditional forms of treatment. Thus, in the eyes of the community, an advisory panel with the local imam's support validates the notion that Islamic and Western concepts and treatments of mental illness are not at odds (see Rosenberg, 2000).

Nurturing Relationships between Muslims and Non-Muslim Mental Health Providers   Outreach to imams by non-Muslim mental health providers may help to not only develop relationships across groups, but importantly, this act can contribute to the actual healing process of individual Muslim clients. As has been documented for other minority groups such as Latinos (Rosenberg, 2000) and Asian Americans (Grigg-Saito et al., 2008; Nguyen et al., 2008), the use of traditional and religious healers is the typical route sought to relieve distress. Therefore, successful treatment relies on respecting this belief and ultimately incorporating it within typically Western treatment plans (Abu-Ras & Abu-Bader, 2008; Grigg-Saito et al., 2008; Rosenberg, 2000; see also Ahmed & Reddy, 2007). Accordingly, culturally competent mental health providers "may find new and creative ways to incorporate clients' personal beliefs into varying psychotherapeutic techniques to build better rapport with these particular clients" (Khan, 2006, p. 36).

Regarding the Muslim community, mosques, having embraced the importance of mental well-being, should invite non-Muslim practitioners to mosque-hosted events such as *iftar*[2] during the holy month of Ramadan. The benefit of doing so is three-fold: (1) to connect with non-Muslim mental health providers by inviting them into the Muslim community, (2) to increase the exposure of the congregation to the notion of mental health treatment, and (3) to introduce Muslims to local non-Muslim providers.

---

[2] During Ramadan, Muslims observe a daily fast from sunrise to sunset. *Iftar* is the breaking of the fast at sunset and is typically seen as a way for friends and community to bond.

Table 9.1 Suggestions for Ways Non-Muslim Mental Health Providers Can Foster a Relationship with Their Local Mosque

1. Request a meeting with key individuals within the mosque (e.g., imam, board, community outreach coordinator, community leaders, etc.) to introduce yourself and identify your organization and reasons why it is important to connect with the Muslim community.
2. Dress appropriately. Women should wear a headscarf (this can be loosely tied) and arms and legs should be covered to wrists and ankles, respectively. Clothing should be loose fitting and should not reveal any silhouette or undergarments. Men should also wear pants, not shorts, so that their legs are covered.
3. Offer to give a talk to the membership. Provide several topics from which the imam and board can chose.
4. Make an effort to invite the leadership of the mosque to appropriate events (without alcohol consumption) hosted by your organization.
5. Connect with the mosque on a regular basis, especially during the holy month of Ramadan when the community comes together to bond.

Additionally, mosques can take the initiative to invite non-Muslim providers to give lectures and host psychoeducational workshops for their members. Regarding non-Muslim mental health practitioners, obviously exhibiting a willingness to learn about and connect with the community in a nonjudgmental way is the key to building trust. A list of simple steps that can be taken for mental health providers to engage their local mosque is presented in Table 9.1.

Databases Identifying Culturally Competent Mental Health Providers As mentioned earlier, a database of mental health providers identified as trained or having experience working with the Muslim community has myriad benefits. A database of culturally competent mental health providers already exits (www.muslimmentalhealth.com) and is a powerful resource not only for individuals seeking treatment, but individuals listed within the database can serve as a resource for each other when a challenging client arises. We propose that such a directory be updated regularly and expanded to include non-Muslim providers who have undergone cultural competence training through work with their local mosque, for example. We also encourage the creation of local databases that can cater more specifically to the unique needs of the surrounding Muslim population. Awareness of these kinds of databases as an important mental health resource can be raised using the community outreach strategies previously discussed so that it may be accessed by the Muslim community, hospitals, general practitioners, social service agencies (e.g., shelters), public and religious schools, and mosques, to name a few.

Prototype of a Community Outreach Program

Although there is a dearth of programs dedicated to addressing the mental health needs of Muslims, several organizations in the Northeastern United States have begun addressing the mental health and social service needs of this population. We were fortunate enough to be a part of a community-based intervention whose goal it was to bring mental health services to a predominantly Muslim Arab-American community. This task force, created by a non-Muslim professional mental health association, was composed of key community figures, non-Muslim mental health providers, as well as representatives of the mosque, to name a few. In the interest of conserving space, the objectives of the task force and strategies used to achieve its goals are detailed in Table 9.2.

As was done with this task force, intervention programs targeting Muslims and mental health should include all aspects of the Islamic community (families, imams, schools, etc.) and aim to nurture ties within the population, as well as with non-Muslim mental health providers. For the task force, this was achieved primarily through meetings, inclusion of non-Muslim mental health providers at community events, and hosting educational workshops—with anonymous question and answer sessions—aimed at the Muslim community. Endorsement by the mosque was a pivotal point for the task force, because only then did Muslim clients in need of service begin to seek treatment. Without doubt, the necessity for such services is present and the Muslim community is likely to be both afraid and unaware that such services exist (Abu-Ras et al., 2008; Aloud & Rathur, 2009). Stated most simply, education and trust are keys to opening doors for Muslims to access services.

Conclusion and Future Directions

Our suggestions for prevention and intervention strategies aimed at improving the mental well-being of Muslims and their available treatment options are the first of their kind.

In this chapter we highlighted some suggestions on how the Muslim community and the community of non-Muslim mental health providers can work both separately and collaboratively to achieve this goal. Only when both entities work effectively together can the task of de-stigmatizing mental illness begin to occur, thereby opening the door to treatment.

In terms of future directions, our hope is for mosques to integrate mental health services with the religious and in many cases social services that are already provided. In terms of non-Muslim mental health practitioners, greater effort to connect with local Islamic centers is clearly a necessary first step toward developing a trusting relationship with the community and ultimately providing effective treatment. Moreover, we fully expect that the awareness of Muslim mental health issues will continue its movement

Table 9.2 Prototype of a Community Outreach Effort Targeting a Predominantly Muslim Arab-American Community

Created by	A non-Muslim mental health association in an area highly populated with Muslim Arab-Americans
Purpose	To forge a connection with the Arab-American community to improve mental illness identification and treatment
Composition of the Task Force	Community outreach coordinator of local mosque, representative from the Christian-Arab community, board members of domestic violence shelter targeting Arab community, family members of mentally ill, representatives of non-Arab social service agencies, and representatives from local hospitals and schools

Goal	How Achieved
1. Create a dialogue between non-Arab mental health professionals and Arab community about cultural perception of mental illness and treatment	• Non-Arab providers held a series of workshops at mosque with anonymous question-and-answer sessions • Arab providers presented at hospitals regarding culture and mental illness
2. Obtain the mosque's endorsement of the non-Muslim network of mental health providers	• Several meetings held with board of mosque • Mosque hosted an *iftar* and invited non-Arab mental health providers
3. Mental Health Association to hire a masters-level mental health clinician	• Connections with the mosque created such enthusiasm that the community became central in creating this position • This position was funded by a grant from the New Jersey Division of Mental Health Services
4. Spark an ongoing interest in mental wellness within the Arab community	• The task force created connections within the community, which ultimately led to opening a mental health and social service agency for Arab-Americans

beyond the Islamic community, into the treatment and research centers, and make its way into professional conferences and emerge as a special focus in the training of interested mental health providers.

The Muslim community possesses great strengths: a robust sense of family and community, a desire for knowledge, and a responsibility to care for one's health as well as others'. Such assets need to be drawn upon in order to de-stigmatize mental illness and reframe it in terms of its place on the spectrum of mental well-being. Critical to this process are two factors: the role that mosques must take on in supporting this goal, and the willingness of the community of non-Muslim mental health providers to learn about and engage the Muslim community. Existing community outreach efforts already in place are laudable; however, a great deal more is necessary to improve the view of mental illness within the Muslim community, as well as to highlight the availability of effective and appropriate treatment for this population.

Acknowledgment

We would like to acknowledge Anne Law for her thoughtful feedback on our chapter. Her insights contributed substantively to the final version of this work and we are deeply appreciative of that.

References

Abu-Ras, W., & Abu-Bader, S. H. (2008). The impact of the September 11, 2001, attacks on the well-being of Arab Americans in New York City. *Journal of Muslim Mental Health, 3,* 217–239.

Abu-Ras, W., Gheith, A., & Cournos, F. (2008). The imam's role in mental health promotion: A study of 22 mosques in New York City's Muslim community. *Journal of Muslim Mental Health, 3,* 155–176.

Ahmed, S., & Reddy, L. A. (2007). Understanding the mental health needs of American Muslims: Recommendations and considerations for practice. *Journal of Multicultural Counseling and Development, 35,* 207–218.

Al-Bukhari, Sahih. Volume 7, Hadith 552.

Ali, O. M., Milstein, G., & Marzuk, P. M. (2005). The imam's role in meeting the counseling needs of Muslim communities in the United States. *Psychiatric Services, 56,* 202–205.

Al-Krenawi, A., & Graham, J. R. (2000). Culturally sensitive social work practice with Arab clients in mental health settings. *Health and Social Work, 25,* 9–22.

Al-Krenawi, A., Graham, J. R., Dean, Y. Z., & Eltaiba, N. (2004). Cross national study of attitudes towards seeking professional help: Jordan, United Arab Emirates (UAE) and Arabs in Israel. *International Journal of Social Psychiatry, 50,* 102–114.

Aloud, N., & Rathur, A. (2009). Factors affecting attitudes toward seeking and using formal mental health and psychological services among Arab Muslim population. *Journal of Muslim Mental Health, 4,* 79–103.

American Psychological Association (APA). (2003). Guidelines on multicultural education, training, research, practice, and organizational change for psychologists. *American Psychologist, 58,* 377–402.

Bronfenbrenner, U., & Morris, P. A. (2006). The Bioecological Model of Human Development. In R. M. Lerner & W. Damon (Eds.), *Handbook of child psychology: Vol. 1, Theoretical models of human development* (6th ed., pp. 793–828). Hoboken, NJ: Wiley.

Chao, S. D., Chang, E. T., Le, P. V., Prapong, W., Kiernan, M., & So, S. K. S. (2009). The Jade Ribbon Campaign: A model program for community outreach and education to prevent liver cancer in Asian Americans. *Journal of Immigrant and Minority Health, 11,* 281–290.

Chen, H., Kramer, E. J., Chen, T., & Chung, H. (2005). Engaging Asian Americans for mental health research: Challenges and solutions. *Journal of Immigrant Health, 7,* 109–116.

Council on American-Islamic Relations (CAIR). (2010). *About Islam and American Muslims.* Retrieved from http://www.cair.com/AboutIslam/IslamBasics.aspx on June 20, 2010.

Delphin, M. E., & Rowe, M. (2008). Continuing education in cultural competence for community mental health practitioners. *Professional Psychology: Research and Practice, 39,* 182–191.

Dwairy, M. (1998). *Cross-cultural counseling: The Arab-Palestinian case.* Binghamton, NY: The Haworth Press.

Grigg-Saito, D., Och, S., Liang, S., Toof, R., & Silka, L. (2008). Building on the strengths of a Cambodian refugee community through community-based outreach. *Health Promotion Practice, 9,* 415–425.

Hedayat-Diba, Z. (2000). Psychotherapy with Muslims. In P. S. Richards & A. E. Bergen (Eds.), *Handbook of psychotherapy with religious diversity* (pp. 289–314). Washington, DC: American Psychological Association.

Khan, Z. (2006). Attitudes toward counseling and alternative support among Muslims in Toledo, Ohio. *Journal of Muslim Mental Health, 1,* 21–42.

Khawaja, N. G. (2007). An investigation of the psychological distress of Muslim migrants in Australia. *Journal of Muslim Mental Health, 2,* 39–56.

Kobeisy, A. N. (2006). Faith-based practice: An introduction. *Journal of Muslim Mental Health, 1,* 57–63.

McGinnis, S. L., & Zoske, F. M. (2008). The emerging role of faith community nurses in prevention and management of chronic disease. *Policy, Politics, & Nursing Practice, 9,* 173–180.

McGraw Schuchman, D., & McDonald, C. (2004). Somali mental health. *Bildhaan: An International Journal of Somali Studies, 4,* 65–77.

Nguyen, T.-U. N., Tanjasiri, S. P., Kagawa-Singer, M., Tran, J. H., & Foo, M. (2008). Community health navigators for breast- and cervical-cancer screening among Cambodian and Laotian women: Intervention strategies and relationship-building processes. *Health Promotion Practice, 9,* 356–367.

Qureshi, A., Collazos, F., Ramos, M., & Casas, M. (2008). Cultural competency training in psychiatry. *European Psychiatry, 23,* S49–S58.

Randhawa, G., & Stein, S. (2007). An exploratory study examining attitudes toward mental health and mental health services among young South Asians in the United Kingdom. *Journal of Muslim Mental Health, 2,* 21–37.

Rassool, G. H. (2000). The crescent and Islam: Healing, nursing and the spiritual dimension. Some considerations towards an understanding of the Islamic perspectives on caring. *Journal of Advanced Nursing, 32,* 1476–1484.

Rosenberg, S. J. (2000). Providing mental health services in a culture other than one's own. *Reflections: Narratives of Professional Helping, 6,* 32–41.

Starkey, M. T., Lee, H. K., Tu, C., Netland, J., Goh, M., McGraw Schuchman, D., & Yusuf, A. (2008). "Only Allah can heal": A cultural formulation of the psychological, religious, and cultural experiences of a Somali man. *Journal of Muslim Mental Health, 3,* 145–153.

Appendix: Muslim Culture and Mental Health Service Scale

All cultures value certain beliefs and practices that can impact the seeking of mental health services, as well as the relationship between client and mental health provider. Following is a set of statements that may or may not be valued by Muslim clients during the therapeutic process. *Use the scale below each question to rate your level of agreement on how important you think each statement would be to a Muslim client. Please choose only ONE response per question.*

For Muslims . . .

1. in crisis, religious leaders are typically sought out for guidance as a last resort.

Strongly Disagree	Disagree	Neutral	Agree	Strongly Agree
1	2	3	4	5

2. . . . undergoing mental health treatment, inclusion of the imam (religious leader) can contribute greatly to healing.

Strongly Disagree	Disagree	Neutral	Agree	Strongly Agree
1	2	3	4	5

3. shame can be brought upon one's family as a result of undergoing mental health treatment.

Strongly Disagree	Disagree	Neutral	Agree	Strongly Agree
1	2	3	4	5

4. the same gender treatment provider is not important in a therapeutic setting.

Strongly Disagree	Disagree	Neutral	Agree	Strongly Agree
1	2	3	4	5

5. approval of mental health services by an imam or religious leader is unimportant.

Strongly Disagree	Disagree	Neutral	Agree	Strongly Agree
1	2	3	4	5

6. mental illness is thought to be caused by a weakness in faith in God.

Strongly Disagree	Disagree	Neutral	Agree	Strongly Agree
1	2	3	4	5

7. it can be offensive if a female therapist wears clothing that excessively reveals arms, legs, and chest.

Strongly Disagree	Disagree	Neutral	Agree	Strongly Agree
1	2	3	4	5

8. who are single and suffer from a mental illness, their chances of getting married are much lower if the Muslim community is aware of the illness.

Strongly Disagree	Disagree	Neutral	Agree	Strongly Agree
1	2	3	4	5

9. discussing personal information to people outside of family comes easily.

Strongly Disagree	Disagree	Neutral	Agree	Strongly Agree
1	2	3	4	5

10. in treatment, an individual's right to follow Muslim law and customs is more important than free will.

Strongly Disagree	Disagree	Neutral	Agree	Strongly Agree
1	2	3	4	5

11. there is nothing shameful about having a mental illness.

Strongly Disagree	Disagree	Neutral	Agree	Strongly Agree
1	2	3	4	5

12. mental illness is thought to be caused by evil spirits invading an individual's body.

Strongly Disagree	Disagree	Neutral	Agree	Strongly Agree
1	2	3	4	5

13. the idea of treatment by a non-Muslim provider can elicit feelings of mistrust, causing an aversion to treatment.

Strongly Disagree	Disagree	Neutral	Agree	Strongly Agree
1	2	3	4	5

14. having a mental illness can bring dishonor to one's family.

Strongly Disagree	Disagree	Neutral	Agree	Strongly Agree
1	2	3	4	5

15. in crisis, advice from religious leaders to address distress will often consist of reading certain passages of the Qur'an (Islamic holy book).

Strongly Disagree	Disagree	Neutral	Agree	Strongly Agree
1	2	3	4	5

16. in therapy, it is important to acknowledge the powerful role of the father in a family.

Strongly Disagree	Disagree	Neutral	Agree	Strongly Agree
1	2	3	4	5

Scoring

Higher scores reflect greater knowledge of Muslim beliefs and practices in each of the areas. Asterisked items should be reverse scored. For the following subscales, sum across the items in each. *Importance of Religious Leader in Treatment subscale*: 1*, 2, 5*, 15. *Community Perceptions of Mental Illness subscale*: 6, 8, 11*, 12, 14. *Beliefs Regarding Therapy subscale*: 3, 4*, 7, 9*, 10, 13, 16.

PART **III**
Service Settings

CHAPTER 10
Inpatient Psychiatric Units

SARAH MOHIUDDIN and SABA MAROOF

Psychiatric inpatient settings inherently serve a more acute population. Patients are often admitted for acute suicidality, homicidality, inability to manage activities of daily living, first-episode or worsening psychosis, catatonia, or other such conditions that come with significant functional impairment and cannot be managed in outpatient settings. Patients may be involuntarily admitted to psychiatric units, resulting in loss of freedom of movement and ability to make personal choices. In such settings, patients may also be admitted for prolonged periods of time; therefore, understanding and accommodating religious practices are often very important. This chapter attempts to familiarize the clinician with the day-to-day practices and issues that may be relevant when treating Muslim patients in inpatient psychiatric units.

According to the Pew Research Center, there are an estimated 2.5 million Muslims of varying ethnic origins living within the United States (Miller, 2009). It is estimated that approximately 30% of Muslims in the United States are African-American, 33% are of South Asian origin, and 25% are of Arabic origin (Al-Mateen & Afzal, 2004). There are also converts to Islam from almost every ethnic and racial group in the United States. Thus, Muslims in the United States vary greatly in their background. For this reason, adherence to specific Islamic practices may vary depending on the cultural or ethnic background of individuals. Culture influences religion and vice versa; however, qualitative investigations often overlook the connection between cultural expression and religious dictates (Padela &

Rodriguez del Pozo, 2010). General principles such as modesty and cleanliness are overarching, but cultural aspects influence practice as well. Also, an individual or family may be considered devout, conservative, moderate, or liberal in regard to their adherence to Islamic teachings. Such differences contribute to further variation in presentation.

Few studies have specifically addressed the religious and spiritual needs of Muslims in psychiatric settings; however, this lack of knowledge and resources may not be limited to Muslims alone. In general, psychiatric patients may desire religious or spiritual care just as medical or surgical patients, but may find that their needs are less often met. A study conducted by Fitchett, Burton, and Sivan (1997) found that 88% of psychiatric inpatients reported three or more current religious needs. Although they found no differences in religious needs between the psychiatric and medical/surgical inpatients, they did find that psychiatric inpatients had less access to religious resources. They also found that psychiatric inpatients had lower spiritual well-being scores and were less likely to have spoken with their clergy. This is most likely due to the fact that clergy are not usually present in freestanding psychiatric hospitals, as they are in medical centers. Additionally, psychiatric units may not have a chapel or meditation area where patients may pray or attend religious services. Given these differences in access to religious/spiritual resources within psychiatric units, more attention is needed to understand and address these needs. This is of particular importance for religious minorities, such as Muslim patients, as psychiatric clinicians may be even less familiar with what their needs would be.

Patient–Provider Relationship and Communication while in the Hospital

Understanding Muslim Families

According to a review article by Al-Mateen and Afzal in 2004, immigrant Muslim families from Eastern cultures often value the community and family above the individual. They describe the Muslim family as one in which the autonomy of the individual may be sacrificed to maintain the unity of the family. They also describe Muslim parents as more likely to be authoritarian, with little encouragement of discussion. This trend may be changing with second-generation Muslims. The immigrant Muslim family may use a more restrained and indirect type of communication, with less confrontation and more inference, in contrast to American society. Additionally, immigrant families may appear enmeshed. These are all issues that should be duly noted by practitioners caring for Muslim patients, both in psychiatric and medical settings (Al-Mateen & Afzal, 2004).

Islamic teachings encourage the Muslim community to visit the sick (Al-Jibaly, 1998), and therefore Muslim patients may get many visitors during hospitalization. This may also pose significant challenges to maintaining issues of safety and patient confidentiality on a psychiatric unit, as the number of visitors may exceed what can be accommodated. Communicating with Muslim families about boundaries and limitations surrounding visitation early in the hospitalization may be important.

Involuntary Commitment

Muslim patients of any origin may be hesitant seeking mental health treatment, mainly due to stigma. Mental health providers may be viewed as "individuals who discard religious values and fail to see these values as a genuine source of solace and healing" (Al-Krenawi & Graham, 2000). Additionally, family members may have difficulty recognizing pathology. A study conducted by Stein, Christie, Shah, Dabney, and Wolport in 2003 found that mothers of Pakistani children living in the United Kingdom were less likely to recognize the difference between emotional and behavioral problems in comparison to their British counterparts and were thus less likely to seek help for behavioral problems. Muslims may also vary in health care–seeking behaviors in general because of post-9/11 discrimination and abuse that led to increased psychological distress and mistrust (Padela & Rodriguez del Pozo, 2010). Because of these reasons, treatment may be delayed until symptoms become very serious, which may result in involuntary commitment.

Involuntary (or court-ordered) treatment poses special issues for Muslim patients, particularly those who have nuclear and extended families who wish to be intimately involved in their care (see Case 10.1). Both patients and families may not understand why the patient is receiving medications or treatment without their expressed consent. Additionally, they may be unfamiliar with the legal process of involuntary treatment. Language barriers or previous experiences with involuntary treatment in other countries may compound this. Having a separate family meeting to discuss the specific guidelines of involuntary treatment soon after admission will often be very helpful in assuaging some of these concerns and build a more collaborative alliance.

CASE 10.1

A 25-year-old African-American Muslim patient with a history of medication noncompliance was involuntarily admitted after becoming aggressive during an acute manic episode. He received multiple doses of intramuscular haloperidol and lorezapam to manage his agitation prior to his court hearing and refused to consent for standing medication dosing. During the hearing, the judge mandated the patient to both inpatient and outpatient psychiatric treatment. His extended family was informed of the hearing after it took place and was very upset that the patient underwent a legal hearing without the family being present. Social work and physician staff met with the family to discuss the process of involuntary treatment including discussion of state law requiring a court hearing within three days of hospitalization. They also discussed in detail the process by which the court order for treatment would be reviewed and maintained. The family informed staff of their prior attempts to have the patient maintain medication compliance. They reported that as the patient still lives with his parents at home, his parents have remained very involved in obtaining his medications and watching him take his medications every evening. They expressed concerns that medication changes would take place through the court order without their knowledge, which would then result in difficulty for the parents to monitor medication compliance at home. After the staff had increased their awareness of parental involvement, they maintained close communication with the parents about medication changes and his final discharge regimen.

The Use of Interpreters

Language barriers often pose a significant barrier to patient–provider communication in a hospital setting. It is often better to involve an interpreter in acute psychiatric settings, as limitations in language comprehension may be compounded by acute psychiatric illness. As with all cases of interpreter use, it is essential to use a trained professional. This again is especially true in psychiatric settings due to the sensitivity of information. The use of family members for this purpose can create tension and may create barriers of communication between providers and patients. Family members may also omit important information, and patients may not be forthcoming with aspects of their history, such as suicidal thoughts, sexual abuse or deviance, and substance abuse, when having to relay this information through a family member. Family members may also try to summarize information in a more acceptable way and therefore may not translate content literally. Thus, markers of disturbed thought process such as disorganization, neologisms, flight of ideas, or loose associations may be missed. In a study conducted by Marcus in 1979, it was found that interpreters who were relatives of the patient tended to either minimize or emphasize psychopathology. Both can be problematic as this can influence diagnosis and treatment. The author also observed that relatives tended to answer clinicians' questions without actually asking the patient.

Other times, family members ascribe their own opinions upon the patient. Because of these issues, it is essential that a translator competent in both languages be utilized. Clinicians may also consider meeting separately with the interpreter to outline the goals of the interview, sensitive areas to be discussed, the dangers of "making sense" of statements made by the patient, and confidentiality (Marcus, 1979).

Diagnosis and Psychoeducation

Providing a diagnosis in an acute psychiatric setting can often be a difficult experience for clinicians and patients alike. Diagnoses given in an inpatient setting are often those associated with poorer prognosis such as bipolar disorder and schizophrenia. Psychiatric inpatient providers must often quickly diagnose patients soon after the initial assessment. Clinicians may find themselves in a position of having to discuss long-term treatment options and prognosis with perplexed patients and families after only one or two brief interactions. This is compounded with the lack of collateral information and time to build rapport with the patient and families.

Muslim patients, regardless of cultural or ethnic background, may have more difficulty accepting psychiatric diagnosis and treatment due to general stigma in the community. Stigma may be compounded by beliefs that religious practice should protect against emotional problems and that mental distress is a sign of weak faith. Hardships and problems may be considered "God's will" or a "punishment" and a person is expected to adjust and learn from the situation (Al-Azayem, 1994). Muslims are often encouraged to seek help within the family support or through religious outlets such as a praying or speaking with a religious leader (Daneshpour, 1998). Many Arabs and Muslims in general are fatalistic, believing that some events are simply God's will (Nobles & Sciarra, 2000). This thinking often does not correlate with the patient's educational level (Al-Azayem, 1994). Muslim patients may also be more likely to seek a religious or spiritual solution to a psychiatric condition, particularly if the diagnosis carries a poorer prognosis (see Case 10.2). Depending on the patient and family, it may be helpful to involve religious clergy that the family trusts in the discussion of the treatment plan and long-term prognosis to aid in treatment adherence and overall coping for the family unit.

CASE 10.2

A 19-year-old Pakistani college student was admitted to a psychiatric hospital after being found psychotic and disorganized by his roommate. He had predominant auditory hallucinations and religious delusions regarding being able to communicate with God. After two weeks in the hospital, he was diagnosed with a primary psychotic disorder.

His mother and father, who had flown in from Pakistan after their son was hospitalized, were skeptical of the diagnosis, stating that no one in their family had ever previously been diagnosed with a mental illness. After meeting with their son, the family did acknowledge that the patient was acting bizarrely, but felt that the patient's report of communicating with God could represent a heightened religious state. They were hesitant to begin antipsychotic medications, reporting a preference for religious intervention. They then asked staff to discharge their son so that he could be taken back to Pakistan for treatment.

Muslims may also feel discomfort discussing treatment and prognosis with practitioners from outside their faith group (Stein et al., 2003). This discomfort may stem from the fear that members from outside the religious group may not understand them. Particularly since the events of September 11, 2001, many Muslims assume that non-Muslims view them as aggressive and violent. Muslim women may feel that others assume they are uneducated or suppressed, and Muslim men may assume that others view them as dominating, crass, uncaring, or volatile. Also after September 11th, there have been reports of FBI tappings, threats of deportation, or being accused of terrorism within the general Muslim community. These experiences may significantly impact patient–provider relationships, as Muslim patients may be more wary about providing sensitive psychiatric information. Having frank discussions with Muslim patients about whether they have concerns seeking care outside of their faith and asking them to describe what these concerns are may help clinicians understand and address these concerns.

Informed Consent and Patient Confidentiality

When dealing with informed consent and confidentiality, there are a number of issues unique to inpatient psychiatric settings that may not be unique to Muslims alone. Given the acute nature of illness during a psychiatric hospitalization, many families new to the inpatient psychiatric experience may expect ongoing involvement in decision making, particularly those involving medications. Families may expect communication standards similar to those in medical/surgical hospitalizations, where family members often remain at the bedside throughout the patient stay. This may lead to difficulty in inpatient settings, where families are often not present when these decisions are made between patients and providers.

These issues may be compounded when dealing with Muslim patients and their families. Muslim families often rely heavily on extended family involvement (Al-Mateen & Afzal, 2004). They may have large numbers of visitors from their extended families and may want to engage many family members in the decision-making process (see Case 10.3). Understanding Muslim family dynamics will also be very important when psychiatric inpatients are unable to give consent for treatment, given a lack of decision-making capacity secondary to acute psychiatric illness. This may become complicated as various family members may have differing views or opinions on the need for psychiatric treatment or medications. Encouraging families to appoint a single person early in the hospitalization to handle daily communication between families and providers can be helpful in preventing frustration between providers and family members. Including these key family members in discussions regarding risks and benefits of treatment options will often be important in patient compliance with treatment plans.

CASE 10.3

An 8-year-old boy is psychiatrically hospitalized following increasing aggressive behavior at home. During the hospitalization, he is diagnosed with ADHD. His father, who is a physician, is hesitant to start him on a stimulant, citing that the patient's grandmother is adamantly opposed to using a medication to treat what she feels is "bad behavior." Staff held a family meeting including the patient's father and grandmother to provide psychoeducation regarding the standard of care practices and pharmacologic treatment of ADHD. During this meeting, the patient's father often deferred to the grandmother for decision making. After taking note of this, inpatient staff began asking the grandmother to regularly call to obtain updates on the patient and to attend family meetings. After building further rapport with the patient's grandmother, the team once again approached the idea of beginning pharmacotherapy with the patient's father and grandmother, with which the grandmother was now in agreement. The patient was eventually discharged on a stimulant and a plan to continue behavior management strategies through his outpatient treatment providers.

Patient confidentiality issues also may be complicated by Muslim family dynamics. Patients on inpatient psychiatric units often report information that they want to be kept confidential from family members, including familial/marital discord, sexual activity, and substance use and abuse. These issues, which may seem commonplace to many psychiatric providers, may often be a source of shame or secrecy within Muslim families; therefore, psychiatric providers must take care in referencing this information in conversations with family members (including spouses) without express consent. Also, Muslim family members may not understand the limits of patient confidentiality in psychiatric settings and may expect that they would have access to psychiatric information similar to the way one's family has access to medical information during a hospitalization. Providers should try to have explicit conversations or handouts outlining patient confidentiality to help patients and families understand these boundaries during an inpatient stay.

Modesty/Privacy

All cultures and religions have their own degrees of modesty, and certainly Islam is no exception. In fact, there is a saying of the Prophet Muhammad that states, "Every religion has an innate character, the character of Islam is modesty" (as cited in Siddiqui, 1976). However, Islam is not a monolithic faith, and Muslims themselves vary greatly in how individuals adhere to guidelines. Many Muslim women believe that they are required to cover their body except for their face, hands, and feet in front of nonrelated males. Women may fulfill this requirement by wearing long sleeves and pants or skirts, with a *hijab* or headscarf in front of unrelated males. Muslim men are required to cover from the navel to the knee. Upon seeking admission to a psychiatric hospital, Muslim patients may have concerns about wearing hospital gowns given that such clothing does not adhere to the Islamic standard for modesty (Padela & Rodriguez del Pozo, 2010). Patients should be reassured that often times they can wear nonhospital clothing within inpatient psychiatric units. Also, Muslim women wearing *hijab* will often want to take off their headscarf in the privacy of their own room and therefore may choose to keep the door of their room closed. This may pose problems in a psychiatric unit if the doors have windows or other ways to monitor patients in their rooms. If the patient is eligible based on her psychiatric status, providing a room in which she would be able to have privacy from other male staff, patients, or visitors would likely improve the Muslim female patient's experience in the hospital. Also, it can be very helpful to have a sign on female Muslim patients' doors asking the staff to knock first before entering. This will provide female Muslim patients time to put on their *hijab* prior to the entry of male staff (Padela & Rodriguez del Pozo, 2010). In psychiatric units that require frequent visual checks on patients throughout the day and night, it may be advisable to use a female staff member for ease of dressing and overall comfort for female Muslim patients.

It might be challenging in some cases to balance the need for safety while providing garments that allow for modesty on an inpatient psychiatric unit. For example, the head covering itself is often made of a square or rectangular cloth. Depending on the length of the rectangular cloth, concerns may arise on the potential of its use for self-harm. Some women also use various pins to fasten the scarf, and ordinarily sharp objects are not allowed on inpatient psychiatric units. If there are acute concerns for suicidality or self-harm, such as cutting behavior or self-mutilation, speaking with female patients about using square headscarfs without the use of pins or other sharp objects may be necessary.

Gender separation is another way Muslims maintain modesty. Many Muslim men and women may adhere to guidelines restricting physical contact between men and women and therefore may prefer same-sex providers. Educating staff members to avoid unnecessary touching of opposite-gender Muslim patients will be important. This may become difficult in the context of managing or restraining an aggressive or agitated patient. However, many Muslims adhere to the principal of flexibility in gender separation during times of necessity or life-threatening issues, such as emergency medical care. Both the condition of necessity and life preservation apply in the acute management of an aggressive or agitated patient. Members of the opposite gender may need to get involved when managing acute agitation or aggression to keep patients safe from harming themselves or others.

Dietary Requirements

Islamic teachings provide guidelines for food consumption. Although Muslims may vary in their adherence to these guidelines, it is important for inpatient psychiatric providers to have a basic understanding of these guidelines in order to understand the various dietary requests for which Muslim patients may ask.

According to the Qur'an, Muslims are prohibited from using pork products, animals that are not slaughtered according to Islamic guidelines, and alcohol and other intoxicants (there is a scholarly difference of opinion on the use of tobacco-containing products). These items are considered *haram*, or prohibited. *Halal* signifies all other foods outside of these restrictions. Muslims may also use the term *zabiha*, which refers to meat, other than seafood, that has been slaughtered and prepared according to Islamic law. This involves invoking God's name to reinforce that the animal was killed only for human sustenance and slaughtering occurred in a manner that was of least pain to the animal (Gulam, 2003). If *zabiha* or *halal* food is unavailable in a psychiatric setting, many Muslim patients may opt for seafood or vegetarian options. Some Muslims may also eat food prepared by other Abrahamic traditions, such as the Jewish Kosher food ritual. Some Muslims believe that most food available in Western countries is *halal*, because the populations of these countries are primarily of Christian faith. These ideas are based on Islamic traditions in which the Prophet Muhammad consumed the food of people from the Abrahamic faiths, considering them "People of the Book." However, not only food and beverages fall within the categories of *halal* and *haram*. Products such as mouthwash, soaps, and detergents should also be screened for use, as pork- or alcohol-based ingredients may have been used in the production process. Having an open discussion with Muslim patients about their adherence to Islamic food guidelines will help providers provide an environment that fulfills their patients' dietary needs.

In terms of medications, Muslims will often avoid taking medicines that contain alcohol or pork (or even bovine) by-products unless they are life-saving drugs and no substitutes are available. At a time of necessity, Islamic scholars follow the general rule that "necessity dictates exception." This has been stated in the Qur'an as, "If one is forced (to eat things that are haram), without being deliberate or malicious, then your Lord is Ever-Forgiving, Most Merciful" (Qur'an 6:145). Clinicians should be aware as to whether medications they are prescribing contain alcohol- or pork-based ingredients prior to prescribing them to Muslim patients.

Hygiene

Islam emphasizes both physical and spiritual cleanliness and purity. A verse from the Qur'an reads, "Truly, God loves those who turn to Him in repentance and loves those who purify themselves" (Qur'an 2:222). The Prophet Muhammad once said, "Cleanliness is half of faith" (as cited in Siddiqui, 1976).

Some Muslim scholars divide hygiene into two main areas: ritual washing before prayers and keeping the body, clothing, and environment clean. Ritual washing prior to prayer is called *wudu*. In this, Muslims wash their hands, nostrils, mouth, face, arms, and feet each three times and wipe over their head and ears. *Wudu* can be performed five times daily in preparation for the five daily prayers. Having ready access to bathroom facilities multiple times a day will therefore be very important to a Muslim patient. It is also important to note that often, in performing *wudu*, water may spill on the floor or get on a patient's clothing. This should not be regarded as a sign of uncleanliness or other symptoms (such as obsessive-compulsive behaviors) that may accompany more acute psychiatric illness. If someone is too ill to perform *wudu*, then the patient can perform *tayammum*, a ritual that involves touching a clean area with two hands and wiping over one's face, hands, and forearms.

Muslims also perform a whole-body ritual washing called *ghusl* to cleanse the body in certain circumstances. These times include after sexual intercourse or ejaculation, or the completion of one's menstrual period. After these events, Muslims must perform *ghusl* in order to resume prayer or fasting. This washing is accomplished through taking a shower and performing the *wudu*. Because of this, patients may want to take a shower prior to the dawn prayer or at other various times of the day. It will be important for clinicians to maintain open communication with Muslim patients about their hygiene needs and practices, and psychiatric units should try to accommodate this request whenever possible.

In regard to body, clothing, and environment cleanliness, the Muslim patient may have specific requests for body cleaning after using the toilet. Many Muslims prefer to wash their private parts with running water following urination or defecation and may require a glass or a jug to take with them to the bathroom. For patients who are unable to take care of themselves or are bedridden, they or their families may request special or additional assistance in performing this task.

Prayer

Muslim religious observance includes three main forms of prayer: a ritualized prayer (known as *salah*), supplication (known as *dua'a*), and a congregational Friday prayer (known as *jumu'a*). *Salah* is a ritualized prayer that consists of a series of movements including standing, bowing, and prostrating with various amounts of repetitions of these movements. *Salah* can be performed as often as one likes, but is required to be performed by Muslims at least five times a day during specific circumscribed times. These times include dawn, noon, late afternoon, after sunset, and in the late evening. Verses from the Qur'an and various supplications and praise of God are recited during specific movements of prayer. *Salah* can be performed alone or in a group and can also be performed silently or aloud. There are a number of requirements in performing these five daily prayers, some of which include being in a state of purity through completion of *wudu* (see section on hygiene), wearing clean clothes, performing *salah* in a clean location (which may include the use of a prayer mat), and performing *salah* at the correct time. Optional or supplementary *salah* can be performed throughout the day and are most often performed by more devout Muslims in the late night.

There are a number of issues regarding *salah* that may become more relevant during an inpatient psychiatric stay. One is that the five required *salah* can take anywhere from 5 to 30 minutes to complete, and excess length in performing these prayers may be a sign of hyper-religiosity sometimes seen in patients in acute states of bipolar disorder, psychotic disorders, or obsessive-compulsive disorder. Also, patients who have become hyper-religious secondary to their psychiatric illness may be performing more optional or supplemental prayers during the nighttime. However, the length and frequency in performing *salah* could also increase if a devout Muslim patient chooses to turn to God for help or reliance in a time of crisis and therefore could also be a sign of appropriate coping. As part of a comprehensive psychiatric inpatient evaluation, clinicians should gain an understanding of baseline behaviors regarding prayers to understand how these may be impacted during a more acute psychiatric illness.

Similar to the practice of prayer in Judeo-Christian faiths, Muslims also perform *dua'a* or supplication, which consists of asking or communicating with God. Although many Muslims put more emphasis on the form of prayer known as *salah*, *dua'a* is also an important component of Muslim religious and spiritual life. There are specific *dua'as* for various parts of one's day, such as upon waking, beginning one's meal, etc., but these are considered optional practices. As there are no mandatory rituals or guidelines to perform *dua'a*, individual Muslim practice of *dua'a* may be based on personal preference or cultural values or experiences.

The last type of prayer is the congregational prayer known as *jumu'a* or Friday prayer. *Jumu'a* occurs in between noon and the early afternoon on Fridays and consists of a short sermon and a shortened *salah*. It can occur in any location, although it often takes place in a mosque. Many medical hospitals have also begun having *jumu'a* prayers to accommodate staff and patients. Although *jumu'a* is considered mandatory for all Muslim males, it is not required during times of travel or illness and therefore would not be mandatory for a Muslim patient to attend during an acute hospital stay.

Fasting

Fasting is an important pillar of Islamic religious observance. Fasting in Islamic tradition consists of refraining from food, drink, or sexual intercourse from dawn to dusk. Most Muslim scholars also interpret this to mean that medications cannot be taken during the time of the fast. However, this is merely the physical component of the fast; the spiritual aspects of the fast are also very important and include refraining from gossiping, lying, slandering, and other negative behaviors as well as spending more time in completing good deeds and engaging in charitable acts. The fasting is intended to help teach Muslims self-discipline, self-restraint, and generosity, as well as sympathy for the suffering of the poor. Fasting is mandatory for Muslims during the month of Ramadan (the ninth month of the Islamic Lunar calendar). Muslims may also perform supplementary fasting intermittently throughout the year because many Muslims derive significant spiritual benefit from fasting. Muslims may particularly want to fast when they or their family member is ill to receive spiritual or physical healing.

There are a number of exceptions to the mandatory fasting that occurs during the month of Ramadan. These exceptions include those who are ill, traveling, pregnant, breastfeeding, or menstruating. Those who do not fast during the month of Ramadan due to these reasons must complete the missed fasts once these conditions have resolved. Those with chronic illness who are unable to complete the missed fasts may give charity instead (Sheikh & Gatrad, 2004). Given that an acute illness is most often the reason for acute psychiatric hospitalization, fasting would most likely not be mandatory for Muslim psychiatric inpatients. However, many Muslim patients may choose to fast if they feel that it does not significantly worsen their health and may provide them spiritual benefit. This may cause some difficulty during an inpatient stay, particularly if a patient's medication regimen requires the use of daytime dosing of medications or depot/long-acting injectable medications. If possible, staff should work with Muslim patients to readjust the timing for meals and medications so that they occur outside the time of fasting (i.e., prior to dawn or after dusk) if a patient decides to fast during Ramadan. However, situations may arise in which staff feel that fasting may cause harm to the patient during a psychiatric inpatient stay or interferes with medication compliance. Some patients may insist on fasting against medical advice and may refuse medications. Consulting local Muslim clergy and having a joint meeting with the patient may be helpful in encouraging and negotiating an alternative plan.

Conclusion

Caring for patients during acute inpatient psychiatric stays is inherently challenging; however, caring for Muslim patients in this setting may result in an additional set of challenges. This requires inpatient psychiatric staff to make themselves knowledgeable of the practices and needs of Muslim patients in order to understand how these needs may translate to the specific constraints of an inpatient unit. Muslim family dynamics and Muslim daily life experiences may affect patient–provider relationships, and inpatient psychiatric providers should take care in maintaining open communication with their Muslim patients and families. Doing this will not only enhance rapport and trust with the patient and family, but will also enable psychiatric providers to gather the information needed to make an adequate diagnosis and treatment plan. Clearly, there is an increasing need to understand the mental health needs of Muslim patients. Addressing their inpatient psychiatric needs may be especially important, as this may often be the patient's first encounter with the mental health system. Enhancing one's knowledge about Muslim culture and religion is an important step in the process of providing more culturally competent care in an inpatient psychiatric setting.

References

Al-Azayem, A. (1994). Influence of Islamic ethics on psychiatry. *Integrative Psychiatry, 10*(2), 58–61.
Ali, Y. (2002). *The meaning of the Holy Quran*. Beltsville, MD: Amana Publications.
Al-Jibaly, M. (1998). *The inevitable journey part 1—Sickness: Regulations and exhortations*. Arlington, TX: Al-Kitaab & As-Sunnah Publishing.
Al-Krenawi, A., & Graham J. R. (2000). Culturally sensitive social work practice with Arab clients in mental health settings. *Health Social Work, 25*(1), 9–22.
Al-Mateen, C., & Afzal, A. (2004). The Muslim child, adolescent and family. *Child and Adolescent Psychiatric Clinics, 13,* 183–200.
Daneshpour, M. (1998). Muslim families and family therapy. *Journal of Marital and Family Therapy, 24*(3), 355–390.
Fitchett, G., Burton, L. A., & Sivan, A. B. (1997). The religious needs and resources of psychiatric inpatients. *Journal of Nervous and Mental Disorders, 185*(5), 320–326.
Gulam, H. (2003). Caring for the Muslim patient. *ADF Health, 4,* 81–83.
Marcus, L. R. (1979). Effects of interpreters on the evaluation of psychopathology in non-English-speaking patients. *American Journal of Psychiatry, 136*(2), 171–174.
Miller, T. (2009, October). *Mapping the global Muslim population: A report on the size and distribution of the world's Muslim population*. Pew Research Center. Retrieved from http://pewforum.org/Muslim/Mapping-the-Global-Muslim-Population.aspx
Nobles, A. Y., & Sciarra, D. T. (2000). Cultural determinants in the treatment of Arab Americans: A primer for mainstream therapists. *American Journal of Orthopsychiatry, 70*(2), 182–191.
Padela, A., & Rodriguez del Pozo, P. (2010). Muslim patients and cross-gender interactions in medicine: An Islamic bioethical perspective. *Journal of Medical Ethics*. [Epublication ahead of print], November 1.
Sheikh, A., & Gatrad, A. R. (2004). Caring for Muslim patients. *The International Journal of Health Planning and Management, 19*(4), 401–403.
Siddiqui, A. (1976). *Sahih Muslim*. Chicago, IL: Kazi Publications.
Stein, S. M., Christie, D. Shah, R., Dabney, J., & Wolport, M. (2003). Attitudes to and knowledge of child and adolescent mental services: Differences between Pakistani and British White mothers. *Child and Adolescent Mental Health, 8*(1), 29–33.

CHAPTER 11

Home-Based Social Services

ANEESAH NADIR and CHERYL EL-AMIN

There are a variety of situations in which social workers and other mental health professionals visit homes to provide services, including ongoing child-centered home-based services. The New Mexico Children, Youth, and Families Department (September 2010) defined home-based services as

> Provision of needed service for children and families with special needs in an individual home on a regular basis; services may be delivered by a teacher, counselor, consultant, therapist, or other professional. Home services allow the professional and child to have exclusive time together. (Bolson, 2004, p. 57)

Home-based services may include hospice care, disaster relief, or grief counseling. A crisis involving family violence, child abuse, domestic abuse, or elder abuse may also require home visits. In cases where a family member is experiencing severe depression or threatening to commit suicide, health care professionals may be called to assess or intervene in the situation. Home assessments may be mandated or be *best practice*, as in cases of adoption home studies, working with adjudicated youth, or in discharge planning. Religious belief system(s) have a documented impact in family functioning and response to therapeutic intervention (Boyd-Franklin, 2006; Bailey, 2002). It is imperative that the practitioner or provider of home-based services for Muslim clientele considers the cultural/religious aspects of service delivery. Religious practices, working with the opposite gender, family composition, and cultural forms of dress are some of the items practitioners may need additional information on when dealing with traditional Muslims. This chapter addresses these items, as well as gives a brief description of the demographics and ethnology of American Muslims.

Demographics

American Muslims reside largely in suburban and urban communities, although some are also present in rural communities. According to Gallup's (2009) Muslim West Facts Project, 51% of the Muslim population is married, averaging 1.33 children (under 18 in the home) having a family size of 3.81 persons (p. 25). Pew's research (2007) observed that 26% of the American Muslim population has a household income of $75,000 or more annually. This figure is comparable to the 28% rate for the American public (p. 19). The same report noted a disparity between the general public and the Muslim populations of France, Spain, Germany, and Great Britain. A larger percentage of Muslims in the aforementioned European countries were part of the lower economic strata compared to the general public.

Muslim homes in America, the United Kingdom, and Australia reflect diversity in culture, language, and religiosity (Nadir & Dziegielewski, 2001; Saeed, 2004). The Islamic Social Service Association (ISSA) of the United States observed four broad groups including immigrants, indigenous Muslim converts, refugees, and first-, second-, and third-generation American Muslim descendants of these groups (ISSA, 2003). Gallup's study (2009) reported that Muslim Americans represent the most racially diverse religious group in the United States (35% African-American, 28% White, 18% Asian, 18% other, 1% Hispanic). Practitioners should keep in mind that ethnicity and culture may add another dimension to the diversity in Muslim households.

Muslim family system configurations are varied. The home care professional may find households with multifaith/multicultural members (i.e., Christian, Jewish, Hindu, and nonfaith based; African-American, European-American, biracial, etc.). The composition may be due to conversion, informal adoption, or interfaith or intercultural marriages. Nonrelated persons (fictive kin) may be adopted into the family and be referred to as mom, dad, aunt, uncle, or grandma in some households (Boyd-Franklin, 2006).

Muslim family constellations also differ and may include extended family members, childless households, and families under 30 or over 50 years of age. Although multigenerational families tend to be a norm in many of the Muslim cultures throughout the world, many Muslims in the United States live in nuclear families and may be isolated from extended family and other Muslims. Muslim families may be two-parent or single-parent families due to divorce, deportation, separation, or death of the spouse. Children may be split between households, even countries, living with grandparents or separated parents.

Pew (2007) reported that 65% of Muslim Americans are immigrants, with the indigenous population of American Muslims rising. Demographic studies of American Muslim populations report that the Muslims in the United States tend to be younger than the general American population. Pew's (2007) study reported that 87% of Muslim adults are between 18 and 54 years of age (p. 17). It is posited that the low percentage of elders is due to the fact that foreign-born Muslims are more likely to have parents who continue to reside in their country of origin. As the Muslim population ages in the United States, Muslim adults and their non Muslim American cohorts are also experiencing the challenges of caring for aging and disabled family members (Hosnain & Rana, 2010). Aging issues, family structure, socioeconomic status, culture, and ethnicity are general areas warranting home-based assessment and service provision.

Home-Based Service Provision

The *process* of home-based services for Muslims is generally no different than that for any other group. Although the process for providing home-based services generally follows the same pattern, service delivery to Muslim clients and families does require some knowledge of religious and cultural norms that have the potential to impact service provision.

The following list gives the varying steps when providing competent home-based services. Specific issues pertinent to the home-based care of Muslim clients will be discussed following the description of process in order to aid home-based service providers working with Muslims.

- Rapport Building – The practitioner seeks to establish a trusting, empathic, and genuine relationship with the client/family.
- Data Gathering – The client/family member or members are interviewed to obtain the family's story and perception of the presenting problem, while noting that individual family members may have differing perceptions. The practitioner notes the home environment and the family's interactions.
- Assessment – The practitioner now evaluates and synthesizes the data, assessing the client/family's strengths and challenges.
- Intervention – The practitioner partners with the client/family to determine the best strategy to facilitate change and determine the need and availability of additional resources.

- Evaluation – The practitioner continues to follow up and monitor the effectiveness of the selected intervention(s).
- Termination – As the home-based health care relationship comes to a close, the practitioner and the client/family review the entire processes, noting the gains, challenges, and follow-through strategies for the future. The termination process should begin prior to the last visit.

Rapport Building

Muslims are often distrustful of secular and other faith providers because they fear they will hold Islamophobic views similar to those displayed in much of the U.S. popular media. Nadir and Dziegielewski (2001) cited "blaming of the religion" as a primary reason Muslims do not seek the assistance of mainstream service providers. Alwani and Abugideiri (2003) indicated that "suspicion and distrust may be a result of Muslim women's fear that Western workers are biased toward divorce; guilt about seeking help outside the family or community; and uncertainty about the choices she will be asked to make" (p. 48). As such, outside service provision may be the last avenue sought by Muslims. The practitioner should be sensitive to a Muslim client's reluctance toward interventions, perhaps allowing more time for the client/family and practitioner to become acquainted. Rapport building with Muslim clients may take extra time and effort due to the perceived biases discussed previously. Additional factors to consider when building rapport include conceptual differences in time, social etiquette when entering the home, and the importance of hospitality.

Conceptual Differences in Time Western training and time constraints placed on service providers by insurance companies, grantors, and agency policies may lead practitioners to be somewhat inflexible and task oriented during home visit sessions. While most Western cultures operate on a linear and specific orientation of time, some Muslim cultures may be less structured and more flexible with respect to notions of time. Some cultural groups among Muslims expect a late arrival and feel uncomfortable when the practitioner arrives at the designated time. Other groups are more acclimated and used to a Western time orientation. It is important for the practitioner to be mindful and prepared in case of these differences in time orientations and related expectations.

The traditional one-hour allotted may be insufficient to begin the rapport-building process with Muslims bound by cultural traditions often practiced in their native homeland. New immigrants and refugees may prefer a more relaxed and casual initial meeting involving the entire family. The clients may expect to begin the meeting with light conversation rather than delving into the presenting problem, as is common among task-oriented professionals with an often overloaded caseload. This type of conversation process should not be confused with avoidance, but rather understood to help the client build comfort and trust with the practitioner. Indigenous Muslims, second and third generations or later, or those more acculturated to Western culture are more likely to be acclimated to starting and ending the meeting "on time" and the task-oriented approach of many clinicians.

Social Etiquette when Entering the Home Many Muslims remove their shoes before or upon entering the home. It is believed by some that not wearing shoes in the home eliminates the potential for bringing impurities into the home. Others simply want to keep the family's designated prayer space clean. To honor this tradition the home-based provider should ask ahead of time if removing shoes before entering is important for the family and be prepared to remove shoes, if asked. A visual clue to this practice can be noted upon seeing shoes arranged at the entrance of the home or if no one in the house is wearing shoes. Offering to remove shoes prior to the client's request is a sign of cultural sensitivity and another step toward building trust and rapport. If agency protocol or provider discomfort prevents shoe removal, there are alternatives. It is recommended that professionals/providers carry shoe covers. Informing the client of the provider's willingness to cover the shoes upon entering may work as well as removing the shoes.

Issues related to gender interaction may also impact rapport building. The client may not make direct eye contact with a practitioner of the opposite gender, which may be indicative of how the client demonstrates modest behavior and shows respect for the practitioner. It is often not intended to be a sign of disrespect or unwillingness to be cordial. Muslims are often taught to lower their gaze or be indirect in their eye contact between men and women who are not close family members as a way to avoid a semblance of impropriety between unmarried men and women. Some Muslims may adhere to this practice, while others may not. Some Muslims may lower their gaze, not for religious reasons, but for cultural ones related to respecting authority and deference to elders, which is common in many Asian and Arab cultures.

Casually touching, hugging, holding hands, etc., are a common part of Western mainstream culture; however, Muslims of various backgrounds may avoid touching between unrelated people of the opposite gender, in keeping with Islamic tradition. Some Muslims are very strict about this practice, while other Muslims will not initiate the handshake but may return it to avoid offending the professional. In the event the professional extends his or her hand the Muslim may bow slightly while informing him or her that cross-gender handshaking is not part of their religious practice. Muslims who may not have as much practice with politely refusing handshakes may display discomfort. The professional can assist in making the meeting more comfortable by waiting until the client expresses a greeting gesture. If the individual is comfortable with handshaking, the client will extend his or her hand.

Hospitality Muslim cultures encourage hospitality toward guests, as was the practice of the Prophet Muhammad (PBUH). Family members will typically offer food (from light desserts to a meal) and something to drink to visitors. It is over food that the rapport-building phase may begin. The family may feel obligated to offer food, even if it presents a financial hardship, and may be offended if the food is refused. Agency policy may prevent practitioners from accepting the client's food offering or the practitioner may not like the ethnic food. To avoid this challenge, the home health care practitioner may choose to consult the client prior to the scheduled visit and arrange the home visit outside of meal times.

Data Gathering

Data gathering is an ongoing process during home visits and often begins with the practitioner's observation of the physical surroundings outside and within the home. During the data-gathering stage, the practitioner listens to the client tell his or her story, collecting information about the situation and the client's viewpoint of the problem(s). Noting particular circumstances of the Muslim client's diverse status (i.e., refugee, convert, immigrant, etc.) may provide insight into client/family behavior or perspective. For example, Muslim refugees may commonly experience severe war trauma or post-traumatic stress disorder (PTSD), which may influence the presenting problem(s). In addition, possible concerns related to intergenerational or interfaith conflicts between family members may also exist. As the practitioner and client/family become increasingly acquainted, the meaning and interpretation of the client's story is essential to the success of the next phase of care.

During the data-gathering phase, providers may notice differences in displays of family artifacts. Family photos and memorabilia are commonly displayed in American homes as a way to adorn the home and demonstrate family cohesiveness. These family artifacts commemorate landmark events and provide visual reminders of extended family who may reside outside of the home. Degrees and diplomas may also be displayed to celebrate family accomplishments. A lack of outward display of family photos or memorabilia is not indicative of a lack of family cohesiveness or support. While photos, degrees, and diplomas may be displayed in some Muslim homes, others prefer to emphasize their Muslim identity through wall hangings of

Islamic art or verses of the Qur'an. Some Muslims do not display images of human beings or animals in deference to certain interpretations of *hadith*, or traditions of the Prophet Muhammad (PBUH). The client/family may have photo albums, CDs, or digital photos of friends and family in other locations within the home.

A genogram is a useful data-gathering tool and facilitates dialogue about the family (Lum, 2005). The practitioner can seize the family genogram session as an opportunity to ask to see photos in hard or digital format and hear about the family's history and its many members. Family is often an important part of Muslim life, and looking through family photos may be a means of building the client/practitioner relationship, as well as provide important information about family dynamics. Observation and good listening skills are required of the practitioner during this data-gathering phase. As with other families, much of what is communicated is subtle and nonverbal.

Assessment

During the assessment phase, the practitioner evaluates the information gathered, noting the client's particular situation, strengths, challenges, and the possibilities for positive change. Because the medical model is more widely recognized, the client's strengths and resources are often overlooked. Saleeby (2002) pointed out that every individual, group, family, and community has strengths. He stated that "the strengths perspective is about discerning those resources, and respecting them and the potential they may have for reversing misfortune, countering illness, easing pain, reaching goals and overcoming oppression" (p. 13). The strengths perspective recognizes the talents, resources, and assets that individuals, families, and communities use to surmount insurmountable challenges (Nadir, 2003). The strengths-based perspective can facilitate a sense of empowerment for Muslims who may have overcome many adversities leading to resilience.

Intervention

The intervention phase is the point at which the practitioner partners with the client(s) to develop a plan that will assist in meeting goals and improving quality of life. This follows after a thorough bio/psycho/social/spiritual assessment. Clients' level of religiosity is an important factor as well as their socio/cultural/historical experience. Due to time constraints the practitioner may be tempted to implement a treatment plan before fully establishing rapport, gaining the client's trust, or completing the assessment. Failing to do so may result in a lack of follow through on the client's part that may be misperceived as noncompliance. It is also important for the client and practitioner to be clear on the implementation plan's time frame and process.

Utilizing culturally and spiritually sensitive resources increases the effectiveness of home-based interventions with Muslim clients. If clients feel that the intervention is culturally/spiritually relevant they are more likely to utilize the suggested strategies. Family counseling, spiritually based counseling, and cognitive therapy based on Islamic tenets have been shown to be effective with Muslim clients (Hodge & Nadir, 2008).

Termination

It is important to monitor and evaluate the success or effectiveness of interventions as part of the termination phase and throughout the helping process. The practitioner should keep in mind that Muslims are not generally inclined to seek mental health services and therefore may seek to terminate prior to completion of the intervention plan. If clients terminate prior to realizing the treatment goals, they may not return to what they feel is failed therapy. Successful termination is part of the planning process and should not be overlooked by the practitioner. The practitioner must work with the client and his or her support system (i.e., imam, extended family, members of the client's faith community, etc.) to maintain the gains made during therapy, as well as to determine ways to address challenges the client may experience in the future.

Religious, Cultural, and Social Considerations

The universal tenets of Islam have been outlined in previous chapters of this text. Religiosity or Islamic practice levels within the home and among family members may vary from household to household. Social etiquette may also vary from home to home depending on adherence to cultural and religious traditions. Asking about client traditions and practices before a visit can be helpful preparation for the home visit. This section highlights additional religious, cultural, and social considerations that may assist home-based providers.

Prayer

Prayer is a basic tenet in the religion of Islam. Depending on the level of practice of Muslim family members, prayer may be an established aspect of home life, and for some families a room in the home may be designated specifically for prayer. Prayer may provide strength, comfort, and guidance. Muslim time orientation may revolve around prayer times, which may affect provider visits. Clients may request that the provider adjust afternoon visits and service provision. This may be mistakenly viewed as a lack of commitment or disinterest in addressing the intervention plan, when in fact the clients may simply be trying to maintain their religious obligations.

In households that regularly pray, if the time for prayer comes during the home visit, family members may excuse themselves (one at a time or all together) to conduct prayers, leaving for about 5 to 15 minutes. Some may prefer to delay making the prayer until their visit with the provider has concluded, but depending on the time of the appointment that option may not always be available to the individual. Client respect can be gained through the practitioner's demonstration of religious sensitivity in acknowledging the importance of prayer, as observed by the family.

Modesty

When visiting a Muslim home, the practitioner should be mindful of Islamic notions of modesty. A client's manner of dress and demeanor with those of the opposite gender may vary depending on the client's religiosity and level of adherence to cultural/religious norms. Although the style of dress may be indicative of the level of religiosity, it is not definitive.

Muslim men's guidelines for appropriate dress include being covered at least from the navel to the knees by opaque, loose-fitting garments. Generally, Western Muslim men's casual wear includes loose-fitting slacks and a waist- or tunic-length shirt. However, some may wear an ankle-length shirt or *thobe*, similar to those worn in Arab and African cultures, or a long shirt with pants, *shalwar khameez*, a common dress for individuals originating from the Indian subcontinent. Many Muslim men have adopted the practice of maintaining a beard in keeping with the tradition of the Prophet Muhammad. Other men may wear a kufi (skull cap) or turban as part of their Islamic identity.

Some Muslim women may be distinguished by their head covering, while others may not be identifiable. *Hijab* or *khimar* refers to the manner in which many Muslim women are dressed: covering their head, wearing loose-fitting clothes and opaque outer garments, and only showing their hands, face, and feet. Some Muslims may believe that their feet must also be covered. Muslim women may wear a *niqab* or face veil in which only the eyes are allowed to be seen. The traditional dress, *hijab* and *niqab*, may be worn in public settings and at home if nonfamily men are present.

Notions of modesty also affect interactions with the opposite gender, which may be a clinical consideration in home-based environments. Meetings alone with a provider of the opposite gender may cause discomfort, because of religious rules of gender interaction. Thus clients may prefer to have a family member or friend join them during the home visit. Professionals may find maintaining confidentiality challenging when Muslim tradition dictates that two individuals of the opposite gender should not meet alone behind closed doors. The stigma or community reputation for a man or woman, if an individual of the opposite gender is seen going to his or her home regularly, may lead to suspicions of a premarital or extramarital affair, which could ruin the individual's or family's reputation. Some clients may prefer to arrange the home visit at certain times of the day when the practitioner is less likely to be seen entering or leaving the home, as a way to keep their confidence from the watchful eye of their neighbors. It is always good practice for the practitioner to notify the family/client when en route to the home. Advance notice allows the female client and the other women in the home to put on the *hijab* and outer garment and to arrange for a family member or friend to join them for the visit. It would be disrespectful for the female practitioner to enter a Muslim home, particularly where adult males are present, wearing clothes that are revealing, such as showing cleavage or a skirt above the knee.

Family Dynamics

It is not uncommon to find varied levels of religious practice within the same household. For example, self-identified religious young Muslims may live with their parents who describe themselves as secular Muslims, or as not adhering to traditional Islamic practices, such as daily prayers or Islamic dress. Williams and Vashi (2007) cited an example of a parent's opposition to their second-generation college student's choice to wear the *hijab*, or head covering. Conversely, Muslim parents and grandparents may object to what they perceive to be marginal practice of Islam by their adult children or grandchildren. Some Muslim college students expressed a "dual consciousness," displaying a "normal American" lifestyle on campus, while assuming a more traditional (cultural/Islamic) mannerism at home (El-Amin Naeem, 2008). The practitioner may be called upon to help both parent and child negotiate their differences. Intergenerational conflict about religion and culture is not unique to the Muslim household.

Muslim converts may live with or have extended family members that identify with other traditions (i.e., Christian, Jewish, other faith, or nonreligious). Non-Muslim family members' reactions to a member's conversion to Islam may range from full acceptance to total rejection. The practitioner may find families conflicted about religious practices such as whether or how to celebrate Islamic, Jewish, Christian, or other faith-based holidays within the same household. When making burial arrangements after the loss of a loved one, surviving non Muslim relatives may refuse to bury their Muslim relative because Islamic burial services are generally held within 48 hours of the death and do not include embalming. There are also cases of strained relations due to the convert's rejection of non-Muslim family members. The home-based practitioner must be careful to remain objective while evaluating whether conversion issues have any bearing on the presenting problem.

Decision Making

For many families the Islamic tradition of *shura* or consultation with family members is a natural part of how decisions are made about their careers, health, future, etc. In situations where a female Muslim client defers to male family members, the practitioner may automatically assume that the male figure is oppressive due to negative perceptions of Muslim males as well as females in the media. In these situations it is essential that the practitioner respect and honor a woman's right to self-determination. Clients should have the right to discuss and consult with whomever they feel supports them and can provide them with the best advice regarding their concerns. There is no norm relative to female deference in the Muslim home. Some women are very outspoken and self determined, while others adhere to familial and cultural practices not specific to Islam. Women may attempt to strike a delicate balance in order to maintain family harmony. Although self expression may be preferred, she may defer to her father or husband out of respect.

That being said, it is still important for the practitioner to be delicate and diplomatic while thoroughly assessing the situation. Sometimes this can best be achieved by acknowledging the male as the head of the household and speaking with the female in the presence of the head of the household. Once the head of the house feels respected by the practitioner, he may allow for more flexibility of expression between the practitioner and the client. However, in cases where domestic violence is suspected or known the practitioner must consider the best interest in maintaining the safety of all parties involved. Sometimes professionals acquiesce prematurely and wrongly attribute a practice as "religious or cultural" when it has nothing to do with either.

Ethical Considerations

The following sections highlight numerous ethical considerations that the home-based provider may encounter.

Confidentiality

It is essential to adhere to ethical behavior when working with clients in home-based settings. Although practitioners enter the home as professionals, they are also *guests*. The same honor and respect due for any other family group must be demonstrated for the Muslim family. Ethics related to confidentiality are sometimes difficult to negotiate in Muslim homes that insist on the presence of multiple family members during sessions. Social service practitioners are taught to protect the client's interest by not disclosing the client's personal information without the permission of the client (School Social Work Association of America, 2002). It is important that the practitioner maintain client confidentiality and not disclose personal family business, with the exception of cases of known or potential abuse (i.e., domestic violence, child/elder abuse). However, this may be challenging in home settings where multiple families or generations may live together, as may occur with new immigrants or refugees. The provider may ask the client to complete the usual release form(s) prior to inviting other family members or friends to join the session, as a way to accommodate cultural norms, but also protect the ethics of confidentiality. As previously stated, once rapport and trust have been established, the practitioner may find the family more willing to allow greater privacy in subsequent sessions.

Language Concerns

The Muslim population, as stated, is racially and ethnically diverse. The accompanying languages are equally varied. English may be the first and primary home language for indigenous Muslims born in the United States. First- and second-generation immigrants may use English to transact business in the larger society (i.e., work, school, etc.) but speak their native language in the home. Reverting to the native language is particularly common when relaxing in the company of others who speak the same language or when under stress. Basic English-speaking skills may be lacking for those women, especially older immigrant women, whose interaction is primarily in the home or within cultural enclaves and negotiated in their native language. Refugees and new immigrants may be reticent to practice their newly acquired English abilities due to a lack of confidence and proficiency.

The need for a translator should be assessed early, preferably prior to the initial home visit, if possible. A telephone language line is used by some agencies to assist with translation. Although many different languages can usually be accessed through this venue, the detached third-party nature of the conversation may impede the practitioner's ability to directly build rapport with the family/client. If the need for a translator is determined, family, friends, and neighbors may be very willing to assist and be readily available. Their assistance may prove helpful in emergencies, and when addressing basic concerns like the need for food, housing, or income. However, relying on friends, family, and neighbors for translation during in-depth therapy or in ongoing counseling situations is not recommended. Using children of any age to translate for parents may place the child and parent in an awkward position. Clients may be reluctant to share experiences they would not want their family member, friend, or neighbor to know about. Cox (2009) noted the embarrassment experienced by an adult son and father (patient) when the son had to ask his father about the regularity of his bowel movements. The translator may filter questions or information he or she feels will be embarrassing or unnecessary for the client or practitioner.

Filtering of this sort may distort both the client's ability to understand the practitioner's questions and comments as well as the practitioner's ability to accurately record the data. Given the varied educational levels and experiences of clients and translators, the practitioner should keep in mind that neither the translator nor the client may be versed in health care professional terminology. It is preferred that the translator is bicultural/bilingual, and knowledgeable and understanding of both the client's cultural linguistic nuances and those within the health care profession (Alwani & Abugideiri, 2003; Smart & Smart, 1995).

The close-knit nature of some Muslim communities may result in translators' acquaintance with clients through the mosque, as friends, or through other interactions. Because stigma and embarrassment is a great concern for many Muslim families, it is important to be sensitive to the client's concern about other community members knowing that they are receiving home-based services. It is recommended that the client sign a release noting the name of the particular translator prior to the session.

Those who learned English as a second language may have varied degrees of English comprehension and fluency (Alwani & Abugideiri, 2003). Some may speak English well but still have comprehension gaps when listening to native English speakers, especially if the speaker uses jargon and speaks fast. There may be a limited knowledge and understanding of professional terms and colloquial phrases. Practitioners' use of profanity is likely to have a negative impact on the client–practitioner relationship; religious Muslims, in particular, are likely to be offended. As in most professional relationships, profanity should be avoided. For individuals whose native language is not English, the practitioner should speak slowly, clearly, and limit the use of professional jargon and colloquial phrases. It is helpful to check for understanding periodically throughout the session. It is important to remain aware that the client for whom English is a second language may have educational levels and abilities that vary from limited schooling to postgraduate education.

Challenges to Maintaining Boundaries

Immigrant Muslim clients may be unfamiliar with the professional helping relationship. The practitioner may be viewed as a concerned friend rather than a helping professional. Social services and helping those in need is considered by Muslims to be acts of worship. They may not be cognizant of a need for professional boundaries. In this case, it is important to gently but clearly explain the rationale for differentiating the role of the practitioner from that of a friend. At the same time, it is desirable to have a friendly relationship with the client/family. Asking personal questions, treating the practitioner as a friend, calling or inviting the practitioner to the home outside of home-based service appointments, and gift giving is generally outside the boundaries of the professional relationship. However, it may be necessary for the practitioner to be somewhat flexible in order to build rapport by accepting small gifts or skillfully using self-disclosure. If strict or rigid boundaries are maintained without explanation, the established rapport may be lost or damaged.

Practitioner Bias or Lack of Cultural Awareness

Whether it is because of practitioner bias or a lack of cultural awareness, a provider may at times ignore the cultural issues discussed previously. The result of this can be that no rapport is built and the helping relationship fails to reach its intended goal of making a positive change in the client or family being served. This will only discourage the client/family from seeking services in the future. It is therefore incumbent on practitioners to confront their bias and excuse themselves from working with Muslim clients, if necessary. Often education about diverse cultural, religious, and spiritual beliefs through research or the use of a religious consultant will aid a practitioner in overcoming stereotypes and bias.

Conclusion

Home-based services are among the many ways practitioners provide mental health and other services to Muslims and those of other faiths and traditions. Information learned after reading this chapter may lead the practitioner to be more aware of important considerations related to the home life of Muslim families, as well as increasing the practitioner's effectiveness with Muslim clients. Although this chapter focused primarily on American Muslims, the information provided is applicable to work with Muslims residing in other Western countries.

Muslims are a diverse population with individuals and families from various countries and cultural traditions. Some were born and raised Muslims, while others converted to Islam. Muslims vary in cultural and religious practice and identification, which must be considered when providing service. Working with Muslims in their homes adds an extra layer of complexity for consideration. Practitioners are encouraged to utilize the material provided as a general framework for interactions.

Acknowledgment

The authors would like to acknowledge Denise Selvey for help in preparing this chapter.

References

Alwani, Z., & Abugideiri, S. (2003). *What Islam says about domestic violence: A guide for helping Muslim families.* Herndon, VA: Foundation for Appropriate and Immediate Help.

Bailey, C. (2002). The effect of spiritual beliefs and practices on family functioning: A qualitative study. In T. Carlson & M. Erickson (Eds.), *Spirituality and family therapy* (pp. 127–144). New York, NY: Hawthorne Press, Inc.

Bolson, M. D. (2004). *Children's behavioral health service definition manual.* Children, Youth, and Family Services Dept., New Mexico. Retrieved from http://cyfd.org/content/home-visiting

Boyd-Franklin, N. (2006). *Black families in therapy, understanding the African American experience.* New York, NY: Guilford Press.

Cox, C. (2009). Using relatives as translators creates a barrier to good care, *Nursing Standard, 23*(38), 29.

El-Amin Naeem, Z. (2008). *Jihad of the soul.* New York, NY: The Niyah Company.

Gallup Poll. (2009). Muslim Americans: A national portrait. *The Muslim West Facts Project.* Retrieved from www.PollingReport.com

Hodge, D., & Nadir, A. (2008). Moving toward culturally competent practice with Muslims: Modifying cognitive therapy with Islamic tenets. *Social Work, 53*(1), 31–42.

Hosnain, R., & Rana, S. (2010). Unveiling Muslim voices: Aging parents with disabilities and their adult children and family caregivers in the United States. *Topics in Geriatric Rehabilitation, 26*(1), 46–61.

Islamic Social Services Association (ISSA). (2003). *Muslim culture and faith: A guide for social service providers.* Tempe, AZ: USA Revised Edition.

Lum, D. (2005). *Cultural competence, practice stages, and client systems.* Pacific Grove, CA: Brooks/Cole.

Nadir, A., & Dziegielewski, S. F. (2001). Islam. In M. P. Van Hook, B. Hugen, & M. Aguilar, *Spirituality with religious traditions in social work practice* (pp. 146–162). Pacific Grove, CA: Brooks/Cole.

Nadir, P. (2003). *An act of faith: Voices of young Muslim women in America.* Arizona State University. Unpublished doctoral dissertation,

Pew Research Center. (2007). *Muslim Americans: Middle class and mostly mainstream.* Retrieved from www.pewresearch.org

Saeed, A. (2004). *Muslim Australians: Their beliefs, practices and institutions.* Retrieved from http://www.scribd.com/doc/5742490/Muslim-Australians-THEIR-BELIEFS-PRACTICES-AND-INSTITUTIONS-by-Professor-Abdullah-Saeed

Saleeby, D. (2002). *The strengths perspective in social work practice.* Boston, MA: Allyn and Bacon.

School Social Work Association of America. (2002). School social workers and confidentiality. In R. Constable, S. McDonald, & J. P. Flynn (Eds.), *School social work* (pp. 77–79). Chicago, IL: Lyceum Books, Inc.

Smart, J., & Smart, D. (1995). Using family as translators though convenient has caveats. *The Journal of Rehabilitation, 61*, 21–24.

Williams, R. H., & Vashi, G. (2007). Hijab and American Muslim women: Creating a space for autonomous selves. *Sociology of Religion, 68*(3), 269–287.

CHAPTER 12

University Counseling Centers

MAJEDA HUMEIDAN

Universities established counseling centers in the United States in response to the influx of soldiers returning from World War II. Those returning from deployment had the opportunity to engage in career counseling for readmission into the workforce or psychological counseling for better adjustment to college. Since that time, counseling centers at universities have become commonplace and remain a central point for mental health, as well as career services at university campuses throughout the United States and expanding across the globe. North American and British studies report that over the past decade the issues for which university students have sought counseling have become more complex and students are presenting to colleges with more severe and prevalent mental health issues (Adlaf, Glicksman, Demers, & Newton-Taylor, 2001; Heads of University Counselling Services [HUCS], 2002). Perhaps students see university counseling centers as more accessible than off-campus mental health services, and therefore counseling centers are seeing an increase in demand (Benton, Robertson, Tseng, Newton, & Benton, 2003). Some argue that mental health concerns are on the rise, while others argue that those with chronic mental health issues are more likely to enter universities than they had in years past given the advances in mental health treatment. Still, some might suggest that the stigma to seek counseling is less, and therefore students are seeking counseling in greater numbers. Although it is unclear why the demand for counseling services is higher, university counseling centers often serve to facilitate the educational, career, and psychological development of students.

The rate of Muslim students seeking services at university counseling is not known, and few counseling centers identify the religious identity of clients. However, it may be assumed that the issues for which Muslim students seek counseling might be similar to their peers with regard to clinical symptoms, issues related to age and life stage such as individuation issues, and career exploration concerns. For example, questions related to choice of career or negotiating parental expectations and personal choices are common among college students. Muslims who are ethnic minorities, children of recent immigrants, or international students may also present with issues related to their identities or immigration status. For example, forming support networks in a new college environment is common to many, whereas adjustment related to cultural differences in a new country may pose challenges for some international students who are also Muslim. Muslim students at counseling centers may present with concerns directly related to their religious identity, such as religious practice in a new environment. Muslim college students may experience concerns directly related to their identity, immigration status, or international student status, as well as other clinical issues faced by peers, such as adjustment concerns, affective disturbances, or any other clinical presentation.

A case example of a Muslim college student seeking counseling at a university counseling center in the United States is presented here to highlight potential client or counselor concerns. Where available, literature that supports issues of relevance to counseling Muslim students at university counseling centers is presented. And finally, recommendations for counseling center counselors are presented for those who wish to be more accessible to Muslim students and offer more culturally sensitive counseling services.

CASE SCENARIO

An Asian American counselor conducted an outreach program on women's career issues for the Asian American Student Organization on a university campus. Following the program, a client, Aneesa, self-referred to therapy requesting to meet with a counselor. While completing paperwork, under "ethnicity" she wrote, "South Asian Muslim feminist woman." At intake, Aneesa, who wore an Islamic headscarf or *hijab*, reported feeling distressed over a conflict she had with her parents. The student reported that she had wanted to fast (during Ramadan), which coincided with midterms. Aneesa reported that many students in her new social support network fasted, and she felt this was an important aspect of her religious identity. However, her parents expressed their concern that fasting would negatively impact her studies, so advised her not to do it. She also stated that fasting was not negotiable to her and was not necessarily the topic she wished to discuss, and that her interest was in addressing conflict with family. The client conveyed that she had a similar conflict with her parents over religion when she chose to wear the Muslim headscarf, or *hijab*, as they feared she would be discriminated against and have difficulties gaining employment.

As the counselor was not familiar with Islamic fasting or headdress rules, she considered referring Aneesa to a Muslim counselor in the community whom she thought would be in a better position to understand the client. When the counselor explored this with the client, Aneesa said that a same-religion counselor was not necessary for her, but was open to the referral if the therapist preferred this. The client added that having an Asian American counselor like herself was also beneficial. Aneesa did not share that the Muslim community in her college town was small and that she was worried that she would be referred to someone within her social network; that is, Aneesa had concerns about confidentiality and the social stigma of counseling, which she did not share with the counselor. The counselor also experienced some feelings of discomfort, because she had overlooked the common ethnicity she shared with Aneesa, as she had focused on the more apparent religious differences. For this reason and others, the counselor sought clinical supervision.

The counselor's supervisor reinforced Aneesa's suggestion that a Muslim counselor was not necessary, especially as the counselor was open to exploring issues with her client, consulting with Muslim community leaders as needed, and seeking outside resources. Also, given that the client's presenting concerns (value differences with her parents, familial expectations, and concerns related to being a first-generation university student) were ones the counselor felt competent to address, a decision was made to not refer the client.

As counseling sessions progressed, Aneesa reported that she felt pressure by her parents to pursue a professional career in pharmacy (like her father) or engineering or medicine. They often told Aneesa that she would not have to search for jobs if she pursued such paths, and that they had worked hard for her to be academically prepared for such studies. Aneesa's parents requested that she not engage in political or religious issues at college, and that she focus on her studies. Aneesa attributed her parents' request to minimize outward expressions of her religion to their immigration status, as well as their desire to protect her from discrimination and aggression. The counselor openly explored such issues and Aneesa disclosed her fears that the counselor might also believe that she should not wear the *hijab*. The client also discussed feeling anger and fear as a result of several incidents of hate against her, as well as one of her social support networks, the Muslim Student Organization.

Aneesa moreover presented with symptoms of anxiety related to exams, her future career, and feelings of guilt related to not appeasing her parents. She had reported eating and sleep disturbances, decreased ability to focus on her studies, and increased isolation. The counselor assessed Aneesa for sociocultural stressors, recent triggers, past trauma, and coping strategies, as she offered a thorough assessment for depression and anxiety disorders, and ruled out disordered eating. As Aneesa continued in individual counseling, she also disclosed having experienced several incidents of hate/bias while at university. She had kept these incidents from her family for fear that her family would blame her or worry excessively about her. The counselor explored these assertions further as they relate to Aneesa's dynamics with family.

Additionally, the counselor, who felt she had been actively involved in many "stop-hate" programs on campus, experienced feelings of guilt at not having extended her programming to the Muslim student group, especially after a few well-publicized incidents of hate on campus. For these concerns and others, the counselor sought supervision. The counselor was urged by her supervisor to remain neutral and not become involved in political issues. Although the counselor appreciated the concerns of her supervisor, she wondered about the limits of her social justice training, as well as the impact on Muslim students, including her client, who may become aware that counseling center staff attended other "stop-hate" events but not theirs. She struggled with her center's stance on whether it constituted hypocrisy or a legitimate strategy. The counselor joined a social justice discussion group in the psychology department at campus to explore such issues further.

The following discussion highlights several issues mentioned in this case, with chapter headings guiding the reader through the topics.

Identities and Labels with Muslims in Counseling

Religious identity questions are not commonly included in counseling center demographic or intake questionnaires. Questions about ethnicity only rarely convey information about religious identity. Muslims in the United States, for example, fall under various racial and ethnic categories, such as Asian American, African American, European American, and to a lesser extent Latino American (Gallup, 2009). Many Muslims who are also Arab American may identify as "other" in the absence of a more fitting ethnicity label (McCarus, 1994). Counseling centers are urged to inquire about religious identity and its role in clients' lives. The client in the case scenario, Aneesa, wore a headscarf, and therefore she may have been visibly identifiable as Muslim. Both identities, her religion and ethnicity, are significant to her. Muslims such as Aneesa whose religion is visible could be at risk for incidents of hate. Additionally, she may be more likely to be identified by her religion, rather than her ethnic identity.

Religion may be an identity that is constant or fluctuating in its salience. Those whose religion is more salient to others, or outwardly expressed via Islamic clothing, for example, may have a different experience of their religion on university campuses. But religiosity should not be assumed by such outward expressions, such as beards for men or *hijab* for women. Outward expression or "visibility" should not be assumed to mirror level of religiosity among men and women; the role of religion on religious clients must be assessed in therapy. For some, headdress or type of covering may be a cultural expression of family tradition more than religiosity. However, in the case of Aneesa the *hijab* was a sign of religious expression. For Aneesa, the "Muslim" label intersected with gender, ethnic identity, and other social identities creates a more complex identity.

Although not specific to Muslims, counselors are urged to be attuned to within-group differences and intersecting identities among adolescents holding a religious identity (Magaldi-Dopman & Park-Taylor, 2010) and those seeking counseling services. For example, Arab American Muslims have been found to experience more acculturative stress and less social support than their Christian Arab counterparts (Amer & Hovey, 2007). Furthermore, little is known about Asian American Muslim students, who may ethnically belong to the "model minority" group in the United States with the many stressors and privileges the label carries (Yoo, Burrola, & Steger, 2010) and also identify as "Muslim." Additionally, international Muslim students who travel to the West for further education may have difficulty facing (perhaps for the first time) negative attitudes directed against their religious identity.

In the United States, when people were asked what comes to mind when they hear the word "Muslim" many expressed negative comments, whereas only 2% reported a positive response (Council on American Islamic Relations [CAIR], 2004). Although the survey was conducted in various segments of the U.S. community, it is assumed that such attitudes would similarly be present on college campuses in Western nations. Little research is available in the area; however, students at a large Midwestern college reported subtle forms of discrimination against those with Arabic names (Bushman & Bonacci, 2007). Racist students were less likely to want to help students with Arab names than those with European names. Counselors are encouraged to create a safe space for clients to describe any race-based stress, experiences of discrimination, and other such issues. In Aneesa's case, the client had withheld disclosing such discriminatory experiences from her parents, but felt safe to disclose her experiences to her counselor, which created an opportunity to explore the client's reaction, coping strategies, and impact on her overall mental health and identity issues. In addition, the counselor was prepared to explore her areas of growth in supervision, such as feelings related to the lack of programming with Muslim students.

Little research is available about counselors' attitudes toward Muslims; however, survey research supports that people who were more highly educated in the United States held fewer misperceptions about Arab Americans, but were also more likely to believe that Arab or Arab American women were oppressed by men (Gallup, 2009). Similarly, it is possible that college students and college professors, as well as counselors who have not thoroughly examined their biases, may hold such attitudes. Many Muslim women, on the other hand, find the label "feminist" congruent with their religious identity (Ali, Mahmood, Moel, Hudson, & Leathers, 2008). In the case described, Aneesa also identified as feminist and sought a feminist counselor; however, this was not addressed by the counselor or explored further. Whereas counseling may not be an appropriate place to discuss differences in theoretical issues, including the definition of feminism, those seeking counseling may be concerned about counselors' knowledge about their values, religion, and beliefs, as well as their attitudes toward Muslims, in general.

Presenting Issues

Clients at university counseling centers are most likely to seek counseling for issues related to relationships, anxiety, family issues, educational concerns, depression, and situational issues (Benton et al., 2003). Muslim clients are also likely to present with these clinical concerns. In addition, Muslim international students may also experience adjustment concerns, whereas recent immigrants, or children of recent immigrants, may face acculturative stress (Abu Baker, 1999; Zhou, 1997). It has also been noted that Muslims, in general, may present with higher rates of post-traumatic stress disorder, and Arab Americans may experience a heightened sense of anxiety and feeling unsafe (Abu-Ras & Abu-Bader, 2008). Given that many Muslims have experienced some form of racism (CAIR, 2004), assessment of the impact of such incidents on clients or clients' families is warranted (Carter, 2007). Speight (2007) argues that internalized racism should be examined among ethnic/racial minorities, as it may result in isolation and other negative consequences. Negative experiences associated with negative bias and racism are not uncommon for Muslims in America. Public polling revealed that Muslims reported feelings of anger and sadness more than those of other religious groups (Gallup, 2009). Additionally, Muslims surveyed were also more likely to identify themselves as "struggling" (although this was not specifically defined) more than other religious groups, despite their greater likelihood of being employed or engaged in academic pursuits (Gallup, 2009). Such surveys, although not specific to college students, may offer some insight into Muslim clients of counseling centers seeking career or psychological counseling.

It is not uncommon that Muslims are perceived to be "foreign" regardless of their ethnicity; implications of being perceived as "foreign" may include a sense of being marginalized or glass ceiling effects in the workplace. This would have implications on career counseling with Muslim college students. It should be noted that institutional racism and interpersonal prejudice are more important predictors of job quality than work stressors (Morgan, Beale, Mattis, Stovall, & White, 2000). Little is known about at what rate Muslim students seek counseling to address such concerns; however, counselors working at university counseling centers with students who are in their first jobs or preparing for their careers must be aware of such issues. In the case of Aneesa, for example, her parents were concerned about the potential impact that her outward religious expression (wearing the *hijab*) may have on her future job opportunities and job quality.

Religion and Coping

When clinicians assess the role of religion and levels of religiosity among their clients, they should seek to identify and integrate positive coping strategies from Islam into therapy (Abu Raiya & Pargament, 2010). Some university counseling centers have tailored stigma reduction programs toward various groups, including Muslims on campus, whereas others have modified their outreach related to suicide prevention to address Muslim students. Any such programs must be created in collaboration and consultation with Muslim leaders on campus, mental health professionals, and the target audience. For reference, Ali, Liu, and Humeidan (2004) provide information about the role of Muslim values, gender issues, and cultural/religious variables on trust building and the therapeutic alliance with Muslim clients. Additionally, Dwairy (2006) offers a more comprehensive resource for practitioners working with Muslim (and Arab) clients including concerns related to intergenerational conflict and restoring family "harmony." Most Muslim youth experience their religion as a source of strength and an avenue for social support (Abu Raiya & Pargament, 2010). Pardoxically, Muslims in the United States were more likely than members of other religions to report a lack of social support, and they did not have anyone to rely on in times of need (Gallup, 2009). Perhaps college organizations, student life, or other structured activities may provide a different experience for Muslim college students, offering an avenue of social support not readily available to nonstudents. Counselors should explore whether Muslim students who seek counseling share similar concerns as the more general

Muslim population surveyed with regard to isolation, or if the university environment or group involvement offers protection against such isolation.

Referral Sources and Help-Seeking Behavior

Muslim college students may readily seek medical services, as it is acceptable and encouraged in Islam to seek medical care. Although Aneesa had self-referred to counseling, it would not be unusual for her to have sought medical help for her eating and sleep disturbances and other symptoms prior to seeking counseling. Counselors must be aware that given the acceptance of the medical treatment, Muslim college students may present to counseling via referrals by medical professionals whom they may visit for physical symptoms or psychosomatic concerns. Therefore, counselors must establish strong ties with the medical professionals on campus to facilitate referrals of Muslim students who may benefit from counseling. Additionally, positive relationships with residence hall staff, Muslim chaplains, if any, as well as international student programming may be alternate ways to reach out to Muslim students.

Counseling center staff may be trained to provide services to university students who have various clinical presentations, career concerns, experiences of racism, and feelings of marginalization—all of which are recognized as potential concerns for Muslim students. However, more significantly, clients who experience racism may be less likely to seek counseling when needed (Morgan & Robinson, 2003). Cultural mistrust may impact help seeking among various ethnic minorities, as was recently observed among Filipino Americans (David, 2010). A "stigmatized" identity may also be related to attitudes toward seeking career counseling (Ludwikowski, Vogel, & Armstrong, 2009). At a time when job discrimination against Muslims is high (CAIR, 2004) and as university students are working toward building their careers, Muslim students' need for career counseling may be high. However, counselors must be aware that Muslim students who have internalized stigma related to their identities, and who may benefit from counseling services, including career counseling, may not readily access it.

Outreach and Social Justice

Outreach to various student groups is a component of many counseling centers, and most regard it as a necessary means to educate students about mental health issues and the centers' services and staff. Outreach may also serve as an entry point to students who may not readily seek counseling centers. Aneesa, as described in the case scenario, sought counseling after attending an outreach program provided by the counselor. It is not uncommon for university students, in general, as well as international and Muslim students, in particular, to become more aware of college counseling services and seek counseling following psychoeducational outreach programs.

There are many potentially positive results for outreach/intervention programs with Muslim students. Programs may be presented specifically for Muslim college students or presented in a more general manner, with advertising efforts targeting Muslim students as well as others. For example, a program called "Finding Your Voice in a College Classroom" advertised by the author at a large university resulted in a higher number of Muslim students in attendance than a program called "My Religion, My Strength: Muslim College Student Discussion Group" by the same counselor earlier that month. One may make many assumptions about the reason for the numbers—a reflection on the relevance of the topics to the college students, interest to discuss religious identity with a university counselor, or time and date factors. Further exploration revealed that all of these issues played a role, but also that students noted that the "Muslim Identity" program brought up some safety concerns as it was heavily advertised and students had fear about hate crimes. Also, as the Muslim Student Association was not familiar with the counselor or counseling center, they did not announce or encourage members to attend. Therefore, whereas outreach programs in general (or advertisements for programs, even if unattended) may offer value to university students as they open a door to university counseling centers, programming related to identity issues is best done in consultation with the target groups.

Not only might psychoeducational programming facilitate a climate of trust in the counseling center and staff conducting the program, it may also facilitate student academic success. Research suggests that students who faced racism and engaged in an intervention program to increase their sense of belonging within the academic setting were more likely to have positive engagement in the academic environment (Walton & Cohen, 2007). If the results of the study were generalized to Muslim university students, intervention programs that aim to decrease experiences of marginalization may result in academic success, as well as enhance mental health.

Counselors (such as the one in the case scenario with Aneesa) may be eager to engage in social justice programming, or even to increase their awareness of social justice issues, but may not have received training in this area. Additionally, supervisors may not be equipped to facilitate trainees' growth in the area or feel ambivalent about the role of social advocacy in a counseling center. In the case of Aneesa, the counselor's clinical supervisor urged her to be more neutral and not engage in social advocacy with Muslim students, but Aneesa's counselor had concerns about her inaction. In such a case, Aneesa's counselor and her supervisor may have benefited from further discussion and training opportunities. Urging counseling psychologists to actively engage in combating institutional racism is not a new concept and dates back several decades (Lopez & Cheek, 1977); however, more recently, Kiselica and Robinson (2001) urged counselors to take notice of history and embrace the rise in social justice issues in the counseling profession. Newer or emerging counselors may receive training on social justice issues beginning at the practicum level (Burnes & Singh, 2010; Lewis, 2010). Regardless of training received, counselors would benefit from guidance and supervision when engaging in advocacy programs. Bradley, Lewis, Hendricks, and Crews (2008) offer recommendations for those who provide supervision (a common component of university counseling centers) to enhance their skills related to social justice advocacy. In addition to attention to clinical skills, counselors at university counseling centers must be prepared to apply social justice skills to better access and reach marginalized communities and students. Reaching Muslim students at university campuses would maximize the chances that clients, such as Aneesa, would be open to engaging in counseling services with culturally sensitive therapists.

Recommendations for Culturally Sensitive Counseling with Muslims

Readers are urged to revisit the case scenario described at the opening of this chapter in light of recommendations for counselors described in the following. Those with an interest in building on their skills with Muslims would benefit from reflecting on their assumptions, new insight, or decision-making process as they examine their approach with Aneesa. Counselors at university counseling centers are in a unique position to facilitate counseling accessibility for Muslim clients. They are encouraged to follow the recommendations to help create an environment that is more conducive to a strong therapeutic alliance. Those with an interest in developing their cultural sensitivity with Muslims seeking services at university counseling centers are urged to examine the following suggestions and consider their fit with the mission of their counseling centers:

- Counseling centers often utilize demographic questionnaires at intake that ask about race and gender and other such questions; counseling centers are urged to ask questions about religion and, if relevant to the client, ethnicity and country of origin.
- Counselors must be prepared to educate clients about the counseling process, recognizing that Muslim clients may have confidentiality concerns.
- Counselors must be prepared to examine their attitudes and biases, and explicitly or implicitly address this in supervision as well as with clients in a therapeutic manner, as Muslim clients may assume that counselors have negative assumptions about their religion, ethnicity, or gender.

- Counselors are urged to examine the role of religion and spirituality in their lives and to facilitate self-awareness and recognition of such variables on their clients (Magladi-Dopman & Park-Taylor, 2010).
- Counselors must be prepared to assess for and integrate multiple social identities (Yakushko, Davidson, & Williams, 2009) and be aware of within-group differences of Muslim clients.
- Counselors must express interest in learning about Muslim clients and their culture, while being attuned to the client as an individual and not as a representative of his or her larger community.
- Counselors working with Muslim clients must assess for immigration-related stressors or race-related trauma of clients or in families, when relevant, and assess stages of adjustment of international students, if appropriate.
- Counselors must broaden their cultural perspectives from direct sources, and expand sources of data about Muslims and interact with others from various communities. The political and world news sources are not always good sources of data on culture or client experiences.
- Counselors working with international students or recent immigrants should be aware of or open to learning about current world events that may impact the clients' perspectives.
- Counselors must know when to refer out and/or seek consultation from other mental health professionals or those with knowledge of Muslim client issues.
- Counselors working with Muslim clients must be prepared to seek supervision when their concerns may impede building a therapeutic alliance; they may also be prepared to refer out if they are unable to provide a positive therapeutic environment or withhold biases.
- Counselors must be prepared to validate experiences with and/or implications of racism or oppression among Muslim clients, being careful to avoid directly or indirectly minimizing, justifying, or comparing to other groups, including challenging any incidents of "competitive victimization."
- Counselors must not provide a null environment but seek to actively recognize and counter any negative biases. If not in an advocacy role, counselors should be prepared to offer a positive environment to counteract a discriminatory environment.
- Counselors must be aware of the implications of political events or politics on the institutional/larger university/community climate, and the counseling center's mission statement.
- Counselors who wish to be more accessible to Muslim clients and advocate for them may benefit from social justice training.

Conclusion

Although rarely identified, religion may be a salient identity among counseling center clients. Individuals who identify as "Muslim" may find religion to be an integral aspect of their lives and rely on religion for positive coping strategies. On the other hand, Muslim clients may carry a significant social stigma associated with their religious affiliation or expect the counselor to hold negative attributions; such factors cannot be ignored when providing culturally sensitive therapy on university campuses. Race-based stress and trauma may not be uncommon among Muslims (Abu-Ras & Abu-Bader, 2008), but recent studies have found that integrating positive coping strategies, derived from religion, may facilitate therapeutic outcome (Abu Raiya & Pargament, 2010).

Muslim clients or college-aged individuals may seek counseling for reasons similar to non-Muslim university students. However, given the climate of cultural mistrust and being a member of a misunderstood group, counselors may need to examine the role of the Muslim identity on clients. Religious identity, in general, should form a part of the counseling center's ongoing discussions about access to services, counselor attitudes, and the therapy process. Counselors must be aware of the impact of racism on clients, as well as on themselves. Those living within a climate of "misunderstanding" may not be immune to negative attributions about Muslims. Counselors, however, may possess or access the educational knowledge and tools to counter their biases.

Supervision, consultation, and seeking appropriate sources of knowledge may result in greater awareness of within-group differences and the intersecting social identities of clients. Outreach is also necessary but may not be sufficient to ease Muslim university students' receptiveness to counseling. Therefore, counselors must be aware of the contextual and cultural variables related to counseling Muslims: What is presented on the intake forms? Which magazines are present at the counselor center waiting room? In what ways does the counseling center climate and larger institution facilitate or hinder Muslim students seeking counseling? Social justice training programs are recommended for counseling center counselors; such programs may result in enhanced skills and support for counselors working with clients who have experiences of oppression and racism, including Muslim clients.

References

Abu Baker, (1999). Acculturation and reacculturation influence: Multilayer contexts in therapy. *Clinical Psychology Review, 19,* 951–967.

Abu Raiya, H., & Pargament, K. I. (2010). Religiously integrated psychotherapy with Muslim clients: From research to practice. *Professional Psychology: Research and Practice, 41*, 181–188.

Abu-Ras, W., & Abu-Bader, S. H. (2008). The impact of September 11, 2001 attacks on the well-being of Arab-Americans in New York City. *Journal of Muslim Mental Health, 3*, 217–239.

Adlaf, E., Glicksman, L., Demers, A., & Newton-Taylor, B. (2001). The prevalence of elevated psychological distress among Canadian undergraduates: Findings from the 1998 Canadian campus survey. *Journal of American College Health, 50*, 67–72.

Ali, S. R., Liu, W., & Humeidan, M. (2004). Islam 101: Understanding the religion and therapy implications. *Professional Psychology: Research and Practice, 35*, 635–642.

Ali, S. R., Mahmood, A., Moel, J., Hudson, C., & Leathers, L. (2008). A qualitative investigation of Muslim and Christian women's views of religion and feminism in their lives. *Cultural Diversity and Ethnic Minority Psychology, 14*, 38–46.

Amer, M. A., & Hovey, J. D. (2007). Socio-demographic differences in acculturation and mental health for a sample of 2nd generation/early immigrant Arab Americans. *Journal of Immigrant and Minority Mental Health, 9*, 335–347.

Benton, S. A, Robertson, J. M. Tseng, W.-C., Newton, F. B., & Benton, S. L. (2003). Changes in counseling center client problems across 13 years. *Professional Psychology: Research and Practice*, 66–72.

Bradley, L. J., Lewis, J., Hendricks, B., & Crews, C. R. (2008). *Advocacy: Implications for supervision training.* Alexandria, VA: American Counseling Association.

Burnes, T. R., & Singh, A.A. (2010). Integrating social justice training into the practicum experience for psychology trainees: Starting earlier. *Training and Education in Professional Psychology, 4*, 153–162.

Bushman, B. J., & Bonacci, A. M. (2007). You've got mail: Using e-mail to examine the effect of prejudiced attitudes on discrimination against Arabs. *Journal of Experimental Social Psychology, 40*, 753–759.

Carter, R. (2007). *The Counseling Psychologist, 35*, 144–154.

Council on American Islamic Relations, (CAIR). (2004). *Civil Rights Report.* Retrieved from www.cair.com/CivilRights/CivilRightsReports/2004Report.aspx

David, E. J. (2010). Cultural mistrust and mental health-seeking attitudes among Filipino Americans. *Asian American Journal of Psychology, 1*, 57–66.

Dwairy, M. (2006). *Counseling and psychotherapy with Arabs and Muslims: A culturally sensitive approach.* New York, NY: Teachers University Press.

Gallup. (2009). *Muslim Americans: A national portrait.* Retrieved from http://www.muslimwestfacts.com/mwf/116074/Muslim-Americans-National-Portrait.aspx

Heads of University Counselling Centers (HUCS). (2002). *Survey of medical, psychiatric and counselling provision in higher education.* Retrieved from http://www.hucs.org

Herek, G. M., Gillis, J. R., & Cogan, J. C. (1999). Psychological sequelae of hate crime victimization among lesbian, gay, and bisexual adults. *Journal of Consulting and Clinical Psychology, 67*, 945–951.

Kiselica, M. S., & Robinson, M. (2001). Bringing advocacy counseling to life: The history issues and human dramas of social justice. *Journal of Counseling and Development, 79*, 387–397.

Lewis, B. L. (2010). Social justice in practicum training: Competencies and developmental implications. *Training and Education in Professional Psychology, 4,* 145–152.

Lopez, R. E., & Cheek, D. (1977). The prevention of institutional racism: Training counseling psychologists as agents for change. *The Counseling Psychologist, 7,* 64–88.

Ludwikowski, W. M., Vogel, D., & Armstrong, P. I. (2009). Attitudes toward career counseling: The role of public and self-stigma. *Journal of Counseling Psychology, 56,* 408–416.

Magaldi-Dopman, D., & Park-Taylor, J. (2010). Sacred adolescence: Practical suggestions for psychologists working with adolescents with religious and spiritual identity. *Professional Psychology: Research and Practice, 41,* 382–390.

McCarus, E. N. (Ed.). (1994). *The development of Arab-American identity.* Ann Arbor, MI: University of Michigan Press.

Morgan, L. M., Beale, R. L., Mattis, J. S., Stovall, E. L., & White, D. L. (2000). The combined impact of racism at work, non-racial work stress, and financial stress on Black women's psychological well-being. *African American Research Perspectives, 6,* 41–50.

Morgan, N. T., & Robinson M. (2003). Students' help-seeking behavior. *Canadian Journal of Counselling, 37,* 151–166.

Speight, S.L. (2007). Internalized racism: One more piece of the puzzle. *The Counseling Psychologist, 35,* 126–134.

Walton, G. M., & Cohen, G. L. (2007). A question of belonging: Race, social fit, and achievement. *Journal of Personality and Social Psychology, 92,* 82–96.

Yakushko, O., Davidson, M. M., & Williams, E. N. (2009). Identity salience model: A paradigm for integrating multiple identities into clinical practice. *Psychotherapy: Theory, Research, Practice, Training, 46,* 180–192.

Yoo, H. C., Burrola, K. S., & Steger, M. F. (2010). A preliminary report on a new measure: Internalization of the Model Minority Myth Measure (IM-4) and its psychological correlates among Asian American university students. *Journal of Counseling Psychology, 57,* 114–127.

Zhou, M. (1997). Growing up American: The challenge confronting immigrant children and children of immigrants. *Annual Review of Sociology, 23,* 63–95.

PART IV
Special Populations

CHAPTER 13
Converts to Islam

SAMEERA AHMED

Increasing numbers of people living in Western nations are converting[1] to Islam. The act of conversion is simple and only requires that individuals testify that they believe there is no God but Allah and that Muhammad is His messenger, a declaration known as the *shahadah*. Although conversion is a simple act, the resulting transformation in the convert's life may be monumental.

Muslims who convert to Islam are heterogeneous groups that vary in their religious and racial/ethnic backgrounds, pathways to conversion, as well as interpretation and practice of Islam. As such, conversion can have a differing impact on individuals' lives. For some converts, their new faith can serve as a source of support and solace in times of need and as a response to life challenges. For others, personal or environmental reactions to their conversion will result in additional sources of stress. For some, conversion to Islam can be a response to stress, a cause of stress, a solution to stress, and even all three at the same time. However, for other converts their conversion may have minimal impact, such as conversions to facilitate marriage.[2]

---

[1] Many Muslims who convert prefer to call themselves "reverts" instead of "converts" because of a hadith, or saying of the Prophet, that indicated God created all humans in a pure state of submitting or acknowledging God (i.e., Islam). It is their environment that makes them an individual of another faith. Therefore, many people believe they are reverting back to their natural state and thus prefer the term "revert" to be used. However, given the greater use of the term in the literature, the term "convert" will be used throughout the chapter.

[2] The Qur'an states, "Let there be no compulsion in religion" (2:256). In theory, conversion should not take place unless the individual believes in the faith. However, in reality conversion for marriage reasons does occur, and the clinician should not automatically assume that conversion will necessarily mean that the changes highlighted in this chapter will apply to all converts.

Muslim converts may face many similar problems and mental health difficulties as the general public. They also share many of the challenges that lifelong Muslims face due to having the same beliefs and similar treatment by their environment. Converts may not need to seek counseling; however, those who do may not realize the role that conversion may have on their mental issues. When converts seek treatment, they are not likely to present with questions regarding their faith; for such issues they are likely to seek a religious support person. As such, the clinician working with Muslim converts will need to be able to understand the subtleties that conversion may have within a clinical setting.

This chapter is an attempt to highlight the unique issues and challenges that are specific to Muslim converts. Despite within-group differences among converts, there are many similar issues experienced. The chapter begins by presenting a case study that will be used for purposes of discussion throughout the chapter. Subsequently, the chapter explores possible pathways and processes of conversion. Specific factors that may impact clinical presentation and treatment are identified (i.e., individual, family, and environment) in order to assist clinicians in understanding complicating factors. Finally, religiously sensitive counseling recommendations are offered for clinicians who may be counseling Muslim converts.

CASE STUDY: MARTHA BEECH[3]

Martha is a 35-year-old African American Muslim convert whose infant son was recently taken away by Child Protective Services due to her repeated heroin use. She is the mother of four other children who reside with her, but who may be taken away if she does not end her drug use. Martha is currently enrolled in a drug rehabilitation program that requires her to participate in both individual and group psychotherapy.

In the initial interview, the client reported depressive features such as loss of interest in activities, depressed mood most of the day, loss of energy, feelings of excessive guilt, and diminished ability to think or concentrate during the last three months. Martha also reported inability to get out of bed, constant crying, and daydreaming about her infant son. She is worried about the potential loss of her other children if she does not address her addiction. She presented for treatment wearing *niqab*, a face veil that covers the lower part of the face up to the eyes, and an *abaya*, a loose-fitting full-length robe that covers the entire body.

---

[3] The name and details of the case have been modified for purposes of confidentiality.

The clinical interview revealed a complex family history. When Martha was eight years old, her mother left her and her two younger siblings because of their father's abusive behavior. Martha has not had contact with her mother since then; her paternal aunt subsequently filled in as a maternal figure. Martha described her father as being strict, and he regularly used corporal punishment to discipline them. Martha described being closest to her younger brother, who was a major source of support throughout her life. When she converted two years ago, he also converted. He passed away nine months ago, due to complications associated with AIDS. His death resulted in immense emotional pain, which contributed to her heroin relapse. Martha's younger sister is still alive and is a drug addict who constantly encourages Martha to use drugs.

Martha converted three years ago after she met her husband Malik, an African American Muslim convert of eight years; the two later married. Martha reports that Malik is the first man who has taken care of her, loves her, and respects her as a woman. She reports that he treats her children from previous relationships well and never asks her for money. Martha is afraid of losing Malik because of her drug use, because substance use is prohibited in Islam. She wonders why he stays with her, given her drug use. Malik is in a leadership position within their local urban Muslim community, which causes Martha to be even more embarrassed of her drug use. He has no prior history of drug use and is not familiar with associated signs and symptoms. Malik had assumed that her behaviors were due to postpartum depression. He was unaware of Martha's drug use until their son was taken away from them. Once Malik was informed about Martha's drug use and attempts for recovery, he appeared supportive but did not appear to fully understand the depth of her struggle.

Martha was diagnosed with major depressive disorder and opioid dependence. At the onset of treatment, there are no obvious diagnostic issues related to Martha's conversion. However, through the process of the clinical interview and the course of treatment, varying factors related to her conversion are identified, which will be highlighted throughout the chapter.

Conversion Process

Knowledge of the conversion process—the varied experiences, challenges, and supports—will help clinicians to be more empathic with their clients. In addition, such knowledge can inform a more accurate diagnosis and case formulation, and provide appropriate treatment intervention that can guide the client toward recovery. Given that there is no set conversion process, individuals may become interested in Islam through varying pathways. This section presents possible pathways and reasons for conversion.

Exploratory Phase

Muslim converts are introduced to Islam through varying pathways that may include a specific incident or an internal desire that may slowly unravel over time. Some converts are introduced to Islam by a Muslim, such as a peer, coworker, neighbor, student, romantic partner, or family member (Sulaiman-Hill, 2007; Poston, 1991). In Martha's case, she had been impressed by the mannerisms of her future husband and wished to live a similar life—a life free from substance use, and possessing family structure and closeness to God. Other individuals may become interested in Islam after traveling to Muslim-majority countries or interacting with Muslims. People's interest in Islam may also be piqued due to repetitive news stories, both positive and negative, resulting from global sociopolitical events.

Converts vary in their family history and background, which may or may not influence their conversion. Some converts report having had a religious upbringing (Kose, 1999), while others may not have had prior exposure to religion, as in Martha's case. Converts may come from families that encouraged communication and religious exploration, or they may have a history of interpersonal conflict with their primary sources of support, which can contribute to the reevaluation of their lives (Spalek & El-Hassan, 2006).

Muslim converts may report a process of disenchantment with previous religious beliefs and practices and then choose to differentiate from their faith group (Spalek & El-Hassan, 2006). They may also experience feelings of alienation from their childhood religious community because they are unable to maintain their evolving identity within their childhood social context/system (Kose, 1999). As such, individuals may explore alternative religions and culture, with the hopes of obtaining greater meaning and purpose in life (Kose, 1999). In this process of examining alternative religions, they may attempt to make meaning of personal values and beliefs (Paloutzian, 2005). The period of deliberation before converting may vary for converts in terms of length of time as well as in-depth analysis.

Converts report varying reasons for conversion. Converts may be attracted to Islamic beliefs, such as monotheism, a personal connection to God without intermediaries, as well as rejection of former religious concepts (Sulaiman-Hill, 2007). Islam's emphasis on morality, family values, sense of community, and promotion of the scientific method are also reasons for conversion (Sulaiman-Hill, 2007; Lakhdar, Vinsonneau, Apter, & Mullet, 2007). Individuals may also have been attracted to the social justice elements of Islam, based on prior experience with injustice (Spalek &

El-Hassan, 2006). In addition, some converts experience frustration due to perceived over-secularization or moral permissiveness of their respective religious traditions and feel the need to seek an alternative spiritual pathway (Kose, 1999).

Conversion

Once individuals decide to convert, they begin a process of adjusting or aligning their past beliefs and values with their knowledge and understanding of Islam (McGinty, 2007*)*. For individuals from Christian and Judaic backgrounds, this process may be easier because Islam acknowledges familiar religious texts and historical figures, and shares basic beliefs of morality. For example, the Qur'an highlights the exemplar character of the Virgin Mary and the Prophet Jesus, as well as the struggles of the Prophets Joseph, Moses, Aaron, David, and Solomon and encourages Muslims to live up to their morals and examples. As such, converts from Abrahamic backgrounds are able to maintain previous figures but modify their understanding of them.

Converts may describe the initial years of conversion as tumultuous with many high and low points. The conversion to Islam can be spiritually comforting, intellectually satisfying, and give converts a sense of purpose in life. However, it can be tempered by challenges adjusting to their new religion. The challenges may be related to individual issues and those related to family, friends, and community, as well as adjusting to sociopolitical realities, such as Islamophobia. The time frame and degree of change in lifestyle, as well as individual and environmental supports, will impact the experience of a Muslim convert. Some converts may join different organizations or ideological groups in an attempt to learn about Islam and develop a sense of belonging, while other converts may become overwhelmed by the stressors and decide to leave Islam altogether. The number of Muslims and the types of Islamic services that the Muslim convert has access to can also affect their postconversion experience.

In Martha's case, she is still in the early years of conversion. Although she has firm faith, she is still learning about Islam, while simultaneously addressing past issues, which proves to be challenging. Martha did not realize the influence her conversion had on her symptoms. Because Martha had mentioned being embarrassed of her heroin use due to Islam's prohibition, the clinician took the opportunity to educate Martha regarding Islam's gradual prohibition of substance use.[4] In addition, the clinician

---

[4] The order of Qur'anic revelation on substance use is as follows: 16:67, 2:219, 4:43, 5:90. This gradual revelation highlights an example of behavior modification used in the Qur'an.

shared with Martha the example of an early Muslim *sahaba*[5] who had struggled with addiction and was loved by God, because he was sincere in his struggle to make change. With an increase in religious knowledge, Martha was more hopeful about her addiction and her status with God. The stigma associated with substance use among Muslims also made it difficult for Martha to connect with Muslim peers who could have assisted her in gaining religious knowledge on the topic. Instead, she had been struggling individually with her desire to practice Islam, despite her difficulty with addiction.

Factors Impacting Clinical Presentation

Once the clinician understands the conversion experience, the next step is to understand if and how conversion may influence the symptom presentation. Understanding the varying factors that may serve as stressors or supports is useful to the clinician. This section discusses individual, family, and environmental factors that may positively or negatively impact the convert.

Individual Factors

Individual factors such as previous mental health issues, Islamic values and beliefs, and ethnic and racial background may potentially influence the convert's experience and impact clinical presentation and treatment intervention.

Mental Health Conversion may result in a new worldview, but the convert may continue to have mental health issues that were present prior to the conversion or arise thereafter. In these situations, conversion can serve as a source of distress, comfort, or both. The clinician should seek to understand if and how the client's conversion influences symptom presentation. In Martha's case, the recent death of her brother, which resulted in an intense emotional reaction, had not been addressed. In addition, she had unresolved issues related to her mother's abandonment of her and her siblings that may have resurfaced as a result of Child Protective Services taking away her infant son after testing positive for drug use. Prior to her conversion, she had learned to cope with difficulties by turning to drugs to self-medicate. Without learning a new coping mechanism to address emotional distress, Martha relapsed and began using heroin once again. However, her decision to use heroin after conversion resulted in additional pain, shame, and loneliness, because of its prohibition in Islam, as Martha explains:

---

[5] *Sahaba,* or Companion, refers to an individual who was alive and interacted with the Prophet Muhammad.

I hid my [heroin] use from my husband. He had never used, so he could never tell that I had been using. But I felt terrible about doing this. How could I, the wife of the muezzin [caller to prayer] be using? I was always worried about being exposed, I was jumpy, irritable, and it really messed up our marriage. I felt like a total loser, a failure as a mom, a wife, and as a Muslim. I never went out and never wanted to interact with anyone, because I was afraid they'd be able to see right through me! I just wanted to crawl back into bed and forget about how terrible I felt.

Islamic beliefs can also be a source of support and be used to motivate the convert toward change. With the help of her therapist, Martha was able to reframe her addiction as a test from God and a method of self-purification. She was able to realize that God knew how difficult the challenge toward recovery would be and took solace in the belief that God would reward her sincere intentions and efforts to change her life. In addition, she was able to find hope that God could provide her with assistance and make the process of change easier, such that she could change the direction of her life. The reframing gave her a new perspective, renewed energy, and motivation to make the necessary changes.

Islamic Beliefs and Practices   Converts will vary in their beliefs, practices, and the extent to which they draw upon the religious teachings of Islam. Islam is not a monolithic, dogmatic religion, but one that allows for a variety of interpretations and practice, depending on textual evidence, specific circumstances, cultural contexts, and priorities. In addition, clinicians should be aware that Islamic teachings and the way Muslims implement Islam may not always be the same.

The initial years of conversion may be overwhelming, confusing, and isolating for some converts because of the varying interpretations that people may have of Islam and try to introduce to the convert. Paradoxically, other converts may be left alone, marginalized, and given no direction or assistance on how to incorporate their new faith into their life, which can be a lonely, confusing, and isolating experience. Converts may be susceptible to ideological extremes, internalize interpretations of Islam that are culturally alien, or move to different Muslim organizations in search for an approach that best fits with their understanding of Islam. At the same time, converts may be better equipped to sort through the varying ideologies presented because they may be more willing to engage in critical thinking and not carry the cultural baggage that lifelong Muslims may carry.

The ideological perspective adopted also influences the identity of a convert. Some converts may integrate their new faith with positive aspects of their former identity, culture, and lifestyle and are able to operate in varying contexts comfortably (i.e., Muslim, non-Muslim, family, friends, work, and society). As they integrate Islam into their lives, other converts may reject their former identity and culture, and instead may adopt immigrant cultural norms. Many other converts may continue to struggle to develop a coherent sense of self that integrates their religious and cultural identities.

The convert's interpretation of Islam and level of practice can result in minimal to major changes in the person's life. Converts may need to reorganize their daily schedule to include prayer times and adjust to dietary changes, such as eliminating pork from meals. Individuals may choose to only eat *halal* meat,[6] which, depending on geographic location, may limit food choice at restaurants. Financial practices may also change based on ideological beliefs and degree of practice. Islamic texts and religious scholars indicate that that use of *riba*, or interest, is considered prohibited in Islam, due to the lack of social justice and equitability to all parties involved. As a result, how the convert interprets the issue of *riba* in Western contexts has implications for mortgages, student loans, and banking accounts (all involving interest), which can have major implications on the convert's life. Another significant change may be in appearance, where Muslim converts may grow beards or wear religiously identifiable clothing, such as a *hijab*[7] or *thobe*.[8] Clinicians should strive to understand the changes that have taken place, the time frame these changes were made, as well as how it has impacted the convert's life, relationships, and environment.

In Martha and her husband's case, they interpreted modesty in Islam as requiring Malik to wear a *thobe* and Martha a *niqab* and *abaya*. Her choice of clothing appears to interact with symptom-related behaviors. For example, Martha would take off her *abaya* before going to buy heroin because she felt it would be disrespectful to her faith if she were to wear religiously identified attire to engage in behaviors prohibited in Islam. The fact that she took off her *abaya*, even temporarily, was also contributing to her negative sense of self.

---

[6] *Halal* means "permissible" and the concept itself has a wide application. When referring to food it usually refers to meat that has been slaughtered according to Islamic guidelines. However, there are different scholarly opinions that allow Muslims to eat commonly available meat, with the assumption that someone who was either a Christian or a Jew (i.e., "people of the book") slaughtered the meat, and hence it would be lawful for consumption.

[7] In Arabic, *hijab* literally means to cover. It refers to an aspect of modesty, which has implications on clothing and gender interaction, and is applicable to both men and women. However, it is commonly referred to as the headscarf worn by Muslim women and will be referred to as such throughout the chapter.

[8] A *thobe* is a long, flowing robe worn by men in traditional Arab cultures.

Ethnic or Racial Background   Converts' ethnic or racial background can also impact their conversion experience. Converts of European ancestry may be more celebrated and accepted than converts of other backgrounds, but there may be more suspicion toward them because of fear that they may be government agents seeking information or trying to entrap Muslims. Converts of European descent may also find it challenging to become a minority, due to changing one's religious beliefs, as they would not have experienced minority status previously.

In the case of converts of African descent, they may have a unique challenge of being a double minority. They are not only a racial minority in their society and likely experience historical, cultural, and institutional oppression and discrimination, but they are now also a religious minority and therefore may experience additional scrutiny and distrust from society and other individuals of African descent. They may also experience racism within the Muslim immigrant community, much to their disillusionment, given Islam's opposition to racism. However, becoming Muslim can be an empowering experience for converts of African descent, because of famous role models like Malcolm X (El Hajj Malik Shabazz) and social justice elements of Islam, and feel that they are reclaiming the intellectual, scientific, cultural legacy of African Muslims. Converts of other ethnicities may also have varied experiences due to their ethnic and racial backgrounds.

Depending on locality, Muslim converts may find particular ethnic groups dominating in the general Muslim community, including the mosques and services available. Some Muslim converts may live in an area where there is a concentration of one ethnic group, which can significantly influence the conversion experience; as such the information and advice given about the implementation of Islam in everyday life may take different forms. Depending on the ethnic background of the convert and the cultural heterogeneity of the Muslim community, issues of ethnic or racial background may or may not be of concern. In Martha's case, her Muslim community was African American, so issues of inclusion were not racially based. In her urban, poor, primarily African American neighborhood, Muslims were viewed positively because of the positive transformation Islam has had on African American Muslims, both historically and locally.

Family Life Cycle

Depending on the life stage and dynamics present, the convert's family can have a differing influence on the individual and can serve as a source of support or stress for the Muslim convert. This section highlights challenges that may be encountered based on the convert's family life cycle.

Family of Origin   Clinicians should explore the impact that conversion may have had on the convert's relationship with his or her family of origin. Converts may experience varying reactions from family members regarding their conversion. In some cases, the changes resulting from conversion may be welcomed and families may be supportive. For example, the convert may have previously engaged in antisocial behaviors and the acceptance of Islam resulted in a major transformation, or the convert's parents may be pleased that their child has a sense of purpose and direction. In these cases, the family of origin may have been familiar with Islam, have had positive experiences with Muslims, or tolerate religious exploration. In situations where conversion is positively received, family members may choose to convert to Islam as well, as was the case with Martha's brother. Other families may be indifferent to the conversion as long as overt demonstrations or restrictions of being Muslim are not present.

Some converts report struggling with their family relationships because of their conversion (Rehman & Dziegielewski, 2003; Sulaiman-Hill, 2007). Converts may experience anxiety and fear related to their families' reaction to conversion, which may also be influenced by the person's dependence on his or her family of origin. Converts who live with their parents and are financially dependent on them, such as adolescents and emerging adults, may experience limitations in their religious observance and choose to conceal their conversion in order to reduce tension with their family. For those who declare their conversion, they may practice religious rituals covertly in order not to upset their relatives who may find the practices disturbing and alien. Family and friends can also view the change in faith as a rejection of their faith, heritage, and/or way of life. For example, some Muslims decide to change their name to a more Muslim- or Arabic-sounding name,[9] which can be interpreted by family members as a rejection of their family history and culture, and may in turn result in straining family relationships. Religious holidays and family traditions may be challenging for Muslim converts because they may need to navigate between respecting family traditions and maintaining religious beliefs (Daneshpour, 1998). Refusing traditional foods such as pork, attending holiday dinners where alcohol is served, and negotiating gender interactions are some of the issues that may cause tension with relatives. This may result in guilt for feeling responsible for straining the relationship or causing it to become awkward.

Family members may be concerned or perplexed by the individual's decision to convert, which may manifest in questions about and criticisms

---

[9] It is not a religious requirement for converts to change their name to a Muslim name, but converts may decide to do so for varying reasons including signaling a new beginning, feeling more Muslim, being identified by others as Muslims, or issues related to the rejection of one's past history.

of Islam. Converts may experience such comments as attacks, react negatively, and can develop a strained relationship with relatives. In particular, parents may be concerned when their convert daughters marry a Muslim man, due to the negative portrayal of Muslim men in the media (Sulaiman-Hill, 2007; Van Nieuwkerk, 2004). Parents of Muslim male converts may fear that they are being brainwashed or "radicalized" by terrorist groups who want to use them for pseudo-political purposes. Family members may also encourage the convert to act in ways that are contrary to Islam, which may be stressful for the convert. Martha recalls how her sister helped her relapse after a period of being drug-free:

> I love my sister, but she's bad news. She's the one that made me start usin' again. She gave me the stuff [heroin], covered for me so he [husband] wouldn't know. He says he don't want her around. I don't know what to do. She's all I have left now... but I know she's no good for me.

Marriage Search   Given that Western notions of dating are not acceptable in Islam, converts may struggle to find an Islamically-appropriate way of meeting a potential spouse. Converts may meet their future spouse through shared activities and interests, rely on the informal family and friendship networks, or use matrimonial services to facilitate marriage. Some converts may easily find a potential mate or may be sought after by lifelong Muslims because they may assume that the convert will be more fun, sexually experienced, or not have traditional cultural expectations of them. Other converts, especially non-White converts, may report discrimination by Muslims who refuse marriage requests due to race, preference of marrying individuals of similar cultural background, fear that the convert may leave Islam, unwillingness to deal with non-Muslim in-laws, concerns regarding past sexual history, or fear of community reprisal. In some cases, particularly involving women who do not have adequate support, potential spouses may take advantage of them or not give them their full rights, as required by Islam.

Marriage   In addition to the numerous difficulties encountered by couples in general, married converts may experience difficulty if their partner is not supportive of their conversion. In cases where the nonconverting spouse is not Muslim, the conversion may be viewed with alarm. The spouse may engage in verbal abuse, belittle the convert's new religious beliefs and practices, or threaten loss of child custody, which is emotionally taxing for the convert. The religious background of the convert's spouse may become an issue of stress for which the client should consult with a religious scholar before making life-altering decisions.[10] Thus, the convert faces a difficult choice regarding whether to continue living with their spouse.

For converts married to Muslims, issues that may cause problems may include differences in religious interpretation, degree of practice, and/or ideological adherence. Spouses who are raised as Muslim may not understand the conversion process, desire for critical analysis, and the need for gradualism before adopting Islamic practices. Converts may also become more religious than their spouses, which can result in resentment and marital discord. Muslim spouses may expect the convert to adopt culturally based practices, and the lifelong Muslim's family of origin may impose pressure and cultural restraints on the convert. This may also make it very confusing for the new convert in terms of differentiating between religious and cultural practices.

In Martha's case, she describes how she and her husband's differences impacted the dynamics of her marital relationship:

> He [Malik, her husband] spends most of his time at the *masjid*.[11] He tries to encourage me to come to the *masjid* and get to know the others, but he doesn't want to push me, since I'm a new Muslim. He thinks all of this [depression] is because of the baby. Maaan, if he only knew [about my drug use]. I'm so scared of him finding out. I don't know what he'll do, how he will react. I don't want to lose him. I'm so scared of him finding out and then leaving me. He's the first man that has ever loved me, provided for me, and took care of my kids. All the other guys just want to get on with me, or just use me for my government support. Man . . . Why do I always ruin my life when things are going good?

Parenting Converts who are also parents may encounter parenting challenges related to their conversion. Generally, children who are infants and toddlers at the time of their parents' conversion are able to make the religious transition with relative ease, as long as parents are uniform in their application and support each other's practice. In cases where the

---

[10] According to Islamic teachings, a male convert married to a Christian or Jewish woman may remain married, and must respect his wife's religion and allow her to practice her religion freely. If a male or female convert's spouse is not a Christian or Jew (referred to as "the people of the book," a special designation in Islam), then the spouse is invited to become a Muslim. If he or she refuses after some time, according to Islamic law, the marriage should be dissolved. Female converts are prohibited from being married to non-Muslim males since they may not allow her to practice her religion freely. However, because of the sensitivity of the potential dissolution of marriage, the convert should seek assistance from a religious leader who is familiar with convert issues to determine how best to handle his or her specific situation before acting.

[11] *Masjid* or mosque refers to a Muslim house of worship.

conversion brought about stability and positive changes in parenting and family culture, children may welcome the conversion.

Parental conversion may be more difficult during adolescence. Convert parents may make parenting changes such as adopting new family rules and rituals (e.g., prayer, dress), while abandoning others (e.g., holiday celebrations). Changes in parental expectations, such as gender interaction or requiring children to attend religious schools or educational programs, may cause resentment. Children may experience feelings of frustration and lack of control over their lives, and may rebel. This may result in parental frustration, negative parent–child interactions, and the converts questioning their conversion due to the ensuing family tension. In addition, converts may struggle with balancing the need to maintain family ties and exposing their children to situations that may contradict Islamic teachings. Parents may struggle with how to address un-Islamic behavior of non-Muslim relatives in the presence of their children, without being disrespectful or condoning the behavior.

Converts may have adult children who may have mixed reactions to their parents' conversion. Adult children may express confusion or difficulties supporting their parents' change. Convert parents may struggle to make changes that impact long-held family traditions. For example, older converts may struggle with organizing and maintaining family holiday traditions, such as preparing Christmas dinner and baking Christmas cookies for their children and grandchildren, while feeling uncomfortable promoting a faith with which they do not agree.

Mental health clinicians should consider the phase of conversion and the developmental age of the convert's children when addressing parenting issues. For recent-convert parents with school-age or adolescent children, the clinician may need to help the parent realize that although the convert went through a period of spiritual exploration, his or her child may not have. Therefore, the parent may be encouraged to communicate values and beliefs prior to making changes in lifestyle in order to help ease the adjustment process. The clinician may help the parent(s) maintain open communication with their children and identify more effective ways to pass on their beliefs and values, and assist children in verbalizing their feelings in a respectful manner.

Environmental Context

The manner in which converts interact and experience their environment can also contribute to symptom presentation and treatment outcome. This section highlights three important areas that clinicians should explore: friends, Muslim community, and sociopolitical context.

Friends Conversion may impact friendships that were made prior to religious exploration. Converts who choose to wear overtly Muslim clothing, such as the *hijab*, may encounter friends who are uncomfortable with their outward manifestation of their faith (Rehman & Dziegielewski, 2003).

Depending on the convert's ideological understanding of appropriate gender interaction in Islam, conversion may strain a convert's relationship with friends of the opposite gender. Some converts may interpret Islamic beliefs to include the total segregation of genders, while others may interpret gender interaction rules as not being alone with the opposite gender. If, prior to conversion, the convert had close friends of the opposite gender and was accustomed to giving friendly hugs and kisses, conversion may greatly impact behaviors. Friends may not understand the changes, feel alienated, and long for the friend they once knew. As such, the process of developing religiously and culturally appropriate boundaries can be a struggle for converts.

Converts may need to adjust leisure activities if they are contrary to Islamic beliefs. For example, individuals who may have previously spent leisure time with their peers at dance clubs and bars would no longer be able to socialize with their friends at these locations, given the Islamic prohibition of alcohol and rules of gender interaction (Sulaiman-Hill, 2007). However, if the convert can maintain shared interests and activities, such as sports, with their friends there is a greater possibility of maintaining their friendships.

In the process of conversion, converts may also gain friends. These friends, both Muslim and others, can serve to help the convert with adjustment issues, provide spiritual guidance, and develop new social and leisure activities that are congruent with their faith. Some converts report that lifelong Muslims have difficulty understanding their situation and challenges. If the conversion results in the loss of previous friendships and is not associated with gaining new meaningful friendships that respect and support the convert's faith, the convert may experience a lack of support and feelings of loneliness. During Martha's treatment, she was able to form a supportive relationship with another woman who was also in the drug rehabilitation program. Although the woman was not a Muslim, she had strong religious conviction and encouraged Martha to rely on her faith and make the necessary behavioral changes for recovery.

Muslim Community The clinician should begin by understanding how the convert defines his or her community. The Muslim community that the client identifies with can serve as a source of support and positive influence for the individual, or can negatively impact the convert. For many individuals their community may refer to worshippers at a local mosque.

However, converts may also identify informal social networks, organizations, or Internet-based groups as their Muslim community.

Supportive communities offer converts social support through friendship opportunities, involvement in activities, and assistance with their spiritual and cultural exploration through educational and social programs. Communities that are able to integrate the convert's cultural identity and heritage with Islam are often helpful in supporting the conversion process. Communities that provide social activities during Islamic holidays help converts integrate more into the community. Converts may be leaving close-knit religious communities, previous sets of rituals, and traditions associated with religious holidays, and may have difficulty forming new traditions that are both culturally and religiously relevant to them.

The Muslim community can also serve as a stressor when the convert experiences a lack of social support, language or cultural barriers, or fellow Muslims' expectations of immediate change in beliefs, behaviors, and dress. Community members may automatically assume that a convert lacks knowledge of Islam, which can be offensive. In addition, the community may promote culturally rather than religiously based Islamic norms pertaining to such issues as dress, gender interaction, gender roles, music, and entertainment, which may make adjustment difficult for new converts. Convert adaptation of ethnic cultural norms of culturally based Muslim communities may result in social distancing from the convert's traditional sources of emotional and social support. In addition, the lack of practice and passion for Islam exhibited by lifelong Muslims may be demoralizing for converts. If the experience of being part of a Muslim community is emotionally exhausting, some converts may choose to withdraw from their Muslim community and even leave Islam.

Sociopolitical Context   Societal response to converts can also be a source of stress and impact the client's worldview. In many Western nations, where ethnicity is tied to nationality and ethno-nationality is tied to religious identity, converts may experience negative responses from their fellow citizens. Muslims are often not considered truly natives, and are assumed to be immigrants despite living in a country for generations. As such, when the individual converts, he or she may be considered a traitor and experience rejection (Van Nieuwkerk, 2004). This feeling of betrayal is enhanced by the wider geopolitical context of living in a post-9/11 climate where some citizens consider Muslims the enemy, and conversion to Islam is seen as becoming a traitor. For example, women who wear the *hijab* may report feeling that strangers assume they are foreigners and belittle them. The negative reaction is partly due to the public misconception of the *hijab* as a symbol of oppression, as well as a marker of what society deems as incongruent with the national identity (McGinty, 2007; Franks, 2000). Despite the negative experiences encountered, converts wearing *hijab* report that they felt liberated, respected, and stronger about their Islamic identity (Franks, 2000).

Ignorance about Islam has resulted in an increase in Islamophobia impacting converts' feeling of safety in their own country. After the 9/11, London, Madrid, and Swedish bombings, Muslims may be afraid to go out in public for fear of being assaulted as revenge for the tragic events. Converts may find themselves in a precarious position of having once felt safe in their own country but now fear being targeted by their fellow citizens, depending on the extent to which they are visibly Muslim (Rehman & Dziegielewski, 2003). Yet converts, like Muslims in general, continue to engage their environment to help dispel misconceptions.

Converts may also experience discrimination. A growing movement in Europe is resulting in governments banning *hijab* for students, employees, and individuals seeking services in educational and government buildings. As a result, the government is perceived as forcing women to choose between practicing their religious beliefs and the pursuit of educational and economic opportunity. Such laws alienate Muslims and sow seeds of resentment toward their nation.

Counseling Muslim Converts

The previous section highlighted numerous factors that may impact the conversion, symptom presentation, and treatment interventions of individuals converting to Islam for religious reasons.[12] This section covers therapeutic considerations in order to effectively assist Muslim converts in treatment.

Assessment

A religiously and culturally based assessment that links diagnostic information to treatment interventions is necessary. Clinicians may rely on formal testing as well as an in-depth clinical interview in order to assess the presenting problem. In cases where formal assessment measures are administered, the clinician should consider religious beliefs and practices that may warrant adjustment in the testing environment. For example, some clients may express discomfort if the test administrator and client are of opposite genders in closed environments, due to gender interaction rules in Islam. A list of potential clinical interview questions correlating to the issues highlighted in this chapter can be found in Table 13.1.

---

[12] As opposed to individuals who may convert for social reasons, such as marriage.

Table 13.1 Potential Convert Assessment Questions

Introductory Questions
- Do you consider yourself a religious or spiritual person?
- Do you identify with a religious group?
- What role, if any, does Islam have in your life?
- Have you always been a Muslim?

   For some people conversion can have a major impact on their life. I would like to ask you more detailed questions about your conversion process to better understand how it may have influenced your life. Understanding this process may help us identify if it plays a role in the issues you are concerned about. In addition, having this knowledge will help me identify sources of support that may help tailor the most effective treatment intervention for your situation.

Conversion Process
- Can you describe your conversion?
- How were you introduced to Islam (individual, experience, etc.)?
- What were the factors and/or beliefs that contributed to your acceptance of Islam? How has this changed over time?
- When did you convert to Islam? How many years have you been a Muslim?
- Can you describe both the positive and negative experiences associated with conversion?
- Can you describe the different types of behavioral changes you made as a result of your conversion (social, spiritual, work, leisure, etc.)?
- How different are your current beliefs and practices compared to your beliefs prior to becoming a Muslim?

Factors Impacting Clinical Presentation
- In your opinion, what role, if any, does your faith play in the problem you are experiencing today (both positive as well as negative)?
- Can you describe if or how your current symptoms may be experienced differently because you are a Muslim? A convert?
- Has your race or ethnicity impacted your conversion experience? Your experience with other Muslims? With general society?
- What is your current level of interaction with your family of origin? How has your relationship with them been affected by your conversion?
- How has your conversion affected your marital relationship?
- How has your conversion impacted your parenting?
- How do your children feel about your conversion?
- What role, if any, do your friends have in your life?
- Describe any changes (interpersonal, leisure activities, etc.) in your friendships that may have resulted from your conversion.
- Can you describe what or who you define as your Muslim community?
- What are the supportive aspects of your Muslim community? What are the challenges you experience?
- How does the sociopolitical environment impact you as a Muslim? Your presenting symptoms?
- How does being a Muslim help you with your life problems?

Gathering History As clinicians gather information during the intake session, it is important that they ask all clients about the role of the client's spiritual, cultural, and personal beliefs. Not every convert will be easily identifiable as a Muslim by his or her name, clothing, or behaviors. Thus, the clinician may not know that a client is Muslim unless the client is specifically asked. For clients who indicate that they are Muslim, the clinician should clarify if the individual was raised a Muslim or converted to Islam. Clinicians should not assume religious upbringing based on ethnic or racial characteristics. For clients indicating that they have converted to Islam, the clinician should explore the client's conversion process and possible implications of conversion. Converts may experience detailed questions about their conversion as inappropriate and intrusive. They may also fear that the clinician may unnecessarily pathologize them because of their conversion. Clinicians can alleviate these concerns by explaining that conversion can be a life-transforming experience and understanding the process, pathways, support, and stressors encountered not only is part of a client's history, but may also identify influences on symptoms and treatment interventions. Even after identifying a client as a Muslim convert, it is important to remember that Islam may not play an integral role, or the convert may not practice all aspects of Islam or may adopt a particular interpretation of Islam that may not be considered mainstream.

Mental Health Attribution Converts may attribute mental health symptoms to a variety of causes, which is important for the clinician to understand in order to develop effective treatment interventions. Converts may attribute their mental health problems to weakness in faith or as a test from God and thus turn to religious sources for coping. They may attribute their symptoms to biological causes and seek medical or alternative approaches for treatment. In addition, converts may attribute mental health issues to situational or environmental factors, or a combination of these factors. In Martha's case, she attributed her relapse to the emotional pain caused by her brother's death. In order to decrease and avoid pain, she chose to use heroin, which eventually led to the loss of her infant son.

Help-Seeking Approaches The convert's attribution of mental health symptoms will likely influence help-seeking approaches. Converts may seek guidance from religious texts or sources of knowledge. Converts may seek solace in reading the Qur'an, the Muslim Book of Guidance, and *sunnah*, the sayings and actions of the Prophet Muhammad. In addition, converts may find comfort in studying the *seerah*, the history of Prophet Muhammad's life. Given that the initial Muslims were converts who experienced similar situational challenges, converts may choose to find inspiration and lessons in learning about the lives of the early Muslims, referred to as the *sahabi*. Individuals may also turn to friends or religious leaders in order to obtain support, advice, and knowledge on dealing with their situation and/or mental health symptoms.

For situational factors related to conversion, such as issues related to family, friends, and community, converts may turn to convert groups for support. In cities with a large population of Muslims, converts may organize their own study circles, retreats, and events during holidays in order to meet their social, emotional, and religious needs. The Internet is also increasingly becoming a source of support for converts through the exchange of ideas, sharing frustration, and providing support. Internet groups, blogs, and websites may help converts feel less isolated in their experiences, and may empower them through the exchange of perspectives. However, Internet resources can also cause confusion because participating converts may be at different phases of conversion and from diverse ideological backgrounds, and may reside within different sociocultural contexts.

Muslim converts may avoid seeking mental health services because they may worry that non-Muslim clinicians may attribute their mental health issues to their conversion. They may also feel that Islam should automatically improve their mental health. Converts are more likely than immigrants to consider seeking counseling services because of the greater familiarity with and awareness of psychotherapy in most Western cultures (Ahmed & Reddy, 2007). However, some converts may believe that Western mental health basic assumptions are contrary to Islamic belief systems. These individuals are more likely to reject counseling and only present for services when forced to by a loved one or in an inpatient setting.

Understanding the history of clients and their conversion process, as well as sources of stress and support, will enable clinicians to identify factors to consider in clinical intervention. Similarly, awareness of mental health attribution and resulting help-seeking approaches used may inform therapeutic interventions. Finally, clinicians should ask clients if they would like to incorporate important religious elements into treatment in order to design a more effective intervention. During the assessment phase of treatment, Martha indicated that her religion was important to her but that she was not sure how it could be incorporated into her treatment. Cooperation between the client and the clinician may enable religion-based solutions to be identified.

Treatment

Like other populations, there is no one particular treatment approach that should be used with converts. The nature of treatment will depend on the symptom presentation and the individual's strength, personality, and needs. However, clinicians should incorporate religious consultants and resources as well as consider the role of transference and countertransference in the therapeutic process.

Religious Consultants and Resources   In order to be able to effectively incorporate culturally and spiritually meaningful resources, clinicians must develop a collaborative relationship with religious and community leaders. Converts may encounter religious moral dilemmas that require balancing numerous factors and religious priorities that may confound the average practicing Muslim. A clinician who has a relationship with a religious consultant with Islamic textual knowledge as well as familiarity with the complexities of conversion can be helpful. Alternatively, the client could be referred to the consultant in order to address religious dilemmas of nonclinical relevance. In addition, the clinician can work with the religious consultant in order to integrate Islamic concepts and practices within the treatment process. In Martha's case, an *imam*, or religious leader, was contacted to help identify historical incidents involving Muslims who had struggled with substance use and had been elevated in religious status for their sincere repentance and attempts to change. The *imam* was able to identify a *hadith*, or saying of the Prophet Muhammad, that helped to instill hope within Martha.

Clinicians must exhibit an attitude and approach to therapy that respects, draws upon, and uses the client's cultural and spiritual resources in order for the treatment to be meaningful. Clinicians unfamiliar with Islam would need to work with a religious consultant or work with the client to explore possible faith-based interventions.

In Martha's case the therapist was able to reframe intervention within her religious context. For example, the client was encouraged to break her day into five components, corresponding with the five daily prayers required of Muslims. Her initial success was measured by the ability to get from one prayer to the next without using drugs. When she was able to get to the prayer without using, she was also able to use her prayer as an opportunity to thank God for her success, as well as ask Him for help as she attempted to get to the next prayer.

Transference and Countertransference   Clinicians should be cognizant of transference and countertransference issues that may impact treatment, particularly sociopolitical events. Like other Muslims, converts may feel hesitant about seeking services from professionals who are not familiar with Islam due to fear of the counselor's lack of religious and cultural sensitivity. Converts may experience discomfort discussing challenges such as frustrations with other Muslims, issues of faith, and marital problems with

Conclusion

For Muslim converts, their conversion to Islam may be a life-changing decision that will often be central to their sense of selfhood, determine how they respond to life challenges, and influence their perspective on various issues. Muslim converts form a unique subgroup within the Muslim population that can often serve as a bridge between their nation and other Muslim subgroups. They may be diverse in their religious upbringing, ethnic and racial backgrounds, conversion experience, and levels of practice. The clinician must conduct an in-depth clinical interview assessing mental health attribution, help-seeking approaches, possible roles of the conversion process, and factors that may influence symptom presentations. Clinicians are encouraged to use the information gathered during the clinical interview and draw upon spiritually meaningful resources in collaboration with religious consultants. Clinicians who are able to integrate the concepts and issues discussed in this chapter and make the therapy process more spiritually meaningful will likely be more effective in treatment.

Acknowledgments

I would like to thank Aisha Shillingford, Leon Moosavi, and Bhawana Kamil for their assistance and thoughtful comments while preparing this chapter.

CHAPTER 14
Adolescents and Emerging Adults

SAMEERA AHMED

Muslim adolescents and emerging adults make up the largest segment of Muslim communities in Western nations (Open Society Institute [OSI], 2005; Zogby, 2001). They are often scrutinized for fear of being the next homegrown terrorists and experience pressures of Islamophobia during an already challenging developmental period. As such, they may be at higher risk for mental health issues and may present with symptoms that are imbedded within a particular sociocultural-religious context. As such, clinicians need to understand issues facing Muslim youth so that they can conduct effective religious and culturally sensitive treatment interventions.

This chapter uses human ecological theory (Bronfenbrenner, 1977) to present different factors that may influence the development of Muslim adolescents and emerging adults. Human ecological theory posits that development is an ongoing interaction that occurs between growing individuals and their constantly changing environment (Bronfenbrenner, 1977). The immediate setting, as well as the larger social context in which the development is nested, influences this process of development. The interaction of these factors impacts development, self-understanding, interactions with the world, and the relationships and connections formed. The interaction is mutually shaping, in which the individual is affected by the environment and the environment is influenced by the individual (Bronfenbrenner, 1977).

This chapter examines different ecological contexts that impact Muslim youths' development. The chapter reviews factors that may influence adolescent development including biological, identity, spiritual, and behavioral. In addition, the importance of understanding the young person's immediate setting, namely family, peers, school, and community, is highlighted. Given that clinicians can have the greatest impact on the developing person and his or her immediate settings, the chapter explores these sections in greater detail. Also important is the interaction between the varying settings, namely family–school collaboration, socioeconomic status, and acculturation. Important social structures that may influence Muslim youth development, such as the creative arts, the Internet, media, and racism are highlighted. Subsequently, institutional patterns, such as global events and the political environment, as they influence Muslim adolescent and emerging adult development, are discussed. Each section highlights potential factors influencing development followed by a case study illustrating how the factors may interact with one another in order to offer clinicians practical examples.

Developing Adolescents and Emerging Adults

Even in seemingly identical environments, such as with identical twins, variances naturally emerge. These divergences can be attributed to the individual differences and how the person chooses to interact with his or her environment. This section highlights factors such as biological changes, identity development, spiritual development, and risk-taking behaviors that may influence the developmental trajectories of Muslim adolescents and emerging adults.

Biological Changes

Although puberty is biological in nature, it also has sociocultural and religious implications for Muslim youth. With the onset of puberty, the individual becomes accountable for one's actions before God, or Allah. This means that religious practices such as prayer, fasting, and almsgiving become obligatory. Additionally, the onset of puberty is associated with the religious requirement of wearing the *hijab*[1] or headscarf for women. For some young women it is a religious mandate that results in donning of the *hijab*. For other young women, it is not a clear mandate and they may choose not to wear the *hijab* for varying reasons, including, but not limited to, personal beliefs, ethnic culture, pressure from family and friends, government rules, and/or fear of persecution. Depending on the sociocultural subcontext of the individual, the decision for wearing the *hijab* may catapult young women into exploring issues of identity.

---

[1] In Arabic *hijab* literally means to cover. It refers to the concept of modesty, which is applicable to both men and women. However, it is commonly referred to as the headscarf worn by Muslim women and will be referred to as such throughout the chapter.

Sexual Development Muslim parents may not talk to their children about sexual issues due to cultural conceptions of modesty, discomfort, and/or beliefs that the information is not relevant to their children (Al-Mateen & Afzal, 2004). For Muslim youth in Western countries, media and peer pressure may promote sexual exploration and activity, whereas Islamic religious and cultural beliefs limit sexual activity to one's marital relationship.

Despite prohibition, Muslim adolescents and emerging adults are sexually active. Young Muslims are increasingly engaging in fellatio, seeking hymen reconstruction, or requesting virginity certificates from physicians before marriage in order to mask their sexual activity (Bekker, 1996). Recent studies in the United States indicate that almost half of college-aged Muslims have had sexual intercourse (Ahmed, Arfken, & Abu Ras, 2010; Ahmed, Sharrief, & Arfken, 2009). Parents may be unaware or in denial about their child's sexual activity and therefore unable to address the issue in an appropriate manner. As such, it is important for clinicians to assess the young Muslim's sexual history separate from his or her parents. When premarital sexual activity is endorsed, clinicians should explore the implications within the individual's belief system and religious, cultural, familial, and social context.

Identity

Adolescence is a period of increased cognitive complexity often resulting in the young person's need for introspection and exploring issues such as identity. Identity exploration is a major developmental task in adolescence (Erikson, 1968). Issues of identity such as "Who am I?" and "Do I matter?" are basic questions of adolescents. During this period, young people may express a greater need for privacy, need for differentiation, and independence in efforts to establish their own identity. Parents may perceive this process of separation as a rejection of them and their values, especially immigrant parents from collectivist cultures where such behaviors may not have been commonly observed.[2]

Identity development is also influenced by the young person's interaction with his or her environment and results in the formation of an ever-changing, fluid set of multiple social identities that may include their religious, ethnic/racial/cultural, national, and gender identity. Muslim youth may attempt to develop a cohesive identity by blending their varying social identities (Ahmed et al., 2009; Britto, 2008; Sirin, Bikmen, Mir, Zaal, Fine, & Katsiaficas, 2008). Given that Islam consists of general principles that can

---

[2] Parents may not have observed such adolescent behaviors while living in their home countries. However, with globalization, facilitated by television and the Internet, it is believed that young people living in Muslim-majority countries are increasingly engaging in more Western-like adolescent behaviors.

be adapted to any culture, Muslim youth may choose to identify more with their religious identity. Their religious identity may allow them to integrate their varying social identities (i.e., ethnic, racial, gender, etc.) into a cohesive identity (Archer, 2001; Chaudhury & Miller, 2008; Kibria, 2008).

Young people's identity is also influenced by their gender. For young Muslim women, gender norms of family, ethnic, and religious community may influence their identification with Islam and ethnic or racial culture. Young women may experience greater pressure than their male counterparts to maintain ethnic dress, language, and behaviors (Dwyer, 2000). Restriction in activities and patriarchal or cultural interpretations of Islam may result in different interpretations about the role of women in Islam and serve as a source of tension between parents and their daughters (Abu-Ali & Reisen, 1999). As such some young Muslim women may develop an aversion to both Islam and their ethnic culture. Other young women may choose to embrace their religious identity because they perceive it as giving them more opportunities than their ethnic culture (Archer, 2002; Dwyer, 2000).

Much less is known about the impact of gender role expectations on the development of Muslim men. They have been painted by the media as aggressive, chauvinistic, militant, and fundamentalist people who are not to be trusted (Shaheen, 2003; Archer, 2001). Young Muslim men believe they are often scrutinized by people in public settings such as on airplanes, subways, or in government buildings over concerns that they may be potential terrorists. Muslim males of African descent report experiencing the additional negative stereotype of being a "Black male." This negative stereotype appears to influence their identities, sense of self, and how they interact with their environment (Ahmed et al., 2009). The lack of acceptance by society, traditionally minimal monitoring of males by parents, and less religious socialization compared to their female counterparts may result in greater numbers of young men choosing to assimilate into society and abandon traditional religious and cultural practices.

Spiritual Development

Individuals commonly begin exploring their spiritual beliefs during adolescence and emerging adulthood due to cognitive changes coupled with new experiences. Researchers note that young Muslims are increasingly engaging in a revivalist approach to Islam, one that is considered a movement toward modernity, rather than hostility toward Western culture (Kibria, 2008). According to Jacobsen (1997), young Muslims may use a revivalist approach to Islam in order to assert their independence from their parents and reject cultural restrictions placed on them. Family and ethnic/religious community members may encourage or resist an increase in the religious behaviors of Muslim adolescents depending on the social, political, and cultural context (Kibria, 2008).

Young Muslims' interaction with their environment and social scrutiny may result in differing trajectories. Some young people may be propelled to explore their spiritual beliefs in greater depth (Ahmed, 2009). Religion can serve as a positive force for young people, providing them with purpose and meaning in life, clear messages of socially appropriate behaviors, development of self-regulatory abilities, and avoidance of health-compromising behaviors. However, in rare cases, young people who perceive discrimination or social exclusion, are not socially bonded to society, do not identify viable mechanisms to address social grievances, and lack functional Islamic literacy[3] may be more susceptible to radicalization. Other young people may be more inclined to focus on Western culture and non-Muslim peers because they are perceived as having a higher status than Muslim peers.

Approximately one-fourth to one-third of Muslim youth in the United States and the United Kingdom report that they have difficulty maintaining their values and beliefs (Ahmed & Akhter, 2006; Federation of Student Islamic Societies [FOSIS], 2005). Difficulties are attributed to peer pressure, social pressure, struggle with identity, lack of religious contextualization,[4] and leisure alternatives (Ahmed & Akhter, 2006; Khan & Ahmed, 2010). In addition, Muslim youth identified their personal lack of knowledge and understanding of Islam as an obstacle for their spiritual development. Muslim youth report learning about Islam through their local mosque or their family (Muslim Public Affairs Council [MPAC], 2007). However, these sources often do not contextualize Islam to Western culture and often lack relevancy. As such, increasingly, the Internet is being utilized as a means for young Muslims to learn about Islam and connect with religious figures who are able to begin the process of contextualizing Islam in the West.

Risky Behaviors

As young Muslims develop and interact with their environment they may choose varying developmental pathways. Of particular concern to clinicians is when adolescents and emerging adults engage in risky behaviors. This may be the reason why a young person may be referred to a clinician.

---

[3] Functional Islamic literacy refers to basic knowledge of Islamic beliefs, practices, and priorities.
[4] Islam can be understood as a set of principles to be applied in daily life. The application of some of these principles will vary depending on the local culture and circumstances. However, in many Muslim communities in the West, the application of Islam is based on Eastern cultures. As a result, Muslim youth who identify with Western culture have difficulty with the lack of contextualization of their faith within Western norms or 'urf. For a detailed discussion on this topic, refer to the work of Tariq Ramadan, namely *To Be a European Muslim* (1999) and *Western Muslims and the Future of Islam* (2004).

Muslim youth, like their non-Muslim peers, engage in self-injurious behaviors, substance use, and criminal activity. Their behaviors may be due to experimentation, negative peer pressure, or underlying mental health issues, which the clinician should explore.

Self-Injurious Behaviors In Islam, suicide or harming one's body is strongly prohibited. However, evidence of suicidal behavior among young Muslims in the United Kingdom found no difference in rates of suicidal ideation and attempts between Muslim youth and their Hindu peers (Kamal & Loewenthal, 2002). Muslim Youth Helpline, a U.K. peer-counseling service, reported that approximately 7% of its clients expressed suicidal ideation (Muslim Youth Helpline [MYH], 2007).

> **BOX 14.1**
>
> **Muslim Youth Helpline** (**MYH**; myh.org.uk) is a peer-counseling service that aims to provide religiously and culturally sensitive service to Muslim youth in the United Kingdom. It has provided services via telephone, e-mail, and chat options since 2001. Males and females between the ages of 18 and 28 are trained to be peer counselors and are provided with ongoing specialized training. Peer counselors report addressing numerous mental health needs such as suicidal ideation and self-injury, depression, anxiety, identity issues, problems with interpersonal relationships (romantic, marriage, family, peers), and issues related to sexuality (lesbian, gay, bisexual, transgender [LGBT], pregnancy and abortion, sexual impulses). MYH has received over 15,000 calls as of 2007 (MYH, 2007).

Common issues that may prompt suicidal attempts include interpersonal stress, academic problems, and shame. Some Muslim youth may exhibit similar warning signs as their peers including depression, suicidal ideation, preoccupation with death, and increased substance use. Other young Muslims may verbalize their preoccupation with death to surrounding people, but may not be taken seriously because of the prohibition of such behaviors. In some cases their verbalizations may be misinterpreted as being extremely religious and preparing for the life of the Hereafter. Muslim youth may also choose not to verbalize their suicidal ideation due to the prohibition in Islam, unless directly asked. The clinician may need to engage in passive or indirect questioning when suicidal ideation is suspected through questions like, "Do you ever wish God would take your life to help ease your pain?" or "Have you ever taken more medication than you were supposed to?"

Nonsuicidal injurious behaviors among Muslim adolescents are also prevalent. Counselors working with Muslim youth indicate that at least 10% of individuals calling Muslim peer-counseling services reported self-injurious behaviors, and this is considered to be an under-representation of the actual phenomenon (MYH, 2007). Young Muslim women engaging in cutting behaviors may go unnoticed by others, especially if they adhere to religious clothing requirements of covering their bodies in public settings. Like their peers, young Muslims may engage in such behaviors in order to gain a sense of relief and control over their bodies, to help regulate and/or distract themselves from strong emotions, to express emotions that they find difficulty in verbalizing, or to punish themselves. Exploring the underlying causes of self-injurious behaviors and factors than maintain the behavior is an important part of the assessment process. Educating clients and parents regarding self-injurious behavior, helping the young Muslim understand the emotional triggers that initiate cutting, and developing alternative ways to regulate tension and conflict within significant relationships are important therapeutic interventions.

Substance Use   In Islam, any substance use, including alcohol, is prohibited and associated with social stigma (Maalouf & Arfken, 2009). Despite prohibition, U.S. Muslim youth report alcohol use in the range of 47% to 71% (Abu-Ras, Ahmed, & Arfken, 2010; Ahmed et al., 2009). Most individuals began drinking prior to entering college, and their reasons for use did not differ from their peers. Surprisingly, there were no significant gender differences observed in rates of consumption. One prominent risk factor included the youths' report of parental approval of alcohol use (Abu-Ras et al., 2010).

Muslim youth reported a range of illegal drug use between 25% to 48% (Ahmed et al., 2009, 2010), cigarette use from 37% to 50% (Ahmed et al., 2010; Islam & Johnson, 2003), with Muslim males having a higher risk for use than their non-Muslim peers (Ahmed et al., 2010). Predictors of tobacco use include peer norms of smoking behavior, mother born in the United States, having a sibling who smoked, and positive beliefs about smoking (Rice, Templin, & Kulwicku, 2003; Islam & Johnson, 2003). In a national random sample of college students, 22% of Muslim students reported having used alcohol, illegal drugs, and cigarettes in the past year (Ahmed et al., 2010).

Given the religious prohibition against substance use, the adolescent or young adult's decision to use substances may be a symptom of internal conflict, peer pressure, rejection of parental values and expectations, or mental health issues. In such cases, clinicians may need to provide psychoeducation for parents, explore underlying issues of substance use, and identify emotional triggers that maintain use, as well as cultural, religious, and social implications of substance use.

Criminal Activity   Although there is minimal data on Muslim adolescent and emerging adult criminal behavior, young Muslims' involvement in criminal activity is of increasing concern. England's prison population is 11% Muslim (Offender Management Caseload Statistics, 2008), many of whom are Muslim youth. In Europe, adolescent and emerging adult criminal activity has been attributed to discrimination, high rates of unemployment, poverty, disparities in housing and education, and lack of social mobility for minorities (Yeager, 1996; OSI, 2010). However, in countries like Australia, there is a perception that a disproportionate number of young Muslims are involved in criminal activity, reflecting negative media discourse, political opportunism, and racist attitudes (Collins & Reid, 2009).

Clinicians working with young Muslims who engage in harmful behaviors, whether self-injury, substance use, or criminal activity, often encounter numerous challenges. Parents may not understand the extent to which their child is engaging in risk-taking behaviors, either due to the young person's refusal to share information, parental denial, or lack of comprehension. The lack of awareness may result in misattribution of behavior, which can impact parental expectations, rules, and response to the young Muslim. As is common during adolescence, Muslim youth may have limited abilities to project possible risks and negative consequences of current actions, and may need the clinician's help to assess risks, reflect rationally on situations, and learn problem-solving skills. The following case highlights how an emerging adult interacts with her environment and how the individual factors discussed previously may present within a clinical setting.

CASE STUDY 1: USRA AND THE CONTEXT OF THE INDIVIDUAL DEVELOPING PERSON[5]

Usra is a 16-year-old Canadian female of Caribbean origin who had presented for treatment with her parents after an unsuccessful suicide attempt. She reported interpersonal conflict with her parents because of her lack of adherence to Islamic values. In addition, her parents reported being frustrated that she sleeps during the day, stays up at night, and does not help out with family chores. As a result of her sleep cycle, she has been tardy and missed school and is in jeopardy of being held back a year.

---

[5] The names and identifying information of the individuals discussed have been changed in order to protect clients and maintain confidentiality.

During the initial evaluation, Usra reported feelings of anxiety, depression, hopelessness, and helplessness. She has difficulty concentrating in school and is failing many of her classes. Further evaluation revealed that Usra was repeatedly sexually abused by a distant relative during her prepubescent years. Her parents became aware of the abuse several years later. Usra declined to share additional information about the abuse, other than that the abuser no longer had access to her. The parents indicated that Usra had never received counseling for the sexual abuse.

Although Usra was raised in a religious family, she appeared unsure about her current values and beliefs. She occasionally attended the local mosque but avoided other community events. Usra reported that she likes to spend most of her time with her boyfriend, because he "makes me feel safe." Her boyfriend is part of a local gang and has protected her from unwanted sexual attention in the past. Unknown to her parents, Usra reports that she is sexually active with her boyfriend, does not use birth control, and is convinced she will not get pregnant. She denies substance use but admits to self-injurious behavior (cutting) and trichotillomania during her middle school years when her anxiety was worse.

Through the course of therapy, it was clear that Usra continued to struggle with her history of sexual abuse. She was depressed, anxious, and engaged in self-injurious behaviors. Although her parents were frustrated with her for sleeping during the day, the client and her parents were unaware that this was a way to defend against fears of being victimized again at night. It was only during the daytime, when the fear had abated, that Usra was able to feel safe and fall asleep. Through therapy, the connection between past abuse and current behaviors was highlighted for both Usra and her parents. Usra was able to understand her anxiety, and began verbalizing intense emotions and choosing alternative methods of coping. The parents were more understanding of her behavior and tried to support her attempts to feel safer.

In family therapy, both Usra and her parents were able to verbalize the impact of unmet family expectations. For her parents, they felt they had failed their religious obligations as parents, for not protecting their child from the sexual abuse and because Usra did not uphold her religious values. For Usra, parental disappointment in her lack of adherence to Islam resulted in lower self-esteem and depression. She internalized the belief that she was a bad Muslim because of her risky behaviors, but still felt connected to her faith, which resulted in an internal conflict with respect to her religious identity and sense of spirituality. To cope, she avoided spending time with her family. Usra and her parents were able to communicate their feelings of hurt, love, and disappointment and began working toward understanding and supporting each other's needs.

As Usra experienced increased safety within the clinical setting, past sexual abuse was slowly explored. The clinician helped Usra unwrap her past experiences and connect it to current maladaptive behaviors. Through this process the therapist was able to explore Usra's risk-taking behaviors and negative thinking. The clinician assisted Usra in restructuring her negative cognitions and testing out new ways of interacting with those around her. This approach helped her to begin developing positive experiences in her environment and a more positive sense of self.

Among other issues, this case highlights how individual factors, such as sexuality, identity, religiosity, and risk-taking behaviors, may interact with each other.

Microsystem

As individuals develop, they interact with their immediate environment, referred to as their microsystem (Bronfenbrenner, 1977). The microsystem includes settings such as family, peers, school, and communities.

Family Setting

Islamic and Muslim cultures have traditionally given great importance to maintaining close family ties. Unlike many young people in Western nations, Muslim emerging adults traditionally live with their parents until they marry, and parents expect to play a major role in their children's life, regarding clothing choices, friends, social and recreational activities, educational aspirations, and choice of spouse. The process of renegotiating family relationships, rules, and expectations resulting from developmental transitions can be challenging for some Muslim families.

Immigrant parents may struggle with adjusting their cultural expectations. It is common across cultures for parents to get upset over their child's lack of adherence to parental expectations. However, for Muslim youth and their parents this may be more difficult because the child and society may perceive parental expectations as more conservative. Parents may fear that their children will engage in religiously or culturally prohibited behaviors and limit their child's interaction and activities at school and with peers, particularly for their daughters (Buitelaar, 2002), without providing them with adequate social alternatives. These circumstances can result in the young person distancing their relationship with their parents, rebelling against their parents' rules, internalizing anger, and intentionally withholding information or misinforming parents about their activities. Children's behavior may increase parental frustration, stress, and restrictions. Clinicians should explore the personal meaning and implications of unmet expectations for both parents and their children. In addition, parents' history of religious and cultural socialization as well as parenting style can provide insight regarding dynamics being played out in the parent–child relationship.

Refugee Muslim families, a subgroup of immigrant families, often experience additional stressors due to their forced migratory experience. Families may have experienced multiple losses and chaotic circumstances during the migratory process. For some youth, these losses may decrease their ability to structure and integrate their experiences, which may manifest itself in the form of trauma symptoms (Ager, 1996). As a result, refugee youth may report lack of trust, social isolation, difficulties maintaining peer relationships, developmental delays, academic difficulties, and symptoms of depression, anxiety, and distress due to survivor's guilt (Snyder, May, Zulcic, & Gabbard, 2005). Clinicians should explore possible war stressors and traumatic events during development because of their long-term impact on young people's development. In addition, refugee parents may invest their hope for their future in their children's academic achievement, serving as an additional stressor for refugee Muslim youth (Weine, Vojvoda, Hartman, & Hyman, 1997).

Indigenous Muslim families or families of nonimmigrant racial groups, consisting of both converts and Muslims of many generations, may also struggle with family tensions. For convert parents, the age of the child when the parent converted as well as whether or not the child has been raised in another faith tradition are important considerations. Convert parents may struggle with the appropriate level of involvement of non-Muslim family members because of concerns regarding exposure to un-Islamic behaviors. Convert parents may be wary of their children's desire to explore and experiment with alternative beliefs and behaviors, and may be stricter because of their social awareness, which may result in tension between parent and child. Indigenous families often struggle with full acceptance from ethnically based Muslim communities and may be ostracized for integrating mainstream cultural practices, such as Halloween.

In households where one parent is Muslim and the other is of a different religious background, families may experience tension, especially if religious upbringing of children is not discussed prior to the marriage. The lack of clarity in religious guidance may also result in the young person feeling alienated from both religious traditions. A common issue that arises during adolescence is dating. The Muslim parent may object due to religious beliefs, but the non-Muslim parent may support the adolescent because of societal norms. In these cases, coalition between one parent and the young person may result in conflict that can raise issues of parental loyalties and negatively impact the parent–child relationship. These situations can also undermine the marital relationship and result in feelings of rejection, alienation, and isolation.

It is important for clinicians to realize that the concept of family for some Muslims may extend beyond the nuclear family and include cousins, aunts, uncles, and distant relatives. The presence of extended family members living with or close to the individual may help with monitoring, parenting, and religious or cultural socialization. However, the presence of extended family can also potentially be a source of emotional stress, lack of boundaries, and forced maintenance of cultural traditions. As such, it is important for clinicians to recognize that family involvement may entail working with extended family members.

When working with Muslim youth, it is important to include parents or adult figures in treatment because the family is often the context of recovery (Steiner & Feldman, 1996). In the author's experience, issues of confidentiality and ethical responsibility often arise when working with Muslim families. Therapists may encounter situations of adolescents engaging in behaviors that are accepted by society but prohibited in Islam. Negotiating the therapeutic working relationship with the adolescent, while keeping the parents informed and engaged, can be challenging. These factors are further complicated when emerging adults (18 and over) present for treatment, but their parents pay for the cost of treatment and expect to be fully aware and involved in the treatment process. Clinicians may also need to serve as cultural brokers helping parents and children understand each other's perspective, assist families in negotiating new rules and setting appropriate expectations, and providing education as needed.

Peer Influence

New peer environments and changes in peer group compositions may result in increased social complexity for young people. Peer acceptance and feelings of belongingness can help mitigate or increase the stress adolescents and emerging adults experience. Muslim youths' experiences with their peers can vary. Some Muslim youth report that their non-Muslim peers have negative views of Islam and believe that Muslims are terrorists, and they may experience racial and religious discrimination by peers (Khan & Ahmed, 2010). Such reactions may result in young Muslims experiencing feelings of rejection and loneliness, resulting in social withdrawal, or may empower them to change their situation. However, Muslim adolescents and emerging adults also report positive experiences with their peers and believe that their interaction has resulted in an increased familiarity, respect, and understanding of Islam and Muslims (Khan & Ahmed, 2010).

Muslim peers can serve as either a positive or a negative influence. By sharing similar experiences, Muslim peers can serve as an important support system that increases feelings of belonging and support. These supportive relationships may promote activities that help to explore religious and ethnic beliefs, and may help develop a cohesive sense of self. Conversely, Muslim peers may negatively influence the individual to engage in behaviors that are contrary to religious beliefs. As evidence, Muslim youth report consuming alcohol and illegal drugs at similar rates with their Muslim and non-Muslim peers (Ahmed et al., 2009).

Adolescence and early adulthood are particularly challenging for young Muslims because behavioral manifestations in faith become more pronounced. Some young Muslims report strong peer pressure to engage in behaviors that are contrary to Islamic values. These behaviors may include dating, premarital sexual activity, and frequenting bars (Ahmed & Akhter, 2006). Young males in particular are often teased regarding their sexual orientation if they refuse advances by young women or do not talk openly about their interest in the opposite sex. Like all religious groups, this tension of following one's faith or friends is often challenging for Muslim youth. Following one's faith may result in alienation from peers, but following one's friends could result in internal conflict due to lack of adherence to one's faith, community, or familial expectations.

Gender Interaction Muslim youth report that gender interaction and dating are important challenges they struggle with due to social norms and the lack of opportunity to address these issues from a faith-based perspective (Ahmed & Akhter, 2006). Muslim communities, religious scholars, and ethnic and racial cultures address the issue of gender interaction differently. Religious beliefs regarding appropriate gender interaction may vary from total physical and social segregation between genders to adult-supervised interaction.

Individuals who develop and maintain friendships with the opposite gender may experience confusion between the sometimes-blurred lines of friendship and romantic interests common during adolescence and emerging adulthood. As a result, many young Muslims may find themselves in romantic relationships and engaging in sexual activity, thereby going against their religious beliefs. Other youth will avoid the opposite gender and may even develop a persona or role that they present to the outer world in order to protect them from unnecessary interaction through choice of dress, manner of speaking, and communication style (Buitelaar, 2002). These young people may be influenced by religious and/or ethnic influence, fear the loss of honor and reputation, or have concerns regarding finding a future spouse.

Clinicians may need to assist Muslim clients with developing social problem-solving skills as they navigate peer pressure and fulfill their need for peer acceptance, while maintaining their beliefs and values. This may also entail helping them identify positive sources of peer support and alternative leisure activities that do not compromise their faith.

Educational Institutions

Educational institutions, such as schools, colleges, and universities, can potentially serve as socializing agents where Muslim youth can experience feelings of belongingness and connection to society, as well as create opportunities to develop skills and knowledge for social mobility (OSI, 2010). Depending on factors such as socioeconomic status, neighborhood, school funding, and school culture, some youth may experience bullying, poor educational environment, lack of teacher expectation for success, or lack of inclusion and engagement, which contribute to negative experiences with educational institutions (Elsea & Mukhtar, 2000; Zine, 2001).

Negative teacher attitudes and bias, such as teachers assuming that female students are oppressed because of wearing the *hijab*, can impact Muslim youth development (Archer, 2002). Low teacher expectations, bias in educational assessment, and disparaging remarks by teachers about students' religious beliefs and practices may be common experiences for some young Muslims (OSI, 2010). Due to teacher bias or lack of awareness, teachers may present the current geopolitical situation as a clash of civilizations and Muslims as the "other," resulting in young Muslims feeling marginalized (Abu El-Haj, 2005). In addition, teachers and professors may invalidate adolescent and emerging adults' religious beliefs on topics such as homosexuality, abortion, and premarital relationships, resulting in a disempowering learning environment.

Administrative attitudes toward scheduling conflicts can either connect or distance students from schools. For example, Muslim men are required to attend Friday communal prayers. School administrators who work with students to meet their needs by making necessary accommodations so that students complete obligatory daily and Friday prayers are likely to strengthen educational engagement because of the practices of religious sensitivity. Similarly, when teachers and administrators take into account religious holidays, such as the two *Eids*[6] when scheduling exams, young people feel more acknowledged and integrated. In addition, schools and universities can also provide same-gendered physical education classes and instructors in order to provide an alternative and promote feelings of inclusion for observant Muslim students, as well as other students wishing to participate in same-gendered activities.

---

[6] Muslims celebrate two major holidays *Eid ul-Fitr* and *Eid ul-Adha*. *Eid ul-Fitr* is a celebration marking the completion of the month of Ramadan, where Muslims fast daily from sunrise to sunset. *Eid ul-Adha* commemorates Prophet Abraham's sacrifice for God and coincides with the completion of the annual pilgrimage, or hajj.

Clinicians working within a school or college counseling setting should work with administrators, teachers, parents, and students to promote a culturally and religiously sensitive and collaborative learning environment. Such an environment will not only support Muslim students, but can also promote understanding and religious tolerance between all students. School interventions can also help with the prevention and early detection of learning disorders and mental health illness, and can help promote Muslim youth development.

Community Settings

The community context may be an integral setting for young people's development. Although different communities exist, this section focuses on the following community settings that may influence young Muslims: neighborhood/geographic location, Muslim and ethnic communities, and youth-focused community organizations.

Neighborhood and Geographic Location The neighborhood young Muslims reside in can have both a positive or negative impact on their identification with Islam. Rural or less-populated Muslim settings provide for greater opportunities for interfaith experiences and dialogue, greater willingness to rely on support services available outside of the Muslim community, and more opportunities to acculturate into mainstream society. Conversely, in rural settings where Muslims are surrounded by individuals of other cultures and faiths, it may be difficult for Muslim youth to exert their religious and/or ethnic identity. They may have fewer opportunities to interact with other Muslim role models and share religious and cultural experiences, less access to obtain support from Muslim peers and mentors, and fewer resources to increase their knowledge of religious beliefs and practices.[7] In such cases, young Muslims may identify with other minority youth, particularly those of African descent. Identifying with these groups may serve to fulfill a sense of belongingness to a larger group with minority status and experiences of discrimination (Archer, 2001).

In neighborhoods with large concentrations of Muslims, young people may feel power in numbers and shared beliefs and thus may be more likely to identify with their religion and culture. They may have more religion-enhancing activities as well as numerous Muslim peers for socialization and identification. Although they may have greater access to cultural and religious sources of support and development, a neighborhood setting with a greater number of Muslims may have its own problems. Living in

---

[7] However, religious educational opportunities are increasingly becoming available due to the accessibility of the Internet.

mainly Muslim neighborhoods may result in increased pressures to conform to ethnic rather than religious standards, without proper exploration and understanding. Such settings can also limit acculturation and development if the neighborhood context provides few models for economic, religious, and social competence, and they can be constraining for young Muslims who do not identify with their ethnic or religious culture.

Muslim and Ethnic Community Muslim communities within Western nations differ based on ethnic/cultural homogeneity or heterogeneity, geographical location (i.e., rural vs. urban), socioeconomic conditions of its members, level of acculturation, and ideological perspective. The community makeup and culture can influence Muslim youth, their development, and their relationship with the community.

In countries where one ethnic community dominates the overall Muslim community, the ethnic culture often impacts the perspective and practice of Islam, which may be more culturally rather than religiously based. In England, the majority of Muslim residents are of South Asian descent; in the Netherlands the Muslim population consists mainly of individuals of Moroccan and Turkish descent; in France the population consists primarily of individuals of Algerian descent; and in Germany Muslims are mainly of Turkish descent (OSI, 2005, 2010). However, in the United States, Canada, Australia, and Denmark, the Muslim population consists of different ethnic backgrounds. The more intercultural interactions that occur, the more likely it is that young people will be able to tease apart the ethnic influences on religious beliefs and practices. In addition, there are different social and political norms that can affect how Muslims are incorporated into society, such as France's banning of the *hijab* in schools. The interaction of these factors (i.e., ethnic, sociopolitical, socioeconomic) may predict mental health outcomes.

Some young people and their families may identify more with their ethnic community and have minimal to no interaction with their religious community. These individuals may feel more affinity and be guided by norms of their cultural group. As such, some Muslim Arab youth may identify more with their Arab Christian peers, compared to their South Asian Muslim peers.

It is also important to remember that adolescents and emerging adults may experience a lack of connection with their religious and ethnic community (FOSIS, 2005). These differences may be attributed to differences in language, culture, and worldview. Muslim communities may exert strong ethnic pressure that can be constricting to young people. Young people may experience a disconnect with their Muslim community because of its isolation from society, lack of cultural contextualization of Islam to the Western context, and lack of developmentally appropriate recreational and social awareness and activities (Ahmed & Akhter, 2006; Ahmed & Ezzeddine, 2009). In addition, the religious leadership may lack knowledge regarding challenges facing Muslim youth and factors that promote youth development, resulting in an inability to provide effective youth programming. However, some communities are able to successfully engage young people by reaching out and supporting their needs. These communities have mentors to promote youth engagement, create youth-centered physical locations, provide opportunities for youth leadership and development, and attempt to provide contextualized religious education.

Community Youth Organizations In areas of medium to large concentrations of Muslims, Muslim adolescents and emerging adults are organizing groups that aim to meet their needs in school, on campus, within the community, and in areas of interest or specialization. In schools and universities, the presence of student groups enables students to organize themselves, mobilize peers, and meet their social, contribution, and activism needs through political advocacy within the school system. Some examples of political advocacy may include collectively challenging inaccuracies on Islam within the curriculum, changing school policies, and advocating for religious accommodations (Zine, 2001). The ability to make positive change in their environment and negotiate with school administrators can empower young people and serve as a model for social change.

Community-based organizations may be affiliated with a local mosque, youth center, national organization, or simply a virtual network of young people connected by an interest or a cause. Some are led by parents or mentors, whereas other organizations are led by young people themselves. Community organizations may foster social support and a sense of belongingness for Muslim youth, helping them negotiate their identity and assist them in the process of acculturating into society without negating their religious and cultural identity (Ahmed & Ezzeddine, 2009). Muslim youth organizations may attempt to promote religious values and beliefs through positive peer pressure, social and recreational alternatives, and avenues to express their experiences as a religious minority.

Although community organizations may exist, not all young people may choose to participate in their programs. They may participate in non-religious programs because of lack of programs or the poor quality of programming within the Muslim community. In some cases, Muslim youth may not want to identify with other Muslims because they do not practice Islam, may have had negative experiences with "religious" Muslims, or they may be struggling with their own identity. Other youth may not be able to participate because of financial pressures requiring them to maintain after-school jobs (Maira, 2004). In addition, individuals who are not legal citizens may fear that participation could lead to identification and eventual deportation.

Understanding potential sources of community support and stress in the young person's life can help the clinician identify religious and culturally relevant resources that can be integrated into therapy. The clinician should be cognizant that young people and their parents may disagree in their perceptions of support, stress, and degree of identification with the community and this should be considered in treatment. The following is a case study that highlights the role of microsystem settings that a clinician may encounter.

CASE STUDY 2: AHMED AND MICROSYSTEM SETTINGS

A Muslim community leader referred Pakistani working-class, immigrant parents living in England for treatment because of their concerns about their 17-year-old son, Ahmed. Ahmed was struggling in school, displaying greater secrecy about his activities and whereabouts, and increasing in his irritability and anger. In addition, his parents reported Ahmed's poor hygiene, his room always smelled, and that he often masked the smell with excessive amounts of air freshener. The clinician suspected potential drug use; however, the parents reported not knowing what drugs looked like, but they knew their son was spending time with "bad people." The clinician provided psychoeducation about drugs and suggested that if the parents find anything of significance to bring it in, in an attempt to positively identify drug use.

During the next session, the parents brought in "powder" they had found in their son's room, which the therapist informed them was an illegal drug. The clinician discussed treatment options, methods to engage their son in treatment, and supportive services available in the community. In the following session, the parents brought Ahmed to treatment but had not yet informed him about the purpose of his appointment. The parents were afraid to address the topic of concern and expected the clinician to address the issue instead. In session, Ahmed was withdrawn, quiet, and uncommunicative with the clinician. The next day the family's eldest son, Faisal, 21 years of age, stormed into the office infuriated and demanded to see the clinician. He yelled at the clinician and told her to stay out of his family's business. Once the therapist was able to calm down the client's older brother, Faisal began pressing the therapist for information regarding the content of her discussions with his parents and client, which the clinician was unable to address due to issues of confidentiality. After leaving the office, the older brother proceeded to scare his parents by telling them that they would go to jail if they acted on the clinician's instructions. As a result the parents dropped out of treatment, despite the therapist's repeated attempts to reengage the parents.

In this case, Ahmed's parents were unaware of the extent of the issues facing Ahmed until a member of their ethnic and religious community whom they trusted referred them to treatment. The parents were unfamiliar with the social and legal system, and relied on Faisal, the eldest son, to be the cultural broker for the family. However, Faisal used his position to bully his parents and gave inaccurate information about the laws of the land in order to protect his personal interest. It appears that Faisal befriended the neighborhood drug dealer and began working with him. Faisal then introduced Ahmed to the drug market in order to help boost sales in the local high school. Had the parents followed through and contacted the school, Ahmed's sales would have been interrupted. The parents were afraid to contact the school or the police because they did not know what would happen to their son or themselves. The school had not taken any action or expressed any concerns regarding Ahmed's academic difficulties. This case highlights how the family, school, peer, and community factors impact the young person's developmental trajectory.

Mesosystem Interaction

Mesosystems consist of the interrelationships between the major settings of the developing adolescent or emerging adult. These include relationships between the individual's family, school, peer groups, and sometime ethnic or religious community (Bronfenbrenner, 1977). This section addresses the following interactions: family and school collaboration, acculturation, and socioeconomic status because of its salience to young people transitioning to adulthood.

Family–School Collaboration

The interaction between the adolescent's family and school setting can range from collaborative approaches to a relationship filled with mistrust. Schools promoting a collaborative culture with ongoing and open communication with parents and multicultural awareness can engage parents and promote youth development. In economically depressed neighborhoods with large concentrations of Muslims, schools are often stressed because they are underfunded, understaffed, and function with minimal resources. Parents are often less financially stable and may be working multiple jobs and be less available to advocate for their child's needs. Immigrant and refugee parents in particular are less likely to be familiar with the new language, culture, social, and educational systems. The lack of familiarity can result in difficulties engaging parents, despite their commitment to their child's education. When racial or religious bullying and discrimination are perceived in schools and parents do not feel empowered to address the issues with school administrators, the family–school relationship is likely to be tested and more adversarial. The lack of a collaborative working relationship between families and schools often results in diagnosable and preventable symptoms being missed, which can have long-term negative consequences for a young person.

Acculturation

Young Muslims and their parents may choose different acculturative strategies, which can have developmental implications. Immigrant and refugee parents may choose to segregate themselves from the greater society and maintain strong connections with their home country. They may also view adolescent angst, acting out, open disagreement with parents, and identity exploration as alarming due to cultural norms of their country of origin. However, their children are more likely to integrate into society and have their nation, rather than the parent's country, as their frame of reference. The difference in cultural identification and frame of reference may result in a culture gap that may manifest itself in differences in communication, expression of emotions, expectations, and goals, as well as religious, cultural, and social values and beliefs.

Socioeconomic Status

The socioeconomic status of the family also impacts Muslim adolescents and emerging adults. In Europe, Muslim children are more likely to live in economically depressed environments because of the high unemployment rates of Muslim parents, in some cases almost double the national average (OSI, 2010). In France, there is an 85% unemployment rate among youth in mainly immigrant suburbs (Silverstein, 2005), and in England 18% of Muslim emerging adults between the ages of 16 and 24 were unemployed, compared to only 8% of Christian youth (Ethnic Minority Employment Division, 2004). In Europe, the socioeconomic conditions are believed to be related to numerous factors including the migratory history of immigrants,[8] discrimination, Islamophobia, disparity in education and public housing facilities, poor wages and work conditions, and the lack of social mobility or opportunities for change within the social system (OSI, 2010). These conditions may result in young Muslims experiencing feelings of marginalization and lack of hope in the future, resulting in lack of

---

[8] The Muslim community in most European countries initially migrated to fulfill unskilled labor shortages.

investment in education, anger, and frustration. Young people may externalize such feelings toward the government and other entities, as was witnessed with disenfranchised young Muslims during the French Riots of 2005 (Haddad & Balz, 2006).

The socioeconomic condition of Muslims in the United States differs from European countries. Some immigrant and indigenous Muslims live in economically depressed neighborhoods and thus share similar stressors as Muslims in European countries. However, due to immigration reforms during the 1960s and 1970s, an influx of highly educated Muslim immigrants resulted in a large number of Muslims with higher earning potential entering the United States. Their legal standing combined with educational and economic capital empowered this group to contribute to establishing mosques and service organizations, as well as engage U.S. society from a greater position of power than previous groups. In the United States, this has resulted in the emergence of groups of Muslim youth divided by financial realities. Muslim youth from affluent communities may have a greater number of opportunities to attend programs and activities that may support their religious and cultural exploration and development.

Muslim youth living in economically depressed environments often lack community support from the larger Muslim community as well as mainstream society. They often have part-time jobs or other family responsibilities in order to assist their financially stressed parents, thereby lacking time for extracurricular activities, academic enhancement, and opportunities to develop peer support (Maira, 2004). Clinicians working with young Muslims should explore the potential role of socioeconomic status in treatment. The individual's socioeconomic situation may be a limiting factor for treatment because parents may not be able to afford treatment or be unable to participate in sessions due to language barriers, multiple jobs, or other responsibilities. Financial stress may also impact the level of physical stress, physical exhaustion, and quality of relationships in the home environment.

The following case study highlights how mesosystems can influence clinical presentation.

CASE STUDY 3: AICHA AND MESOSYSTEM INTERACTIONS

Aicha is a 20-year-old French emerging adult of Algerian descent who was brought into treatment by her neighbor after expressing suicidal ideation. She reported feeling depressed and expressed feelings of hopelessness, helplessness, and decreased self-esteem. Aicha indicates that her daily activities consist of sleeping most of the day and watching television, and she reported gaining 15 kg in the last two months. Although she has struggled with depression in the past, her recent suicidal ideation was triggered by her decision to divorce her husband of six months and the ensuing opposition she experienced from her family.

Although the focus of Aicha's treatment was to decrease her level of depression and increase her level of support, internalize new coping styles, and restructure her negative cognitions, the clinical interview revealed a number of factors in her mesosytem that had contributed to Aicha's current symptomology. The clinician was able to identify that Aicha had an undiagnosed learning disorder, which led to academic failure and negative self-perception. Aicha recalls a teacher who had expressed academic concern about her and had written a note asking her parents to attend a parent–teacher meeting. Her parents never attended the meeting because her mother did not speak French and her father was unavailable to meet due to working multiple jobs to provide for their family and relatives in Algeria. Her father had considered letting Aicha continue her education; however, because of her poor academic performance and inability to obtain work, he insisted that she get married to help reduce the financial burden at home. Once married, she realized she had agreed to get married because she had felt like a failure and marriage would be a way to redeem herself in her family's eyes. However, in hindsight, she realized she should not have married. Her family was extremely upset at her request for divorce due to the financial burden of the wedding and the inevitable gossip that the divorce will cause among their ethnic community.

In this case, one sees how the varying mesosystem factors—family-school, acculturation, and socioeconomic status—can interact with each other and contribute to Aicha's symptomology.

Exosystem

The exosystem refers to social structures that do not necessarily contain the developing adolescent or emerging adult, but have an indirect impact on the individual or his or her immediate setting (Bronfenbrenner, 1977). Examples of exosystems that may impact the development of Muslim youth include creative arts, the Internet, the mass media, racism, and discrimination.

Creative Arts

Opportunities for creative expression have been known to promote youth development (Larson, Hansen, & Moneta, 2006) and are increasingly becoming popular with Muslim youth, particularly hip-hop and the spoken word. This increase is attributed primarily to a greater number of Muslim artistic role models being popular in the mainstream, as well as within Muslim circles. In addition, an increase in opportunities and venues where young people can exhibit their talents has helped to promote creative arts within young Muslim social circles. The creative arts serve as a mechanism for self-expression, identification, and communication. The arts allow young people to channel their energy and express their struggles with marginalization and discrimination, concerns regarding social justice, and attempts to create multifaceted identities (Miah & Kalra, 2008; Miller, 2010). The opportunities for creative expression have enabled Muslim youth to connect with their non-Muslim peers through a different medium and share with them their challenges while being accepted for their differences. For artistically inclined clients, clinicians may consider encouraging the young person to artistically express his or her struggles, particularly when verbalization may be difficult, uncomfortable, or threatening.

The Internet

The Internet has revolutionized the world and has impacted how young people think, feel, and interact with each other online and in person. Young Muslims are able to increasingly maintain connections with their Muslim peers through social networking sites, which can serve to reduce feelings of loneliness and isolation, and increase a sense of belongingness to the greater Muslim community. This may be particularly important for Muslim youth living in rural areas or smaller Muslim communities. The Internet has allowed young Muslims to exchange ideas and resources, learn from religious scholars, and connect with youth mentors who are able to assist them with the challenges and angst of adolescence.

The accessibility, anonymity, and affordability of the Internet also exposes young people to multiple risks. Muslim youth may be the subject of cyberbullying by peers or may themselves be perpetrators. The sharing of personal information, status updates, and pictures by friends on Facebook and other social networking sites can result in the exposure of socially undesirable behaviors, as deemed by the Muslim community, and can result in individuals being stigmatized from community and support persons. Muslim youth may feel less inhibited with the opposite gender online and may engage in online dating, sex chats, and voyeurism. Approximately 70% of young people between the ages of 10 and 17 have seen some pornographic material on the Internet (Delmonico & Griffin, 2008), and Muslim youth are likely no exception. According to Muslim youth mentors, young Muslims are increasingly reporting pornography addictions. Young people are able to hide their surfing and pornographic images from their parents because many parents do not suspect such behaviors and are not technologically savvy enough to monitor such Internet use by their children.

Parents reporting increased Internet use, isolated use of computers, and secrecy related to the contents of Internet surfing should be encouraged to monitor Internet use (Delmonico & Griffin, 2008). When a young person presents with symptoms of anxiety and depression following Internet use, has periods of lack of Internet use, and/or suffers consequences due to excessive Internet use (e.g., absent/tardy to school, falling grades, loss of social functioning), issues surrounding Internet use should be explored in treatment. Treatment should focus on understanding underlying issues, educating parents, and monitoring online behaviors (Delmonico & Griffin, 2008).

Impact of Media

The media is a significant vehicle for socialization and the dissemination of beliefs and attitudes, and can influence feelings of inclusion and social cohesion. However, an overwhelming majority of Muslim youth in both England and the United States believes that the media plays a critical role in influencing people's negative view of Islam (FOSIS, 2005; MPAC, 2007). Many feel that news outlets have constructed images of Muslim males as militant, aggressive fundamentalists, and present Islam and Muslims as foreign and "enemies of freedom, tolerance, and pluralism" (Abu El-Haj, 2005). In addition, many movies and television sitcoms portray Muslims in a negative light (Shaheen, 2003), with few exceptions, such as the sitcom *Little Mosque on the Prairie*, aired in Canada. Negative representation of Islam in mainstream media can increase levels of anxiety and stress for young people and alienate Muslim youth from society. In addition, many express frustration over the generalized blame and having to repeatedly take responsibility for the actions of a few disturbed Muslims, when the same expectations are not made of individuals of other faiths.

Racism and Discrimination

Emerging adults report that racism and discrimination are a challenge for them (Ahmed & Akhter, 2006). Approximately 70% of American Muslim youth and 47% of British Muslim youth report experiencing negative reactions due to their religious beliefs and practices (MPAC, 2007; FOSIS, 2005), which likely contributes to feelings of alienation. Muslim youth in England reported an 83% increase in religious discrimination after 9/11 (Sheridan, 2006). In addition, 37% of Muslims between the ages of 16 and 24 believed that the U.K. government was not doing enough to protect their civil rights (OSI, 2005). Post 9/11, religious discrimination has increased and may be more implicit than explicit. Examples of implicit forms of discrimination, such as religion-based teasing, insulting or disrespectful comments, and being stared at or ignored, as well as explicit forms, such as assault and racist remarks, may be experienced (Sheridan, 2006). Real or perceived discrimination may be associated with mental health symptoms (Sheridan, 2006). Muslim adolescents and emerging adults may internalize these experiences and feel excluded from society. Such negative experiences can lead to rejection and isolation from society (Archer, 2001; Dwyer, 2000) and increases the possibility of radicalization.

The following case study presents an example of how exosystems can influence presenting symptoms and be integrated into treatment.

CASE STUDY 4: OMAR AND EXOSYSTEM INTERACTIONS

Omar is a 14-year-old Latino boy living in the United States. His primary care physician referred him for treatment due to repetitive hand washing during the last six months that has resulted in severe eczema, causing him great pain and embarrassment. According to Hussain's mother, he has always been an anxious child, but the severity of the anxiety has varied over time. She first noticed an increase in hand washing a few months ago.

An exploration of family dynamics revealed that Omar's parents have a tumultuous relationship, fraught with screaming and yelling, which is anxiety provoking for Omar. He explains that he tries to decrease the fighting between his parents by keeping their house extremely clean and orderly, which his mother validated. He attributes his current anxiety to being the only minority in his high school and fears that he may be picked on by other students because of his ethnicity and religious background, especially given the recent controversy over the building of a new mosque. In addition, he confides with the therapist that he has recently begun watching pornography on the Internet. Although he knows it is against his religion and he is embarrassed by his behavior, he is constantly drawn to the images and does not know what to do.

The client was referred for a psychiatric evaluation and was prescribed medication to decrease his obsessive-compulsive thoughts and behaviors. The clinician began by exploring the underlying issues related to his current hand washing and anxiety. Omar reported that cleaning had been a way to cope with his intense anxiety when he was younger. However, recently when the Islamophobia on the television began as a result of the new mosque being built, it increased his anxiety about being the only Muslim and Latino in his new high school, and he worried about how people would treat him. As a result, he turned to the Internet to avoid the negative newscasts, only to be inundated with pornographic advertisements, which he eventually started exploring. The combined anxiety related to negative media, fears of discrimination at his new school, and watching of pornographic material appear to be the precipitating factors that led to the increased hand washing.

The clinician engaged Omar's parents and provided them psychoeducation about the presenting symptomology and maintaining factors. The parents were referred to couples counseling and were encouraged to monitor their son's Internet use. The clinician worked with Omar to adopt new coping styles in order to address his anxieties. During the clinical interview, Omar had reported an interest in poetry. As a therapeutic intervention he was encouraged to use poetry as a medium to verbalize his struggles, anxieties, and fears that he had been internalizing. Omar was able to effectively use poetry to explore his fears of hate and discrimination. He shared a piece of his poetry with his English teacher, who encouraged him to publish it in the school newspaper, and his peers received it positively. The positive reception in turn helped to decrease his anxieties about acceptance and discrimination.

Macrosystem

The macrosystem refers to the ideology or overall institutional patterns of a culture that may affect the development of the individual. These factors shape the environment in which the adolescent and emerging adult lives and to which he or she responds. This section focuses on areas that often impact young Muslims: global events and the political environment.

Global Events

Like many other youth, Muslim youth's identity is impacted by global events, resulting in a fluid and constantly shifting identity (Chaudhury & Miller, 2009; Hutnik & Street, 2010). Global events may heighten awareness of one's religious minority status and trigger Muslim youth's identity search at an earlier age than their peers (Ahmed, 2009). Events such as 9/11 and the London and Madrid bombings not only impact young Muslims living in those locales, but also Muslim youth living in different parts of the Western world (Sheridan, 2006; Hopkins, 2007). The personalization of events and trauma that results from being identified by fellow citizens as part of a national destabilizing threat is often met with feelings of anger, fear, frustration, and feeling trapped. Muslim youth experience anger at the individuals engaging in criminal behaviors for hijacking their religion. They also experience anger at fellow citizens for questioning their loyalty to their nation and for generalizing and painting all Muslims as potential terrorists. When global events occur, many young Muslims are concerned about their safety and fear being physically attacked by strangers due to religious discrimination.

Political Environment

Global events have also prompted political opportunism that appears to have negatively impacted Muslims living in Western nations. The political discourse of nations impact how members of society view Muslims, how Muslims view themselves, and their willingness to integrate into society. In countries that have traditionally been multicultural and accepting of cultural differences, Muslim youth are observed to better integrate into society, whereas in more homogeneous nations, an increase in racism is experienced and there is a lesser desire to integrate (Kibria, 2008). The recent debates over the banning of the *hijab* or *niqab*[9] in France and other European nations has developed a cultural context of xenophobia, mistrust, and increased animosity between Muslims and the political establishment. Some Muslim youth are harnessing the political power that comes with their status as citizens, while others are disillusioned by the establishment.

Obstacles to inclusion and acceptance also include exclusionary legislation in many countries. Some European countries are adopting tighter immigration policies, targeting individuals from Muslim-majority countries and making it more difficult for them to become citizens. Such actions negatively impact Muslim youths' psyches and willingness to integrate, serve their nation, and can lead to disenfranchisement.

Conclusion

The developmental transition from childhood to adulthood is influenced by numerous individual and contextual factors in a young Muslim's environment. Clinicians who understand the ecological environment their client is imbedded in and how the varying factors may influence the client's life are better able to conceptualize clinical cases and tailor effective therapeutic interventions. As such, it is critical for clinicians to be aware of religious and cultural aspects of symptom presentation, sociocultural implications of behaviors, and potential environmental supports and stressors in order to be effective as clinicians. Like adherents to other religious traditions, it is important to recall that Muslims are heterogeneous in their backgrounds, experiences, situations, levels of religious adherence, and cultural identification. Clinicians are encouraged to exhibit an attitude and approach to therapy that respects, draws upon, and uses religious and culturally meaningful resources. In addition, clinicians unfamiliar with Islam and Muslims are encouraged to develop a collaborative relationship with a religious consultant in order to assist in the treatment process. Appreciating and exploring the complexities in relationships, interactions of settings, and societal impact will help the clinician develop a stronger therapeutic alliance, tailor interventions, and improve treatment outcome.

---

[9] *Niqab* refers to a face veil that covers the lower part of a woman's face up to eyes and is worn by some Muslim women.

References

Abu El-Haj, T. (2005). Global politics, dissent and Palestinian-American identities: Engaging conflict to re-invigorate democratic education. In L. Weis & M. Fine (Eds.), *Beyond silenced voices: Class, race and gender in United States schools* (pp. 119-215). Albany, NY: SUNY Press.

Abu-Ali, A., & Reisen, C. A. (1999). Gender role identity among adolescent Muslim girls living in the U.S. *Current Psychology, 18*(2), 185-192.

Abu-Ras, W., Ahmed, S., & Arfken, C. L. (2010). Alcohol use among U.S. Muslim college students: Risk and protective factors. *Journal of Ethnicity in Substance Abuse, 9*(3), 206-220.

Ager, A. (1996). Children, war, and psychological intervention. In S. C. Carr & J. Schumaker (Eds.), *Psychology and the developing world* (pp. 162-172). New York, NY: Praeger.

Ahmed, S. (2009). Muslim youth: Religiosity and presence of character strengths. *Journal of Muslim Mental Health, 4*(2), 104-123.

Ahmed, S., & Akhter, K. (2006). *When multicultural worlds collide: Understanding and working with Muslim youth.* Invited presentation at the 114th Annual Convention of the American Psychological Association, August 12, New Orleans, Louisiana. Retrieved from http://thefyi.org/publications-presentations

Ahmed, S., Arfken, C., & Abu-Ras, W. (2010). *Risk-taking behaviors of U.S. Muslim college students.* Presented at the 13th Biennial Meeting of the Society for Research on Adolescence, March, 11, Philadelphia, PA. Retrieved from http://thefyi.org/publications-presentations

Ahmed, S., & Ezzeddine, M. (2009). Challenges and opportunities facing American Muslim youth. *Journal of Muslim Mental Health, 4*(2), 159-174.

Ahmed, S., Sharrief, S., & Arfken, C. (2009). *Juggling cultural identities: Challenges for second-generation African American Muslim youth.* Presented at the 117th Annual Convention of the American Psychological Association, August 7, Toronto, Ontario. Retrieved from http://thefyi.org/publications-presentations

Al-Mateen, C. S., & Afzal, A. (2004). The Muslim child, adolescent, and family. *Child and Adolescent Psychiatric Clinics in Northern America, 12*, 183-200.

Archer, L. (2001). "Muslim brothers, Black lads, traditional Asians": British Muslim young men's constructions of race, religion and masculinity. *Feminism Psychology, 11*(1), 79-105.

Archer, L. (2002). Change, culture and tradition: British Muslim pupils talk about Muslim girls' post-16 "choices." *Race Ethnicity and Education, 5*(4), 359-376.

Bekker, M. H. J., Rademakers, J., Mouthaan, I., De Neef, M., Huisman, W. M., Van Zandvoort, H., & Emans, A. (1996). Reconstructing hymens or constructing sexual inequality? Service provision to Islamic young women coping with the demand to be a virgin. *Journal of Community & Applied Social Psychology, 6*, 329-334.

Britto, P. R. (2008). Who am I? Ethnic identity formation of Arab Muslim children in contemporary US society. *Journal of American Academy of Child and Adolescent Psychiatry, 47*(8), 853-857.

Bronfenbrenner, U. (1977). Toward an experimental ecology of human development. *American Psychologist, 32*, 513-531.

Buitelaar, M. W. (2002). Negotiating the rules of chaste behavior: Re-interpretations of the symbolic complex of virginity by young women of Moroccan descent in the Netherlands. *Ethnic and Racial Studies, 25*(3), 465.
Chaudhury, S. R., & Miller, L. (2008). Religious identity formation among Bangladeshi American Muslim adolescents. *Journal of Adolescent Research, 23*(4), 383–410.
Collins, J., & Reid, C. (2009). Minority youth, crime, conflict, and belonging in Australia. *Journal of International Migration and Integration, 10*(4), 377–391.
Delmonico, D. L., & Griffin, E. J. (2008). Cybersex and the e-teen: What marriage and family therapists should know. *Journal of Marital and Family Therapy, 34*(4), 431–444.
Dwyer, C. (2000). Negotiating diasporic identities: Young British South Asian Muslim women. *Women's Studies International Forum, 23*(4), 475–486.
Elsea, M., & Mukhtar, K. (2000). Bullying and racism among Asian schoolchildren in Britain. *Educational Research, 42*, 207–217.
Erikson, E. H. (1968). *Identity: Youth and crisis*. New York, NY: W.W. Norton.
Ethnic Minority Employment Division (2004). Department for Work and Pensions.
Federation of Student Islamic Societies (FOSIS). (2005). *The voice of Muslim students*. Accessed at http://fosis.org.uk/_old/component/docman/cat_view/117-student-affairs-committee
Haddad, Y., & Balz, M. (2006). The October riots in France: A failed immigration policy or the empire strikes back? *International Migration, 44*(2), 23–34.
Hopkins, P. (2007). Global events, national politics, local lives: Young Muslim men in Scotland. *Environment and Planning, 39*, 1119–1133.
Hutnik, N., & Street, R. C. (2010). Profiles of British Muslim identity: Adolescent girls in Birmingham. *Journal of Adolescence, 33*(1), 33–42.
Islam, S., & Johnson, C. (2003). Correlates of smoking behavior among Muslim Arab-American adolescents. *Ethnicity & Health, 8*(4), 319–337.
Jacobsen, J. (1997). Religion and ethnicity: Dual and alternative sources of identity among young British Pakistanis. *Ethnic and Racial Studies, 20*(2), 238–256.
Kamal, Z., & Loewenthal, K. M. (2002). Suicide beliefs and behaviour among young Muslims and Hindus in the UK. *Mental Health, Religion and Culture, 5*, 111–118.
Khan, F., & Ahmed, S. (2010). *Peer relations and risky behaviors of African American Muslim youth*. Presented at the 118th Annual Convention of the American Psychological Association, August 14, San Diego, CA. Retrieved from http://thefyi.org/publications-presentations
Kibria, N. (2008). The "new Islam" and Bangladeshi youth in Britain and the US. *Ethnic and Racial Studies, 31*(2), 243–266.
Larson, R., Hansen, D., & Moneta, G. (2006). Differing profiles of developmental experiences across types of organized youth activities. *Developmental Psychology, 42*(5), 849–863.
Maalouf, W. & Arfken, C. L. (2009). Assessing the Problem of Substance Abuse in the Arab World. *Journal of Muslim Mental Health, 4*, 5–8.
Maira, S. (2004). Youth culture, citizenship and globalization: South Asian Muslim youths in the United States after September 11th. *Comparative Studies of South Asia, Africa and the Middle East, 24*(1), 219–231.

Miah, S., & Kalra, V. S. (2008). Muslim hip-hop: Politicisation of Kool Islam. *South Asian Cultural Studies Journal, 2*(1), 12–25.

Miller, L. (2010). *Muslim youth identities among Beur: An analysis of North African immigrants and self-perception in France*. Unpublished thesis, University of Pittsburgh.

Muslim Public Affairs Council (MPAC). (2007). *The impact of 9/11 on Muslim American young people*. Washington, DC. Available at http://www.mpac.org/publications/policy-papers/impact-of-911-on-muslim-american-young-people.php

Muslim Youth Helpline (MYH). (2007). *Providing faith and culturally sensitive support services to young British Muslims*. The National Youth Agency, UK: Malik, R., Shaikh, A., Suleyman, M. Available at www.ealingcvs.org.uk/documents/575.pdf

Offender Management Caseload Statistics. (2008). Home Office, NOMS RDS.

Open Society Institute (OSI). (2005, October). *Muslims in the U.K.: Policies for engaged citizens*. Gyoma, Hungary: Q.E.D. Publishing.

Open Society Institute (OSI). (2010). *Muslims in Europe: A report on 11 EU cities*. Gyoma, Hungary: Q.E.D. Publishing. Retrieved from http://www.soros.org/initiatives/home/articles_publications/publications/muslims-europe-20091215

Ramadan, T. (1999). *To be a European Muslim*. Leister, UK: The Islamic Foundation.

Ramadan, T. (2004). *Western Muslims and the future of Islam*. Oxford, UK: Oxford University Press.

Rice, V. H., Templin, T., & Kulwicku, A. (2003). Arab-American adolescent tobacco use: Four pilot studies. *Preventive Medicine, 37*, 492–498.

Shaheen, J. G. (2003). Reel bad Arabs: How Hollywood vilifies a people. *The ANNALS of the American Academy of Political and Social Science, 588*(1), 171–193.

Sheridan, L. (2006). Islamophobia pre- and post-September 11th 2001. *Journal of Interpersonal Violence, 21*(3), 317–336.

Silverstein, P. (2005). *Algeria in France*. Bloomington, IN: Indiana University Press, pp. 93–94.

Sirin, S. R., Bikmen, N., Mir, M., Zaal, M., Fine, M., & Katsiaficas, D. (2008). Exploring dual identification among Muslim-American emerging adults: A mixed methods study. *Journal of Adolescence, 31*(2), 259–279.

Snyder, C., May, D., Zulcic, N., & Gabbard, W. (2005). Social work with Bosnian Muslim refugee children and families: A review of the literature. *Child Welfare League of America, 84*(5)607–630.

Steiner, H., & Feldman, S. S. (1996). General principles and special problems in the psychiatric treatment of adolescents. In H. Steiner (Ed.), *Treatment of adolescents*. San Francisco, CA: Jossey-Bass.

Weine, S., Vojvoda, D., Hartman, S., & Hyman, L. (1997). A family survives genocide. *Psychiatry, 60*, 24–39.

Yeager, M. G. (1996). *Immigrants and criminality: A meta survey*. Ottawa, Ontario: Ministry of Citizenship and Immigration. Government of Canada.

Zine, J. (2001). Muslim youth in Canadian schools: Education and the politics of religious identity. *Anthropology & Education Quarterly, 32*(4), 399–423.

Zogby International (2004). *Muslims in the American public square: Shifting Political Winds and Fallout from 9/11, Afghanistan, and Iraq*. Washington, DC. Accesssed at http://explore.georgetown.edu/news/?ID=1310.

CHAPTER 15
Refugees

SAMEERA AHMED and FRIEDA ABOUL-FOTOUH

Large numbers of Muslim refugees continue to immigrate to Western nations as a result of internal tribal, ethnic, religious, sectarian, and political conflicts. Under the 1951 United Nations Convention Relating to the Status of Refugees, a refugee is a person:

> who owing to a well-founded fear of being persecuted for reasons of race, religion, nationality, membership of a particular social group, or political opinion, is outside the country of his nationality, and is unable to or, owing to such fear, is unwilling to avail himself of the protection of that country.

According to 2009 data collected by the U.S. Department of Health and Human Services, 40% of the current refugee population originated from the predominantly Muslim countries of Afghanistan, Iran, Iraq, Pakistan, Somalia, Sudan, and Yemen. Muslim refugees are diverse in their ethnic and racial backgrounds, sociocultural-political histories, reasons for departure from country of origin, and pathways to resettlement. However, they share common religious beliefs and experiences of being religious minorities in Western nations.

There is a growing need for mental health professionals to be familiar with issues facing Muslim refugees. Migratory stress and the resettlement process coupled with differences in faith and culture may complicate symptom presentation encountered by clinicians. This chapter begins by presenting a short case study to highlight the importance of understanding the refugee experience when working with such clients. The chapter then identifies the different phases of the migratory process and explores varying factors that may influence the mental health of Muslim refugees. The impact of these factors on refugee family dynamics is then examined. Subsequently, religious and culturally sensitive mental health interventions are introduced. Finally, the case study is revisited and additional information is presented that incorporates clinical issues discussed in the chapter.

CASE STUDY: AYESHA, PART 1

Ayesha is a 19-year-old female Afghan refugee living in a medium-sized city in the United States. She is referred to treatment because she has lost guardianship of her younger siblings, aged 7 and 9, for having physically and verbally abused them. The children are currently in foster care and Ayesha is court mandated to seek therapy in order to regain custody.

As clinicians, we are often provided preliminary information about our clients and must then begin the process of gathering relevant clinical information, conceptualizing the presenting problem, and developing effective treatment interventions. However, understanding and exploring the underlying factors that may impact the presenting symptoms will increase the accuracy of diagnosis, as well as improve treatment outcomes. The following sections highlight these factors, and the chapter concludes with revisiting Ayesha's case.

Migratory Process

The following sections highlight the migratory factors that are important to understand during the assessment and treatment phases. Specifically, the premigratory, asylum-seeking, and resettlement stages are explored in order to enable clinicians to be more sensitive to their clients' experience, contextualize symptoms, and identify potential client strengths and resources that can be used to augment treatment.

Premigratory Stage

As a first step, the clinician should explore the client's perception of life before the period of instability. Understanding issues related to the refugee's beliefs and values, education, physical setting (urban vs. rural), socioeconomic status, occupational status, community support, and social support will enable the clinician to contextualize the client's resettlement experience. For example, Bosnian refugees with higher levels of education in their country of origin were found to be more objective in their analysis of their current situation and better able to develop a plan of action than refugees with less education (Colic-Peisker & Walker, 2003). It is theorized that higher education may have a cognitive destressing impact and may promote mental health, as well as the ability to access social supports (Colic-Peisker & Walker, 2003).

Physical location, such as whether an individual lived in an urban or rural setting prior to migration, can influence the refugee's resettlement. For example, urban Bosnian refugees were more willing to marry individuals outside their ethnic and religious backgrounds. However, upon resettlement in Western nations, Bosnian families that intermarried with other religious groups were less likely to have a sense of belongingness or obtain support from Bosnian religious or cultural groups (Colic-Peisker & Walker, 2003).

As a second step, the clinician should inquire about the conflict itself because exposure to trauma is often a predictor of psychological presentation (Mollica et al., 1998). Some refugees may have experienced direct forms of trauma (e.g., physical, psychological, or sexual). Trauma may have occurred at a single point in time, repetitively, or been experienced across multiple generations, such as the experience of refugees from Palestine, Kashmir, and Afghanistan. Factors such as the person's role in the conflict (e.g., dissident or bystander) and the presence of secondary trauma, such as witnessing the torture, rape, and humiliation of family members and friends, can be a major stressor (Snyder, May, Zulcic, & Gabbard, 2005). In addition, refugees may have escaped direct trauma but experienced fear and anxiety due to perceived or potential threats, or experienced deprivation of essentials, such as food and shelter, which may have been traumatic.

A refugee's method of departure from his or her country may also be important to explore. The experiences of individuals whose departure was abrupt, without preparation of documentation and belongings, will differ from those who had time to prepare for their departure (Colic-Peisker & Walker, 2003). In addition, separation from family and other social supports, as well as uncertainty about the future, likely impacts a refugee's experience.

Understanding an individual's preconflict context and being able to compare it to the individual's current condition can give the clinician insight into the current stressors experienced, as well as clarify diagnosis and appropriate treatment intervention.

Asylum-Seeking Stage

Upon fleeing their country, refugees must gain asylum in another nation. During the asylum-seeking process, the individual may experience feelings of vulnerability, uncertainty about the future, and limited access to services. Refugees may seek asylum where family and friends are settled or in a refugee camp. Individuals who must wait in a refugee camp for their papers to be processed may experience an impersonal bureaucratic system. They may be confined to detention centers, called by a number, stripped of personal belongings, and repeatedly have to prove their identity to authorities (Bowles & Mehraby, 2007). Some refugees may experience violence and crime within refugee camps, which can leave the individual feeling degraded, having a lack of personal control, feeling powerless, and experiencing a loss of humanity (Colic-Peisker & Walker, 2003; Bowles & Mehraby, 2007). In addition, refugees may experience feelings of hopelessness, hurt, distrust toward others, frustration, and anger. If the refugees require mental health services during the asylum-seeking period, it is unlikely they will verbalize their needs or seek such treatment for fear of being rejected asylum. Instead, they may focus on more acceptable health issues (Watters, 2001).

Resettlement Stage

Upon arrival to the host country, refugees must learn to navigate bureaucracy and interagency communication in order to obtain basic needs (Colic-Peisker & Walker, 2003). During the initial years, the major challenges encountered by refugees are housing, health care, education, financial stability, social support, and acculturation. These issues are explored in detail here in order to provide clinicians with greater insight into potential postmigratory stress.

Housing   Housing is a prominent issue for refugees as they adjust to their host nation. Refugees may experience difficulties finding affordable housing due to a significant level of housing discrimination (Dion, 2001). In addition, some refugees are resettled by agencies in areas far from family members or individuals sharing tribal, ethnic, or sectarian backgrounds. Housing refugees in close proximity to family and community support may help to decrease feelings of isolation, empower refugees to develop new social networks, and serve as sources of support (Ahearn, Loughry, & Ager, 1999).

Health Care   Muslim refugees may experience similar barriers to treatment as refugees of other faiths (e.g., language, transportation, finances, etc.). However, unlike other refugees, for Muslim refugees discrimination and interpersonal backlash due to religious or ethnic affiliation has been associated with negative health outcomes (i.e., blood pressure, neurological, respiratory, and digestive health problems) (Kira et al., 2010). Refugees may have different explanatory models for their symptoms, and some may prefer herbal remedies, such as honey and black seed, because of a *hadith*, or sayings of the Prophet Muhammad, indicating their medicinal properties. In addition, refugees may originate from countries that did not have concepts of wellness visits (Dillman, Pablo, & Wilson, 1993) and may only seek treatment in hospitals at later stages of disease (Garretson et al., 2006). Finally, refugees may be reluctant to be examined by physicians of the opposite gender due to religious and cultural beliefs of modesty and gender interaction in Islam (Padela & Rodriguez del Pozo, 2010).[1]

Education and Language Acquisition   Education is an important tool for social mobilization in many host nations. The inability to speak the national language impacts refugees' ability to navigate the social systems meant to assist their integration into the host culture (Colic-Peisker & Walker, 2003). In addition, the inability to speak the local language can create social isolation, dependency on others, loneliness, depression, and difficulties gaining employment (Casimiro, Hancock, & Northcore, 2007).

Resettlement agencies may offer classes to teach the host nation's language to new refugees; however, these classes may not be accessed for varying reasons. Similar to other refugees, Muslims may not attend classes due to lack of awareness, long waiting periods, conflicts with work schedule, transportation, and childcare issues (Akotia & Naidoo, 1998). Classrooms may consist of individuals from varying educational levels, ranging from college educated to individuals with no formal education. Teachers may not be equipped to help refugees who have recently experienced traumas and are facing a significant cultural change. Classes may evoke feelings of inadequacy, poor self-worth, and helplessness. Refugees who have experienced trauma may have ongoing cognitive difficulties that preclude them from being able to concentrate and learn (Casimiro et al., 2007). Refugees originating from some Muslim cultures may also feel uncomfortable with mixed-gender classes based on cultural and religious beliefs of appropriate gender interaction (Casimiro et al., 2007).[2]

Educational issues are compounded for refugee children. They may reside in poor school systems and attend overcrowded classrooms with

---

[1] Modesty is an important concept in Islam and defines clothing, behavior, and gender interaction between males and females. Within medical settings, Muslims may feel uncomfortable exposing their body to medical staff of the opposite gender; therefore, it is recommended that a professional of the same gender care for observant Muslim patients. However, according to Islamic principles, the preservation of life takes a higher priority than upholding principles of modesty. As such, if medical situations necessitate professionals of the opposite gender to be involved in treatment, it is acceptable and in some cases required.

[2] Religious scholars have varying opinions on the degree of gender interaction. Religious beliefs range from total segregation and isolation between members of the opposite gender to integration and interaction in settings, as long as individuals are able to maintain their faith and practice.

fewer resources. Refugee parents may have difficulty advocating for their child's needs. Students may encounter discrimination from teachers and administrators who may not understand the parents' lack of involvement (Birman, Trickett, & Bacchus, 2001). In addition, some students express feelings of being marginalized due to the peripheral placement of classrooms, poor funding of language acquisition programs (e.g., English as second language), segregation in the lunchroom, and xenophobic beliefs reported by other students (Gitlin, Buendía, Crosland, & Doumbia, 2003). Refugee youth may experience bullying from peers in the form of name calling, social isolation, and physical assault (McBrien, 2008), which can be associated with lowered self-esteem (Kirova, 2001). As a result, students may attempt to avoid peer taunting and stereotypes by dropping out of school (Birman et al., 2001).

Financial Stability and Reemployment Inextricably intertwined with the needs of housing, education, and health care is the refugee's financial stability. Refugees may have left their homes without proof of educational degrees and work experience, making it difficult to obtain employment (Casimiro et al., 2007). Those who are able to gain employment may experience a loss of occupational status, contributing to feelings of shame and inadequacy (Colic-Peisker & Walker, 2003). However, refugees who increase or maintain their previous occupation status may experience positive social identity and may be better able to adjust to the host country (Colic-Peisker & Walker, 2003).

Employers may lack understanding of Islamic beliefs and practices, which may result in discrimination. Documented reports of high levels of discrimination as well as denial of employment among Muslim refugees have been noted (Fozdar & Torezani, 2008; Casimiro et al., 2007). In addition, employers may require Muslim employees to complete religiously mandated daily prayers at home, or repeatedly perform more challenging tasks than their coworkers (Casimiro et al., 2007).

Social Support Forced migration results in a tremendous loss of social support for refugees. The presence or lack of social support in the resettlement community can help transition or hinder the refugee's settlement. The ability to form social support networks may be related to war trauma and breakdown of social trust, as well as the presence of warring factions within the resettlement community (McMichael & Manderson, 2004). For example, McMichael and Manderson (2004) found that Somali refugees were sometimes inhibited from trusting others and creating new relationships because of memories of war atrocities. The scarcity of funds and time also affect the mutual obligations and exchanges that contribute to an erosion of social networks (McMichael & Manderson, 2004). Refugees may work multiple low-paying jobs to meet financial needs, and this may result in the individual having less time as well as opportunity to socialize with others (Colic-Peisker & Walker, 2003).

Refugees may or may not choose to identify with their ethnic or religious group, depending on the social capital gained from such an affiliation (Colic-Peisker & Walker, 2003). Perceived discrimination can increase a sense of isolation, impact adaptation, and decrease refugees' sense of well-being, and is strongly associated with social and psychological adjustment (Lindert, Korzilius, Van de Vijver, Kroon, & Arends-Toth, 2008; Ellis et al., 2010). It is theorized that Bosnian Muslim refugees did not interact with the general Muslim community during the resettlement process because their European ethnicity led to less discrimination than their Islamic identity (Colic-Peisker & Walker, 2003).

Acculturation Acculturation is influenced by different factors including individual and family characteristics, cultural distance from host nation, and geopolitical realities (Colic-Peisker & Walker, 2003). Elderly refugees may have difficulty integrating into the host nation, while children may be better able to integrate into society. A refugee's cultural distance and visibility in the host society can also affect acculturation (Colic-Peisker & Walker, 2003). Refugees who are closer to the host country in culture and racial makeup, such as Bosnians, are able to integrate into the society more readily than refugees who are visible minorities and culturally distant from the host culture, such as Somalis. Islamophobia and economic instability may result in politicians highlighting refugees as a financial burden to the welfare system, which can impact refugees' sense of safety (Aroche & Coello, 2004) and level of acculturation. After 9/11, Muslim refugees in America reported heightened fear of discrimination, feelings of insecurity, depression, and traumatic flashbacks, as well as greater feelings of vulnerability compared to refugees of other faiths (Kinzie, 2004).

Family Dynamics

Refugee families encounter multiple stressors that are experienced differently by each member of the family. Families can be separated during the migratory process, and the delays in family reunification efforts can impact family stability. Once in the host nation, financial instability may affect family cohesiveness, as families may spend less time with each other due to balancing numerous responsibilities (McMichael & Manderson, 2004). This section discusses how resettlement may impact family roles and responsibilities.

Men

Muslim male refugees may come from patriarchal societies where they have been socialized to be the breadwinners and heads of their households. In Islam, men are considered religiously obligated to meet their family's financial needs. Thus, the inability to provide for one's family may be experienced as a loss of one's manhood and can impact a male's sense of self. Significant tension may surface if the wife is able to gain employment while the husband is not. In these situations, men may be requested to participate in childcare and household chores, which may be experienced as shame.

Refugee men may continue to play a protective role and accompany women and children to appointments and outings, as they had done in their country of origin. However, such actions may be viewed in the host country as controlling or intrusive. Husbands may become protective of females for fear of discrimination and perceived negative influences of the host culture, as well as a desire to shield their wife from the financial and social stresses of the host nation (Casimiro et al., 2007). However, such behaviors can also be used as a method to control women in order to deny access to information and available resources, and limit social relationships (Casimiro et al., 2007). Men may take such actions and believe it to be their religious right and responsibility due to their interpretation of the concept of *qawamah*, or family leadership in Islam.

Some men may reframe their resettlement stressors and changes in family dynamics in religious terms that are empowering (Shoeb, Weinstein, & Halpern, 2007), as well as frame their challenges as an opportunity to grow and develop. However, other men may experience grief and difficulty moving forward in their new life. They may exhibit symptoms of depression, isolation, irritability, anger, and violence. In situations where males attribute negative behaviors to religious beliefs, as in the case of not providing household support, and controlling or abusive and controlling behaviors, the clinician is recommended to work with a religious consultant to augment treatment. Religious consultants can reduce the cultural stigma of housework by exploring religious role models, such as the Prophet Muhammad, who was known to be involved in household chores of sewing, cooking, and parenting. In cases where the concept of *qawamah* is used to engage in abusive or controlling behavior, the clinician can work with the client and religious consultant to explore the concept within the family, religious, and Western contexts.[3]

---

[3] Clinicians can refer clients and religious consultants to *Family Leadership: Qawamah* (2009), by M. R. Beshir, as a reference. The book presents varying religious interpretations of the concept, explanations within a Western context, and case examples of appropriate and inappropriate use of the concept of *qawamah*.

Women

Arrival in the host nation can result in changes in roles and responsibilities. For some women, employment options may be experienced positively, granting them intellectual challenge, opportunities, and financial independence. However, other women may feel that they are violating religious and cultural beliefs if required to work. Refugee women may also feel overwhelmed and bewildered by work environment norms, gender interaction, and differences in societal culture, which they may not have previously encountered. Employment is often coupled with the challenge of finding affordable childcare (Colic-Peisker & Walker, 2003) and trying to navigate between old and new cultural expectations and norms (Snyder et al., 2005). For example, women may be asked to contribute financially while still carrying the traditional tasks of child rearing, household responsibilities, and entertaining guests.

Like men, refugee women may also have experienced different types of trauma during the migratory process. Women may have been the victims of rape and sexual abuse, which they may be unwilling to admit for fear of social stigma, and experience symptoms of post-traumatic stress disorder. Women who were impregnated by the rape may have struggled with the decision as to whether or not to seek an abortion or carry the child to term[4] (Snyder et al., 2005). They are often expected to maintain privacy and not discuss problems with outsiders (Snyder et al., 2005).

Clinicians working with refugees who seek treatment should consider cultural contexts. Collaboration with a religious consultant may be helpful. For women who experience discomfort due to beliefs that they are going against religious values, the clinician can help to reframe their situation by encouraging them to discuss with a religious consultant examples of Muslim females living during the Prophetic time period and early Islamic history. A careful review of women in Islamic history can identify individuals who were scholars, businesswomen, healers, and laborers, providing evidence for religious permissibility for women to work.

Children

Refugee children may have experienced multiple losses (e.g., extended family members, friends, and familiar contexts), which may increase their vulnerability and impact their ability to integrate into the host society. They may be challenged with issues of identity related to their religious or

---

[4] Abortion is generally prohibited in Islam, except for certain cases. These cases include situations that may cause harm to the mother or the unborn child. Some scholars consider impregnation from rape as a valid reason for an abortion, but it must take place prior to four months after conception. However, the client may not be aware of religious rulings for such cases.

ethnic identity, which may include frustration due to lack of memories of their home country, attachment to their country of origin at the expense of connecting with peers, or detachment from ethnic culture in attempts to avoid emotional triggers (Berman, Ford-Gilboe, Moutrey, & Cekic, 2001). Parents may also pressure children to maintain cultural norms of country of origin, and children may respond with appeasement, rebellion, or the formation of dual identities (Whittaker, Hardy, Lewis, & Buchan, 2005).

Children may present with different psychological symptoms and presentations. Children may struggle with trust issues as a result of negative cognitions about others, the world, and their future. They may present with attachment difficulties, symptoms of depression, anxiety, and posttraumatic stress disorder. Depressive symptoms in refugee children may present as sadness, survival guilt, pessimism, and suicidal ideation (Snyder et al., 2005). Refugee children may experience anxiety symptoms demonstrated by greater difficulty maintaining attention in the classroom setting (El Habir, Marriage, Littlefield, & Pratt, 1994). They may try to control their bodies through anorexia nervosa and/or developmentally regress as evidenced with nocturnal enuresis (Snyder et al., 2005). Those who have either experienced or observed violence may have difficulty processing those traumatic events (Snyder et al., 2005), which may result in difficulty managing affect, developmental delays, poor academic performance, and depression (O'Shea, Hodes, Down, & Bramley, 2000). Finally, difficulties with social adjustment may manifest as risk-taking behaviors (Snyder et al., 2005) or feelings of loneliness (Halcyon et al., 2004).

Parenting

The numerous difficulties encountered during the migratory process can make parenting a challenging experience. Different rates of child and parent adjustment to host country can exacerbate parenting difficulties. Children often adapt to the host country more quickly than their parents. Parents may feel the stress of being unable to help their children navigate school and peer environments (McMichael & Manderson, 2004). Children's greater familiarity with the host country may result in children becoming cultural brokers for their families and interpreters of the host culture for their parents (Snyder et al., 2005). This may result in parents' increased dependence on their children and a shift in family dynamics. Refugees who once felt competent as parents may become embarrassed and ashamed of their inadequacies. In addition, children may challenge their parents by choosing different norms, values, and friends than those approved by the parents (McMichael & Manderson, 2004).

Parents and children may experience differing levels of trauma, which may impact the parents' pathology, and may manifest itself in difficulties with attachment, inability to monitor children, poor parenting skills, and use of corporal punishment. Despite being religiously abhorred, corporal punishment is a common practice in many Muslim cultures. Parents may also struggle with adjusting their parenting strategies as well as religious and ethnic socialization. Clinicians can encourage clients to increase their knowledge of Islamic-based parenting techniques.[5]

Mental Health Interventions

In this section potential interventions the clinician can use with refugees are offered. Community outreach efforts are discussed as a method of building trust and gaining visibility within the refugee community. Then religious and culturally sensitive approaches to intake screening, orientation, and obtaining refugee history are presented. Finally, treatment interventions and considerations are offered.

Community Outreach

Refugees often experience mental health issues but may not seek treatment due to differing explanatory model for symptoms, the use of religious or cultural coping mechanisms, or fear of stigma. Western notions of psychotherapy are uncommon in many Muslim-populated countries, and mental health issues are often associated with misinformation. Even if the client wants to receive treatment, other factors such as mental health awareness, knowledge of culturally informed therapists, agency location, language barriers, transportation, and finances may serve as barriers to service utilization.

Given the numerous obstacles to treatment, agencies are encouraged to engage in community outreach efforts. Offering programs to orient refugees to their new environment and providing information about community resources in a culturally and religiously appropriate fashion can build trust (Akotia & Naidoo, 1998). Agencies can deliver psychoeducational workshops to address issues that can assist in the resettlement process (Gordon, Taylor, & Sarkisian, 2010) and facilitate employment support groups as well as social support groups to decrease adaptation stress and help reduce social isolation (Akotia & Naidoo, 1998). Psychoeducational programs and agency presence at community events allow for visibility as well as formal and informal consultation within the safety of the refugee's own community (Aroche & Coello, 2004). These interactions can also help the agency identify the needs of the resettlement community, cater services, and connect with possible clientele. Agencies that are flexible and able to meet the needs of the refugee community will be most effective

---

[5] Parents can also be referred to *Parenting in the West* (1998) by Drs. Ekram and Rida Beshir. The book addresses parenting from an Islamic and Western context.

in connecting with those in need of mental health services. In addition, many individuals will only present for treatment if recommended by religious and/or ethnic community leaders, or culturally informed physicians. Establishing a trusting and collaborative relationship with key gatekeepers in the resettlement community can help reduce stigma, assist refugees in obtaining necessary mental health services, and facilitate cultural and religious consultation when tailoring interventions.

Psychotherapy

Intake Screening   The intake process usually begins with the initial contact either by phone or in person with an intake screener and the waiting room experience. The refugee's interaction with the intake screener is often the first impression of the psychotherapy process and may determine whether or not the refugee engages in treatment. A personal approach that asks about the well-being of the individual, conveys empathy, and shows respect for the client is imperative. If staff members are impersonal, bureaucratic, and focused on obtaining necessary details, it may elicit memories of negative experiences associated with bureaucratic agencies that were dehumanizing and disrespectful during the asylum-seeking and resettlement process. Office staff should help put clients at ease by initially providing them with information needed so that clients are informed and feel empowered. Staff members should then explain the information the office will need to collect and put the person at ease in answering questions.

The intake screener should attempt to understand the cultural background, refugee-related issues, and symptomology experienced in order to match the person with an appropriate clinician. The intake screener should be sure to query language needs and ask if the clients would like to speak with someone from their ethnic and/or religious background. In situations where an interpreter is required for treatment, the clinician should be cognizant of the interpreter's effect on the clinician–client dynamic. In addition, the interpreter needs to be trained to communicate exactly what the client has said, as opposed to rephrasing the client's words, in order to identify neologisms, bizarre thought processes, and other cognitive impairments. Families may request that children serve as translators; however, this practice is discouraged due to the potential impact on family dynamics. Although ethnic and language matches between therapist and client is often beneficial, some clients may decline out of concerns of confidentiality.

The screener should also be familiar with religious and cultural norms as well as sociopolitical conflicts that may negatively impact a therapeutic match between a client and therapist. For example, a Palestinian refugee may experience difficulty forming a therapeutic bond with an Israeli therapist, due to the sociopolitical and historical issues. Similarly, refugees may prefer having a clinician of the same gender, due to religious or cultural beliefs of gender interaction. Therefore, cultural competency training for all staff members interacting with clients is essential (Akotia & Naidoo, 1998).

In addition, agencies attempting to meet the needs of refugee clients should attempt to make the waiting room inviting as well as culturally and religiously sensitive in its décor. Having religious symbolism may create discomfort for Muslim refugees who may fear that the agency may try to convert them. Having ethnically oriented reading material, as well as ethnic and religious identifiers in the intake forms, can be more inclusive (Aroche & Coello, 2004).

Clinical Introduction The initial session with the clinician is important and should focus on introducing the client to treatment. The client may have been referred to treatment without understanding the reasons for referral or the nature of psychotherapy. The client may be afraid and confused and may request support persons to be present for the initial session to alleviate anxiety.

Issues to be discussed with the client include the nature and length of treatment, role of clinician and client, confidentiality, and relationship boundaries. Clients may present with varying expectations of therapy, including fears that they may be institutionalized or deported to their country of origin if they are identified as having a mental illness. Clinicians should help reduce anxiety by explaining phases of treatment and how the client may experience these phases. Clients are often confused by psychiatric and psychotherapy services and may expect to be "cured" in a few sessions, or with medication.

Issues of confidentiality are of great concern to many refugees. Refugees may be fleeing totalitarian governments and project those experiences on the agency and clinician. Refugees may be distrustful and resistant to the therapy, which should be acknowledged by the clinician but not be taken personally. Refugees may worry that material discussed in session will be shared with government or resettlement agencies, which could result in denying refugees essential services or even deportation. In addition, if the clinician is from the same ethnic or religious community, the clinician would need to address how to interact in public settings in order to maintain confidentiality.

Relationship boundaries will also need to be addressed at the beginning of treatment to avoid hurt feelings as the treatment progresses. Refugees may confuse the therapeutic relationship with a friendship and invite the clinician to their house for meals, give gifts, and wonder how to repay the clinician for their kindness. A discussion at the onset of treatment about the nature of the therapeutic relationship and benefits of maintaining boundaries to ensure confidentiality and privacy may be helpful.

Rapport Building In the initial session it is essential for clinicians to focus on rapport building and allow clients to express their story, feel heard, and experience an emotionally available clinician. Because refugees come from varying religious, cultural, family, and trauma backgrounds, it is sometimes difficult for clinicians to know the most effective way to build rapport with a particular client. As such, as the clinician is getting to know the client, it is recommended that the clinician match the client's nonverbal body language. In addition, clinicians who express interest and respect for the client's religious and cultural beliefs as well as practices are more likely to understand the client's context. Knowledge about the client's religious and cultural beliefs, norms, and activities will enable the clinician to utilize them as meaningful resources during treatment intervention. Finally, it is important to match the client in speed of language and avoid the use of medical or psychological jargon.

Obtaining History Clinicians should gather relevant information about the client's social, emotional, developmental, family, interpersonal, and migratory histories in order to develop an accurate diagnosis, case conceptualization, and religiously as well as culturally sensitive treatment interventions. The clinician should be careful of under- or over-diagnosis based on a mismatch of cultural perspectives (Bemak, Chung, & Pedersen, 2003). It is important to understand the presenting symptoms within religious and cultural norms as well as cultural interpretations of behaviors.

When obtaining history, clients may become suspicious about the need for detailed information that may appear unrelated to their issue of concern. For refugees who have been interrogated by authority figures in the past, it is important that the therapist does not recreate a similar dynamic during the clinical interview process. As such, the clinician should clarify the possible relevance of areas questioned and provide the client with examples of how seemingly unrelated factors can impact clinical presentation and subsequent interventions. The clinician should document the refugee's experiences within refugee camps or detention centers in order to understand how these experiences may influence the client's sense of self and worldview (Aroche & Coello, 2004). In addition, clinicians can acknowledge that some aspects of the individual's history may be too difficult to talk about at an early stage of therapy. Agreeing to discuss traumatic issues when the client is ready is often experienced positively by the client.

Understanding the client's explanatory model of the symptoms and coping mechanisms used prior to presentation provides the clinician with additional insight and also highlights the potential need for collaboration with other professionals. For example, clients may attribute their symptoms to religious concepts, have sought religious leaders for assistance, have relied on religious parables, or have used the recitation of Qur'an to cope with adversity (Bowles & Mehraby, 2007). Understanding the religious sources of support that are most meaningful can help the clinician later frame treatment interventions that are relevant to the client's explanatory model, as well as determine if collaborating with a religious consultant is necessary.

The clinician should also assess different facets of the client's identity, such as gender, tribal, regional, ethnic, religious, occupational. Although refugees may come from a particular country, clinicians should not assume homogeneity in culture because refugees may identify with different subgroups. Each group will have its own history and experience, which the clinician must take time to understand. The interaction of varying social identities and the migratory experience on the presenting symptoms should be explored.

Clinicians should explore the role of religion in the client's life. Religious beliefs can be a source of support for refugees and may have been instrumental in their coping with migratory stress (Gozdziak, 2002). However, other refugees may have had negative experiences associated with people connected to religion. For these clients, the introduction of Islamic concepts in treatment may be troublesome. The role of faith should not be assumed based on the presence or absence of religious identifiers, such as the *hijab*. It is often best to explore the meaning faith has in the individual's life, how it may influence symptoms, and the client's desire for its role in treatment.

The refugee experience is often viewed within a victim framework. Clinicians should help empower clients by exploring personal strengths that can be used in recovery. In addition, identifying the individual's sources of support (i.e., family, social, and community) and the extent of interaction can clarify the refugee's relationships, sources of support, or degree of isolation. The refugee's physical or virtual[6] proximity to family and community members may play a role in their availability to provide support and meet emotional needs. The refugee's growing relationship with mainstream society will also affect the makeup of the support network.

Case Formulation The information gathered should then be organized into a case formulation, which may guide treatment intervention. Given the complexities often encountered with refugee clients such as missing information, cultural misinterpretations, and discomfort sharing traumatic experiences, clinicians should present their formulation to their clients in order to clarify any religious, cultural, or historical misattribution of information gathered. In addition, it also provides the client an

---

[6] Access to Internet telecommunications (i.e., skype, gchat, msn, etc.) has enabled some families to maintain emotional connections despite physical distance.

opportunity to present additional information that may strengthen or weaken the clinician's working hypothesis and serve to educate the client about his or her symptomology. Details on how to develop a religiously and culturally sensitive case formulation are discussed elsewhere in this book.

Therapeutic Interventions   Once the clinician has a clear working hypothesis of the symptom presentation, treatment interventions should be tailored to the individual's situation and context. When considering treatment intervention, the clinician should consider the nature of symptoms and diagnosis, as well as the individual's strengths and personality, migratory experience, family dynamics, religious and cultural values, and social supports. Western psychological approaches typically focus on personal goals and individual achievements, rather than the person's broader social milieu (Bemak et al., 2003). However, many Muslim refugees originate from collectivist societies, and an individually focused psychological framework may not be the most effective method of treatment. Family, friends, and community may be more intricately linked to one another and the client's goals, decisions, and behaviors. Therefore, depending on the case formulation, different modalities of therapy should be considered. Individual, family, and group therapies have all been shown to be effective with refugee populations (Bemak & Greenberg, 1994; Morris & Silove, 1992). It is important for the therapist to realize that family counseling may include extended relatives and neighbors, as this flexibility will better meet the client's needs. Group and/or family therapy may be considered to help foster interdependence (Morris & Silove, 1992), but would not be helpful when discussing traumas, particularly sexual traumas due to the attached social stigma. Play therapy and other creative approaches to treatment can be effective methods to work through trauma and restore a sense of control in clients' lives, particularly for children. For example, Berman et al. (2001) used photo novellas or picture stories that allowed children to tell stories about their experiences in order to identify themes of life before, during, and after the migratory experience, as well as hopes and dreams for the future.

Regardless of the approach utilized, the following issues should be considered in the process of therapy: psychological safety, religious sources, cultural differences in communication and time, sexual trauma, as well as transference and countertransference issues, which are discussed in greater detail below.

Psychological Safety   Refugees who have experienced threats in their country of origin or harassment in their host nation often have difficulty attaining psychological safety. They may initially present concerns about children's adjustment and resettlement issues because it is less threatening than dealing with the adult refugee's issues. Allowing the focus to remain initially on the children acknowledges the individual's concerns and helps to build trust with the therapist. As the level of trust increases with the clinician, clients will present their own struggles.

In some situations, clients may present with distrust and reticence, which the clinician may view as a survival strategy that was once helpful and required during conflict, but is no longer needed. Strong defense mechanisms may have been erected, and only when the individual feels safe will the refugee be able to address trauma in treatment. The client may avoid painful thoughts and memories. These defenses may result in the individual lacking visible emotions when describing past events, and clients may describe their past trauma in a matter-of-fact fashion. Therapy may initially focus on the here and now, such as identifying and understanding triggers in the current environment, such as news items related to political events that occur in clients' country of origin. One approach to treatment may be to help clients unpackage their experience in smaller doses in order to deal with the intensity of the trauma. As the trauma is acknowledged, skills that were useful in the context of trauma will need to be unlearned, and additional skills can be adopted for the new context.

Religious Resources For clients who are religiously inclined, the use of Qur'anic verses, *hadith*, religious concepts, and Islamic history and personalities can help them reframe their mental health issues. Verses of the Qur'an can be used to help engage clients in change, such as the following verse: "Verily Allah will not change the condition of a people, until they change what is within themselves" (Qur'an 13:11). Similarly, refugee clients struggling with numerous stressors may find solace with *hadiths* or sayings of the Prophet Muhammad: "No Muslim is afflicted with any hurt, even if it is no more than the pricking of a thorn, but Allah wipes off his sins because of it and his sins fall away from him as leaves fall from a tree" (Bukhari, as cited in Sabiq, 1991, p. 1). Islamic history can also be explored, particularly the experience of the early Muslims who endured religious persecution by their tribesmen and sought refuge in the Christian kingdom of Abyssinia (modern-day Ethiopia). In addition, lessons from the *hijrah*, or migration of the Prophet Muhammad and the early Muslims from Makkah to Madina as a result of religious persecution, can provide faith-based examples from which clients can draw.

Clinicians who are unfamiliar with aspects of Islam are encouraged to work with religious consultants to enhance their ability to provide religiously meaningful interventions. In addition, the consultant can serve as a referral source if the client chooses to explore issues of religious concern that are not related to treatment.

Cultural Differences in Communication Understanding the cultural meaning of both verbal and nonverbal communication is important. Interpersonal boundaries may differ between Western culture and the refugee's culture. For example, it is common among some Muslim refugees to hug, hold hands, and kiss the cheek of someone from the same gender. However, they may refuse or experience extreme discomfort with casual touches between opposite genders, such as shaking hands, due to religious rules of gender interaction. However, experiences of trauma may complicate cultural norms and elicit an unexpected emotional reaction.

Some Muslim cultures may encourage indirect communication, whereas the therapist may use a more direct method of communication. Differences in the communication of respect may also occur. In Western cultures, lack of eye contact may be viewed as disrespectful and symptomatic of pathology. However, refugees from certain cultures may believe that eye contact with any individual of authority, including the clinician, is a sign of disrespect. In addition, from a religious perspective, some refugees may also believe it is inappropriate to make eye contact with the opposite gender.[7] Refugees who may have been interrogated, tortured, or experience high levels of anxiety may also have difficulty making and maintaining eye contact.

Given the complexities in cross-cultural communication, the clinician should attempt to match the client's verbal and nonverbal means of communication, as mentioned earlier. A mismatch can result in the client experiencing the clinician as rude, and the clinician may be surprised by the client's negative reaction. Clinicians working with refugees should be conscious of these differences and adjust their communication style to meet the client's needs.

Cultural Differences in Time The concept of time is different between Western cultures and many Muslim cultures. Refugees may have a more relaxed attitude about time, and their day may be organized in terms of prayer times. A common example that clinicians may struggle with is with refugees maintaining their appointments. For example, a client may ask for an appointment at 'Asr time (the afternoon prayer), which he or she may explain to the therapist is at 3 p.m. The clinician would then expect the client to come at 3 p.m. However, from the client's cultural context the same statement would mean that the client will pray the 'Asr prayers *around* 3 p.m. at home and then travel to the appointment, by which time the client may have missed the appointment. The different notions of time may cause tension within the therapeutic relationship. The client may be frustrated by the clinician's perceived inflexibility and lack of religious tolerance, and

---

[7] As the Qur'anic verse 24:30 is understood by some Muslims.

the clinician may experience anger and frustration with the client for not coming to the session on time. The clinician will need to work with the refugee's sense of time and help the client adjust to Western notions of time, so that it does not negatively impact other areas of life, such as work and health. However, it is important for clinicians to differentiate between differences in cultural notions of time and cognitive disorientation resulting from past traumas.

Sexual Trauma Refugee women who present to treatment may have been sexually traumatized and have high rates of post-traumatic stress disorder symptoms, but will not report a sexual assault (Mehraby, 2002). Muslim culture honors virginity and purity, and forbids sex outside of marriage for both men and women. Survivors may worry that they will be judged and blamed for being raped, and may be afraid of being ostracized or abandoned by their family. In cases where a rape is known, men in the family may experience shame and humiliation for not being able to protect their loved one. In situations where men have been sexually traumatized, they may experience humiliation for not being able to prevent such actions and worry about stigma associated with homosexual behaviors. As such, the clinician should be cognizant of cultural stigma when approaching the topic of sexual trauma.

Transference and Countertransference Clinicians should be aware of how the sociopolitical context may influence transference and countertransference issues within the therapeutic relationship. The social, religious, and ethnic groups the client and therapist may identify with can influence the therapeutic relationship. If the refugee has escaped a conflict between two racial or religious groups, the client will likely feel uncomfortable having someone from the other racial/religious group serve as a counselor (Aroche & Coello, 2004). For example, a Bosnian female refugee will likely have difficulty connecting with a Serbian male counselor. Although they may share a similar culture and language, the mass rapes of Bosnian women committed by Serbians will likely elicit negative transference and preclude building a therapeutic relationship.

Similarly, public opinion in the host country may impact countertransference issues experienced by the therapist. The impact of 9/11 and other similar events on the perception of Muslim immigrants has been profound. The clinician should reflect on his or her own conscious or subconscious biases that may impact the treatment of the Muslim refugee. If the clinician shares an ethnic or religious background with the client, countertransference issues, such as testing boundaries, overidentification, and overinvestment in clients, can result in emotional exhaustion or anger toward the client. Clinicians may also experience secondary trauma when working with refugee clients. In these situations it is important to seek clinical supervision.

CASE STUDY: AYESHA, PART 2

Having reviewed the varying factors that may impact a refugee client's experience, we revisit the case of Ayesha presented at the beginning of the chapter.

> Ayesha was referred to treatment by a Christian social service agency that had sponsored her resettlement in America. She had arrived in America at age 17, accompanied by her younger siblings aged 7 and 9. She reported to the resettlement agency that her parents, two older siblings, and other relatives had died during the Afghan wars.
>
> The case manager at the resettlement agency reported that Ayesha was exhibiting numerous behavioral problems. Ayesha was physically abusing her younger siblings and had temporarily lost guardianship. She was depressed about losing her siblings and attempted suicide by overdosing with Tylenol. During supervised meetings with her siblings, the case manager observed that Ayesha vacillated between being emotionally detached and verbally abusive. Unrelated, but of concern to the agency, was that a young Afghan male had begun living with Ayesha. Although there were no Afghan cultural specialists at the agency, the case manager believed her behavior to be both religiously and culturally dystonic and was concerned about social stigma that may result from the client's behaviors. At intake, Ayesha was resistant to therapy and only presented because it was required to facilitate reunification with her younger siblings. Ayesha's description of her premigratory life was vague, providing little information to the therapist. The therapist enlisted Ayesha's case manager and siblings to obtain greater information.
>
> Ayesha was born in northern Afghanistan during the time period when Soviet troops were withdrawing. The clinician was able to integrate the sociopolitical context with her developmental history and realize that Ayesha grew up amid the backdrop of instability and infighting between different Afghan leaders, and the eventual takeover of the Taliban. The constant fighting made her village unsafe and had destroyed the economy and infrastructure of the region, which resulted in their family moving to an overcrowded refugee camp in northern Pakistan. Ayesha grew up with negative associations about Islam, due to the patriarchal and literal interpretation of Islam implemented by the Taliban and Pashtun ethnic group controlling Afghanistan and Northwestern Pakistan.

Ayesha's mother died as a result of a roadside bomb when they still lived in Afghanistan. Although the agency paperwork indicated that her father and two older siblings were deceased, neither Ayesha nor her young siblings would explain how they died, suggesting that Ayesha and her siblings were trying to hide something. Ayesha's younger siblings recalled that she had always been volatile and expressed intense anger over minute issues, had difficulty obeying authority, and would constantly fight with her father and older sisters. Oftentimes she would impulsively leave the house without telling family members where she was going. As a result, her father would routinely physically beat her in hopes that she would behave. On occasion, she would take her younger siblings on her "adventures," where they would visit unfamiliar men. While the siblings played in a separate room and were given candy, Ayesha would be in a separate room with one or more men. It was suggested that she may have been doing sexual favors for them.

Ayesha had applied for asylum to America and was sponsored to come to a medium-sized Midwestern city with a small Muslim population of 20 Afghan families. Upon arrival to America, Ayesha appeared to have formed a social support network within the Afghan community. Ayesha described friendships with numerous males, but no meaningful relationships with other women. Although she denied that she had any sexual relationships with her male friends, when describing her relationships, sexual undertones were present. It is probable that Ayesha was trying to hide her relationships from the therapist because of cultural and religious prohibitions or fear that the information would be given to the resettlement agency and would result in termination of services. When exploring the quality of her relationships, they appeared to be intense, unstable, and highly conflictual. For example, after an argument with one of her male friends, she impulsively drank bleach, which resulted in hospitalization but enabled her to gain the attention and sympathies of the male friend once again.

Ayesha's affect varied from session to session. At times she was engaged, very talkative, and reported an increase in goal-directed behaviors in school, work, and social settings. However, other times, she was more reserved, expressed feelings of emptiness, and was irritated that she was required to attend therapy sessions in order to have her siblings returned to her. The pattern of unstable and intense interpersonal relationships, impulsivity of behavior, volatility and difficulties managing anger, repeated suicidal gestures, and affective instability in the country of origin as well as in the host country indicated that Ayesha likely had a dual diagnosis of bipolar I with mixed episode and borderline personality disorder. Ayesha was referred for a psychiatric evaluation and prescribed medication for symptoms.

Ayesha was initially guarded in therapy so the therapist focused on ways the client could gain custody of her siblings, an issue of personal honor and of grave concern to the client. Occasionally, Ayesha would let her defenses down and talk about feelings of emptiness and display a degree of insight about her intense anger outbursts and how it has affected her current situation. However, these sessions were often followed by missed appointments, which she attributed to misunderstanding or difficulties with transportation. Over time, the therapist was able to create a presence of safety, security, and boundaries to help start the healing process. Once Ayesha was ready to pursue further commitment to treatment, the clinician then referred Ayesha for more intensive dialectical behavioral therapy (DBT) in order for long-term symptom reduction and management. Her adherence to treatment recommendations and change in attitude and behavior toward her siblings resulted in the settlement agency working with Ayesha to help her regain custody of her young siblings.

This case highlights how clinicians can integrate the information presented in the chapter to provide culturally and religiously competent care to Muslim refugees. The use of multiple informants to assess premigratory and asylum-seeking phases helped the clinician to establish a history of bipolar and borderline disorders. In addition, the clinician's awareness of sociocultural history and norms enabled her to identify culturally dystonic behaviors. The clinician was able to understand Ayesha's distrust of her, due to fear that information would be communicated to the resettlement agency, and not allow her behavior to elicit feelings of negative countertransference. The clinician was able to help Ayesha overcome distrust by creating a safe and confidential therapeutic environment, which enabled the client to begin her recovery process.

Conclusion

The growing population of Muslim refugees in Western nations has made it increasingly important for mental health professionals to be sensitive to the needs of this diverse population. Although Muslim refugees are heterogeneous in their backgrounds, they share common religious beliefs, values, and cultures. Clinicians working with refugee clients must adopt an attitude of learning and openness about their clients' religion and cultural beliefs and be willing to integrate these beliefs into treatment, if requested. A thorough history of migratory experience helps clinicians to understand and contextualize the struggles Muslim refugees may experience during resettlement in their host nation. As refugees work to learn a new language, gain financial stability, and meet the basic needs of housing and health care, they may also be adjusting to changes in family and support network (religious, cultural, or other) dynamics. Men, women, and children each face unique challenges. These factors may impact the therapeutic process. As such, mental health agencies should be cognizant of factors in the therapeutic process that can enhance cultural sensitivity in order to build a positive therapeutic relationship with Muslim refugee clients and help formulate religiously and culturally sensitive interventions.

References

Ahearn, F., Loughry, M., & Ager, A. (1999). The experience of refugee children. In A. Ager (Ed.), *Refugees: Perspectives on the experience of forced migration* (pp. 215–236). London: Continuum.

Akotia, C., & Naidoo, J. (1998). Positive and negative experiences of refugees in accessing a settlement service in southern Ontario, Canada. *IFE Psychologia: An International Journal, 6*(2), 152–169.

Aroche, J., and Coello, M. (2004). Ethnocultural considerations in the treatment of refugees and asylum seekers. In J. Wilson and B. Drozdek (Eds.), *Broken spirits: The treatment of traumatized asylum seekers, refugees, war and torture victims* (pp. 53–79). New York, NY: Brunner-Routledge.

Bemak, F., Chung, R., & Pedersen, P. (2003). *Counseling refugees: A psychosocial approach to innovative multicultural interventions*. Westport, CT: Greenwood Press.

Bemak, F., & Greenberg, B. (1994). Southeast Asian refugee adolescents: Implications for counseling. *Journal of Multicultural Counseling and Development, 22*(2), 115–124.

Berman, H., Ford-Gilboe, M., Moutrey, B., & Cekic, S. (2001). Portraits of pain and promise: A photographic study of Bosnian youth. *CJNR: Canadian Journal of Nursing Research, 32*(4), 21–41.

Beshir, E., & Beshir, M. R. (1998). *Meeting the challenges of parenting in the West*. Beltsville, MD: Amana Publications.

Beshir, M. R. (2009). *Family leadership (Qawamah): An obligation to fulfill, not an excuse to abuse*. Beltsville, MD: Amana Publications.

Birman, D., Trickett, E. J., & Bacchus, N. (2001). *Somali refugee youth in Maryland: A needs assessment*. Maryland Department of Human Resources. Retrieved from http://www.dhr.maryland.gov/mora/pdf/somali.pdf

Bowles, R., & Mehraby, N. (2007). Lost in limbo: Cultural dimensions in psychotherapy and supervision with a temporary protection visa holder from Afghanistan. In B. Drozdek and J. Wilson (Eds.), *Voices of trauma: Treating survivors across cultures* (pp. 295–320). New York, NY: Springer.

Casimiro, S., Hancock, P., & Northcore, J. (2007). Isolation and insecurity: Resettlement issues among Muslim refugee women in Perth, Western Australia. *Australian Journal of Social Issues 42*(1), 55–69.

Colic-Peisker, V., & Walker, I. (2003). Human capital, acculturation and social identity: Bosnian refugees in Australia. *Journal of Community & Applied Social Psychology, 13*(5), 337–360.

Dillman, E., Pablo, R., & Wilson, A. (1993). Patterns of health problems observed among newly arrived refugees to Canada. In R. Masi, L. L. Mensah, & K. A. McLeod (Eds.), *Health and cultures: Programs, services and care* (vol. 2, pp. 253–262). Buffalo, NY: Mosaic Press.

Dion, K. L. (2001). Immigrants' perceptions of housing discrimination in Toronto: The housing new Canadians project. *Journal of Social Issues, 57*(3), 523–539.

El Habir, E., Marriage, K., Littlefield, L., & Pratt, K. (1994). Teachers' perception of maladaptive behavior in Lebanese refugee children. *Australian and New Zealand Journal of Psychiatry, 28,* 100–105.

Ellis, B. H., MacDonald, H. Z., Klink-Gillis, J., Lincoln, A., Strain, L., & Caporal, H. (2010). Discrimination and mental health among Somali refugee adolescents: The role of acculturation and gender. *American Journal of Orthopsychiatry, 80*(4), 564–575.

Fozdar, F., & Torezani, S. (2008). Discrimination and well-being: Perceptions of refugees in western Australia. *International Migration Review, 42*(1), 30–63.

Garretson, A. A., Barmen, I., Deville, W., Van Willie, L. H., Hoven, J. E., & Van Der Pole, H. M. (2006). Use of health care services by Afghan, Iranian, and Somali refugees and asylum seekers living in the Netherlands. *European Journal of Public Health, 16*(4), 394–399.

Gitlin, A., Buendía, E., Crosland, K., & Doumbia, F. (2003). The production of margin and center: Welcoming-unwelcoming of immigrant students. *American Educational Research Journal, 40*(1), 91–122.

Gordon, R. D., Taylor, R., & Sarkisian, G. V. (2010). Psychoeducational workshops as a practical tool to facilitate resettlement with Iraqi refugees and anchor relatives. *Journal of Muslim Mental Health, 5*(1), 82–98.

Gozdziak, E. (2002). Spiritual emergency room: The role of spirituality and religion in the resettlement of Kosovar Albanians. *Journal of Refugee Studies, 15*(2), 136–152.

Halcyon, L., Robertson, C., Slavic, K., Johnson, D., Spring, M., Butcher, J., Westermeyer, J., & Jarsonson, J. (2004). Trauma and coping in Somali and Oromo refugee youth. *Journal of Adolescent Health, 35,* 17–25.

Kinzie, J. D. (2004). Some of the effects of terrorism on refugees. *Journal of Aggression, Maltreatment & Trauma, 9*(3/4), 411–420.

Kira, I. A., Lewandowski, L., Templin, T., Ramaswany, V., Ozkan, B., & Mohanesh, J. (2010). The effects of perceived discrimination and backlash on Iraqi refugees' mental and physical health, *Journal of Muslim Mental Health, 5,* 59–81.

Kirova, A. (2001). Loneliness in immigrant children: Implications for classroom practice. *Childhood Education, 77*(5), 260–267.

Lindert, A. T., Korzilius, H., Van de Vijver, J. R., Kroon, S., & Arends-Toth, J. (2008). Perceived discrimination and acculturation among Iranian refugees in the Netherlands. *Journal of Intercultural Relations, 32*(6), 578–588.

McBrien, J. L. (2008). The world at America's doorstep: Service learning in preparation to teach global students. *Journal of Transformative Education, 6*(4), 270–285.

McMichael, C., & Manderson, L. (2004). Somali women and well-being: Social networks and social capital among immigrant women in Australia. *Human Organization, 63*(1), 88–99.

Mehraby, N. (2002). Counseling Afghanistan torture and trauma survivors. *Psychotherapy in Australia, 8*(3), 12–18.

Mollica, R., McInnes, K., Pham, T., Smith Fawzi, M., Murphy, E., & Lin, L. (1998). The dose-effect relationships between torture and psychiatric symptoms in Vietnamese ex-political detainees and a comparison group. *Journal of Nervous & Mental Disease, 186*(9), 543–553.

Morris, P., & Silove, D. 1992. Cultural influences in psychotherapy with refugee survivors of torture and trauma. *Hospital and Community Psychiatry, 43,* 820–824.

O'Shea, B., Hodes, M., Down, G., & Bramley, J. (2000). A school-based mental health service for refugee children. *Clinical Child Psychology and Psychiatry, 5*(2), 189–201.

Padela, A. I., & Rodriguez del Pozo, P. (2010). Muslim patients in cross-gender interactions in medicine: An Islamic bio-ethical perspective. *Journal of Medical Ethics, 37*(1), 40–44.

Sabiq, A. (1991). *Fiqh us Sunnah: Funerals and Dhikr* (vol. 4). Indianapolis, IN: American Trust Publications.

Shoeb, M., Weinstein, H. M., & Halpern, J. (2007). Living in religious time and space: Iraqi refugees in Dearborn, Michigan. *Journal of Refugee Studies, 20*(3), 441–460.

Snyder, C., May, D., Zulcic, N., & Gabbard, W. (2005). Social work with Bosnian Muslim refugee children and families: A review of the literature. *Child Welfare League of America, 84*(5), 607–630.

U.N. General Assembly. (1951, July 28). Convention Relating to the Status of Refugees. United Nations, Treaty Series (vol. 189, p. 137). U.N. Refugee Agency. Retrieved from http://www.unhcr.org/refworld/docid/3be01b964.html

U.S. Department of Health and Human Services. (2009). *Fiscal Year 2009 Refugee Arrivals.* Retrieved from http://www.acf.hhs.gov/programs/orr/ data/refugee_arrival_data.htm

Watters, C. (2001). Emerging paradigms in the mental health care of refugees. *Social Science of Medicine, 52*(11), 1709–1718.

Whittaker, S., Hardy, G., Lewis, K., & Buchan, L. (2005). An exploration of psychological well-being with young Somali refugee and asylum-seeker women. *Clinical Child Psychology and Psychiatry, 10*(2), 177–196.

PART V
Special Issues

CHAPTER **16**
Domestic Violence

SALMA ELKADI ABUGIDEIRI

Treating Muslim individuals and families affected by domestic violence necessitates an exploration of multiple factors that contribute to how the issue is perceived, why it occurs, and how it is dealt with. Despite presumptions among some professionals that Muslims are more prone to family violence than other populations, as well as misconceptions among Muslims that they are immune from this social and public health issue, Muslims, like any other group of people, are affected by domestic violence. The biases and stereotypes carried by both the treatment provider and the client are important to identify, assess, and process in order to provide the most effective treatment (Alwani & Abugideiri, 2003).

Domestic violence is also referred to as intimate partner abuse or violence, family violence or abuse, and maltreatment. Here, the term "domestic violence," which itself has no single agreed-upon definition, will be used to refer to a pattern of behavior used by one person in an intimate relationship to have power or control over another person in the relationship. Although this term will be used in its broadest sense to include the abuse of any family member by another member of the household, the primary focus of this chapter is spousal abuse. The violent behavior can include physical abuse (hitting, shoving, pulling hair, biting, using a weapon); verbal abuse (name-calling, insults); psychological abuse (threats, intimidation, humiliation, isolation, stalking, etc.); sexual abuse (forced sexual acts, forced pornography viewing, withholding sex); financial abuse (deprivation from access to money); and spiritual abuse (misusing religious teachings to manipulate behavior, interfering with worship practices).

Domestic violence and mental health issues tend to co-occur, with abuse increasing the risk for mental illness. At the same time, living with a mental illness increases the risk for being abused. Physical and sexual abuse may lead to a wide range of health problems, including physical injury, gynecological disorders, gastrointestinal disorders, poor health, and a range of mental health disorders such as depression, anxiety, phobias, post-traumatic stress disorder, suicidality, substance abuse, and psychosomatic disorders (Abugideiri, 2007; Douki, Nacef, Belhadj, Bouasker, & Ghachem, 2003; Ellsberg, Jansen, Heise, Watts, & Garcia-Moreno, 2008).

Many factors have been identified as contributing to domestic violence. Feminist studies have highlighted the significant role of patriarchy (Krahé, Bieneck, & Möller, 2005), as well as other factors such as unemployment, globalization, life events stress, and substance use (DeKeseredy & Dragiewicz, 2007). Additional contributing factors in the international literature include socioeconomic variables, gender roles, and the normative acceptance of aggression in a given society (Krahé et al., 2005). Although there is not enough research to date regarding Muslims and domestic violence, it seems reasonable to conclude that because asymmetrical decision making has been found to be a causal factor in domestic violence (Krahé et al., 2005), in Muslim families whose original cultures are heavily patriarchal, women are more likely than men to be victims of family violence (Kulwicki & Miller, 1999; S. Alkhateeb, 1999).

Islamic Paradigm

It is important to distinguish between the lived culture of Muslims and the religious teachings of Islam (Hassouneh-Phillips, 2003). Religious texts and teachings can be interpreted in many different ways, depending on factors such as historical and cultural contexts, as well as individual experiences and personalities (Douki et al., 2003). There are many references in the Qur'an and *hadith* to different forms of abuse, all of which are prohibited under the broad category of oppression (*zulm*) (Alwani & Abugideiri, 2003). According to the Qur'an, men and women were created from a single soul (Qur'an 4:1; 49:13), suggesting an inherent equality in their nature. Their purpose in life is the same: to worship the Creator and to serve as His vicegerent on earth (Qur'an 2:30; 51:56). Believing men and believing women are described as mutual friends and protectors who work together to enjoin good and forbid evil (Qur'an 9:71), and who serve as garments for one another as spouses (Qur'an 2:187).

Marriage is based on love and compassion (*mawaddah*) and mercy (*rahmah*), with mutual tranquility (*sakeenah*) being the desired outcome

(Qur'an 30:21). In terms of gender roles, the Qur'an assigns financial responsibility to men (Qur'an 4:34). Many Qur'anic verses dealing with marriage are directed toward men, warning them to treat women kindly and to avoid behaviors that could be emotionally abusive (Eid, 2005; Qur'an 2:225–227; 2:231; 4:19–21; 65:6).

These teachings are exemplified in the life of the Prophet Muhammad (peace be on him[1]). His interactions with his wives illustrate relationships that are mutually respectful and tolerant. He modeled a collaborative type of leadership in which he engaged in mutual consultation (*shura*) to arrive at decisions; he took part in the household chores; and he openly expressed his love and affection for his family (Alwani & Abugideiri, 2003; Ibrahim & Abdallah, 2010). A holistic reading of the Qur'an, in conjunction with a study of the Prophet Muhammad's lifestyle, which together form the basis for Islamic jurisprudence, clearly leave no room for any type of abuse.

BOX 16.1 AN ABUSED VERSE FROM THE QUR'AN

Husbands are the protectors and maintainers of their wives, because Allah has given the one more (strength) than the other, and because they support them from their means. Therefore the righteous women are devoutly obedient, and guard in (the husband's) absence what Allah would have them guard. As to those women on whose part ye fear disloyalty and ill-conduct, admonish them (first), (Next), refuse to share their beds, (And last) spank them (lightly); but if they return to obedience, seek not against them Means (of annoyance): For Allah is Most High, great (above you all). (Qur'an 4:34, as translated by Ali, 1989)

This translation of the Qur'anic verse 4:34 is representative of the cultural influences that have led to misleading and even erroneous interpretations of Islamic teachings. In-depth study of the verse in its original Arabic,[1] within the context of the Islamic paradigm, reveals that it is a verse intended to regulate men's behavior to prevent them from reacting violently in the event of suspecting the wife of behavior that might undermine the integrity of the marriage. Scholars have differed about the meanings of key individual words in the verse, leading to interpretations that range from permitting the husband to use a gentle tap when his wife has not responded to the first

---

[1] Muslims regard only the original revelation in Arabic to be divine and indisputable. The Qur'an has been translated into most of the world languages, with multiple translations or interpretations within these languages.

---

[1] Muslims say this phrase after mentioning or hearing the name of Prophet Muhammad.

> two steps (talking to her, then sleeping separately) to suggesting that husbands separate from their wives when there has been no positive response to the first two steps. In no case does a scholar suggest that this verse makes wife beating or any form of abuse acceptable or permissible (Alwani, 2007; Ammar, 2007; Douki et al., 2003; Eid, 2005; FaithTrust Institute & Gargiulo, 2007; Ibrahim & Abdallah, 2010).

Accountability is an extremely relevant element of the Islamic paradigm. Men and women are equally accountable to God for their actions (Qur'an 9:72; 33:35) and cannot blame others for their own actions (Qur'an 4:112; 6:164). This is an important concept when helping victims realize they cannot be blamed for being abused, and in confronting perpetrators when they insist they were provoked.

Domestic Violence in the Muslim Community[2]

Similar to other faith communities, Muslim leaders have been reluctant to address the issue of domestic violence and to accept that families of faith are not immune to domestic violence (Alkhateeb & Abugideiri, 2007; Nason-Clark, 2000). Literature addressing the issue of domestic violence among Muslims in Western countries can be divided into ethnically focused studies (Abraham, 1999; Ahmad, Riaz, Barata, & Stewart, 2004; Ayyub, 2000; Dasgupta, 2000; Halabu, 2006; Kulwicki & Miller, 1999; Raj & Silverman, 2002) and studies that focus on the primary identity of "Muslim" across ethnic divides (Abdallah, 2007; Abugideiri, 2007; M. B. Alkhateeb, 2009; S. Alkhateeb, 1999; Hassouneh-Phillips, 2003). As Muslim communities become increasingly comprised of second and third generations, as well as indigenous converts, the Muslim identity may often be more meaningful than the original ethnicity (Abdul-Karim & Kiely-Froude, 2009; Abugideiri, 2007). Therefore, in addition to considering the intersection of race, class, and gender (Sokoloff & Dupont, 2005), the intersection of culture and religion may have unique implications.

Prevalence

In a WHO multicountry study, 15% to 71% of women surveyed reported experiencing some form of physical or sexual violence by an intimate partner (not necessarily a spouse) (Ellsberg et al., 2008). To date, research regarding domestic violence among Muslims has consisted of more qualitative than quantitative research using small sample sizes, convenience samples, and a

---

[2] Examples of specific clients will be used throughout the paper. All names are fictional; other identifying characteristics have been changed to preserve confidentiality.

variety of measures. Preliminary surveys of Muslims in the United States indicate that 10% to 18% of the respondents reported physical abuse by a spouse, and approximately 30% reported having experienced some form of emotional abuse in the marriage (S. Alkhateeb, 1999; Ghayyur, 2009).

Exacerbating Factors

Many factors can increase the risk for domestic violence, even though they may not be causal factors in and of themselves. Although Muslims are an extremely diverse group in terms of culture and history, a large number of Muslims come from cultures and histories of oppression. Whether it is the immigrant Muslims coming from oppressive regimes and colonization experiences, or the African American Muslims' experience of slavery and societal oppression, these experiences can increase the stress levels in the family, blur the lines of what constitutes abusive behavior, and interfere with help-seeking behavior (Abdul-Karim & Kiely-Froude, 2009; S. Alkhateeb, 1999; Kasturirangan, Krishnan, & Riger, 2004). As one Somali war survivor who had witnessed family members being slain and who was raped in a refugee camp said to me, "My husband and I were both tortured in the camp. If he pushes me or hits me occasionally, it is nothing compared to what we have been through."

For Muslims coming from South Asian and Arab cultures, the contrast between individualistic and collectivist cultures can be quite difficult to navigate. Immigration and acculturation-related stressors may include loss of socioeconomic status, lack of language and job skills, role reversal when women are more easily employed, loss of the extended family support network, and women's quicker acculturation in terms of shifting gender roles. In attempting to protect their families from perceived external threats to the family, and in response to shifting power dynamics as the role of breadwinner and head of household changes, men might resort to violence to regain their authority and masculinity (Ahmad et al., 2004; Baobaid, 2002; Kasturirangan et al., 2004).

Current and historical geopolitical circumstances are possible exacerbating factors, as well as potential barriers, to seeking services (Ammar, 2000). Muslims often have family members who are directly being impacted by the wars in Afghanistan and Iraq, as well as by the Israeli-Palestinian conflicts. They may be watching news coverage of the violence on a daily basis. Furthermore, it is public knowledge that Muslims have been profiled as potential terrorists post 9/11, and even further after the Madrid train bombing in 2004 and the London underground bombing in 2005, and that as a result of laws such as the U.S. Patriot Act, Muslims have been detained, deported, and investigated, often with little or no cause. Muslims in many cities live under increased stress and anxiety, believing that they are being watched and that they may be falsely charged if anyone feels that their behavior is "suspicious."

Second- and third-generation Muslims in Western countries face their own unique struggles related to living between two or more cultures, often with contradictory messages about gender roles and family structure. Young couples in my practice struggle to figure out their roles and a balance of power that may look very different from what they observed in their parents' relationships. More and more young couples seem to be experiencing mutual violence as gender roles have become more equitable and women have become less likely to willingly remain in a passive or submissive role. In the case of one professional couple in their 30s, Yasmine complained that during arguments, Adam would pin her against a wall or hold her down. Adam reported that he had received stitches in his arm due to being cut by a vase she hurled at him, and that during arguments he had to dodge her cell phone to avoid being hit on the head with it.

Female converts (or "reverts") to Islam may experience an increased risk for domestic violence because of their vulnerable position (Abdallah, 2007). Many times they lose their family support upon conversion, becoming quite isolated, thus relying heavily on their husbands for guidance as they learn about their new religion and navigate unfamiliar cultures. Men who are abusive may exploit their eagerness to learn and their dependence.

Contributing Cultural Values

In addition to the inter- and intragroup variability among Muslims, their diverse cultures contain contradictory values that can either be supportive of abusive practices or liberating from abusive practices. The existence of patriarchal values within a culture does not necessarily mean that violence against women is explicitly accepted (Kasturirangan et al., 2004; Raj & Silverman, 2002; Sokoloff & Dupont, 2005). An example of contradictory values is the seemingly inferior status of women in the family in Arab culture, while Arab women have been able to conduct their own business, own property, and enter contracts for over 1400 years (Ammar, 2000).

Many Muslim immigrant families come from patriarchal, collectivist societies that traditionally prescribe fairly rigid but complementary gender roles. Men may take pride in taking good care of their family members and may feel responsible for ensuring their security (financial and otherwise). At the same time, the inherent power given to men in the family and broader systems, as well as women's financial dependence on men, can contribute to abuse and make it very difficult for abused women to seek resources or to get out of abusive relationships (Ayyub, 2000; Baobaid, 2002; Raj & Silverman, 2002).

The deeply entrenched values regarding family honor in South Asian and Arab cultures can further complicate the situation. Collectivist cultures tend to view individual accomplishments and successes, as well as individual failures, as reflections on the entire family. Violations of acceptable behaviors can create shame for the entire family and may lead to disciplinary action to redeem the family honor, especially if the guilty party is female (Ayyub, 2000; Baobaid, 2002; Hassouneh-Phillips, 2001a).

Both male and female immigrants may view hitting a wife as justified if she does not live up to her traditional role, is unfaithful, refuses to have sex with her husband, disobeys him, undermines his authority, insults him, or challenges his masculinity (Abu Ras, 2007; Baobaid, 2002; Douki et al., 2003; Kulwicki & Miller, 1999). Sexual abuse can occur as a result of attitudes supporting male prerogative to control women's sexuality and her reproductive choices, as well as cultural beliefs that husbands have absolute sexual access to their wives (Abraham, 1999).

A tendency to interpret Muslims' cultural behaviors as Islamic leads many converts to Islam to adopt some of the underlying cultural attitudes of immigrant Muslims. Although their identity as Muslim may often take priority over their ethnic identity, it is important to be aware of the cultural and historical factors that can impact converts' perceptions of, and responses to, abuse. For example, African American women may struggle with a mistrust of services that are offered, a desire to avoid contributing to negative stereotypes about African American men, and a belief that seeking help is a sign of weakness. The intersection of their Islamic identity with their historical socialization to be strong and even physically retaliate against physical abuse may lead to conflicting feelings on how to respond to their abusers (Abdul-Karim & Kiely-Froude, 2009).

Culture-Specific Manifestations of Domestic Violence

In addition to the general types of abuse that can occur in any population, there may be some culture-specific manifestations of abuse and control tactics that are experienced by Muslim victims as more severe than physical abuse (Hassouneh-Phillips, 2001a; Sokoloff & Dupont, 2005). These may include threats to ruin a woman's reputation, falsely accusing her of adultery or promiscuous behavior, or threats to ruin her family's reputation (Dasgupta, 2000). Many of my clients who have experienced severe physical and sexual abuse report that the most painful abuse they endured was the repeated pronouncements of divorce[3] and the forced sex-

---

[3] In Islamic law, men initiate divorce by pronouncing the word *talaaq*, which means divorce. If the necessary conditions outlined in Islamic law are met, the couple continues to reside in the same home without engaging in sexual relations for three months to ensure that there is no pregnancy. At the end of the three months, the divorce is complete. The couple can reconcile and may go through the same process up to three times, after which point the divorce is irrevocable. Women may also initiate divorce, with a slightly different process, which is called *khul'*. In this process, women must return all gifts received from the husband during marriage and waive their right to maintenance in order to be released from the marriage when there are no grounds for divorce. In cases where there are grounds for divorce, such as abuse, a judge may grant a form of *talaaq* if the husband refuses to initiate it (Alwani & Abugideiri, 2003).

ual activity after such a pronouncement because of the belief that sex is no longer religiously permissible.

Various types of abuse can occur around marriage and divorce practices, including pressuring or forcing young women to get married or arranging a forced arranged marriage as a means to interrupt rebellious teenage girls' behavior (Ayyub, 2000; Hassouneh-Phillips, 2003). In abusive joint family systems, it is not uncommon for the perpetrator of abuse to be someone other than, or in addition to, the husband (Dasgupta, 2000; Halabu, 2006). For example, after several years of being hit and deprived of money to buy milk and diapers for the kids, Zeinah complained to her brother who told her that if she did not comply with her husband's wishes, then the brother would beat her himself.

While Islamic conditions of marriage require the consent of both parties, as well as a marriage contract with terms that can be specified by either party, these conditions are sometimes violated in abusive relationships. Although either party can initiate the dissolution of the marriage, in order for women to retain their marital assets and the right to maintenance, they must be divorced by their husbands through *talaaq* (as mentioned in previous footnote). An abusive man may withhold the *talaaq*, in attempts to prevent his wife from remarriage (Eid, 2005; Hassouneh-Phillips, 2001a).

A minority of Muslims practice polygyny. Statistics for the prevalence of this practice among Muslims in Western countries are not available; however, polygyny is practiced among 5% to 12% of Muslims in Arab nations according to one somewhat dated reference (Chamie, 1986). In and of itself, polygyny is not a form of abuse; however, it can sometimes be a vehicle for abuse to occur. Examples of abuse include threatening to take a co-wife as a control tactic; keeping the second marriage secret, which increases isolation; co-wives being forced to watch their husband engaging in sexual relations with another wife; or co-wives actually perpetrating verbal and physical abuse against each other (Eid, 2005; Hassouneh-Phillips, 2001b; Magid, 2007). Wives whose marriages are not registered in court are more vulnerable to abuse because there is no legal protection of marital rights, including the provision of *mahr* (gift given by the groom to the bride). All of these abusive acts are completely prohibited by Islamic teachings.

Role of Religion

Religion is very difficult to separate from culture, because religious teachings are often interpreted through cultural and historical lenses, and the practice of religion can be shaped by local culture. The intersection of religion and domestic violence can be quite complex, with religious teachings sometimes serving as a means to maintain the abuse, and at other times serving as a source of liberation from abuse (Ayyub, 2000; Halabu, 2006).

There is often confusion about religious teachings and gender that can occur among Muslim women whose cultural norms may seem to support male dominance, or who rely on their abusive husbands to interpret Islam for them, especially if those husbands are somehow justifying the abuse through religious teachings, usually by taking teachings out of context (S. Alkhateeb, 1999; Eid, 2005; Magid, 2007).

The experience of being abused can create a crisis of meaning that will likely be expressed in religious terms (Fortune, 2001). Common questions include, "Why did God let this happen to me?" and "Where was God when I called out to Him?" Religious beliefs that encourage saving the marriage, compounded with cultural beliefs that divorce is shameful, can lead to significant feelings of guilt if the survivor is contemplating leaving the marriage. Similarly, cultural attitudes about family privacy may be intertwined with Islamic prohibitions of speaking ill of others' flaws (which do not apply in cases where injustice has occurred). Guilt around these issues may be verbalized as, "Will God forgive me?" or "If I were a better Muslim wife, I would have been able to make the marriage work."

Furthermore, many victims develop negative self-cognitions as a result of the abuser's messages, as well as broader cultural messages that blame the victim for the abuse. These cognitions may be expressed as, "God must be punishing me for being a bad Muslim," or "If I were more patient, or stronger in my faith, I would not be here." One of the more debilitating interpretations of the abuse is when victims (and their families) believe that the maltreatment is their destiny (*qadar* in Arabic; *kismet* in Farsi, Turkish, and Urdu) (Ayyub, 2000; Dasgupta, 2000; Eid, 2005), because there is more likelihood of remaining in the relationship and enduring the abuse. The abuse itself, as well as the responses to seeking help, may lead women to retain the same quality of faith as before the abuse, reinterpret Islamic teachings as a result of having to critique the initial understanding, or completely reject their faith (Hassouneh-Phillips, 2003).

The Islamic values of patience and forgiveness are often used in unhelpful ways with women of various faith traditions in abusive relationships by pressuring them to endure the abuse and to forgive the abuser (Eid, 2005; Hassouneh-Phillips, 2003; Nason-Clark, 2000; Sweifach & Heft-LaPorte, 2007). When used appropriately, these concepts can actually facilitate, rather than inhibit, an abused person's journey toward health and safety (Alwani & Abugideiri, 2003). Patience and perseverance (*sabr*) can help women to endure the challenges and obstacles they must face as they reach out for help, deal with many types of helpful and unhelpful responses from family and community members, struggle to make the right decision, and do their utmost to fulfill their Islamic duty (Qur'an 4:97–99; 42:39–43) to free themselves from oppression, if at all possible. In this way, patience becomes an active stance that provides strength and perseverance along the often-difficult path to healing. Forgiveness often comes near the end of this journey, once some sort of justice and accountability for the abuser has taken place (Alwani & Abugideiri, 2003; Fortune, 1991; Magid, 2007). Religion and spirituality may have healing effects as they have been correlated with lower rates of depression and post-traumatic stress symptoms among abused women (Watlington & Murphy, 2006).

Victim and Community Responses to Domestic Violence

Victim Responses

Muslim victims of domestic violence may be caught up in a conspiracy of silence (Douki et al., 2003), which may be caused by a combination of beliefs about the importance of keeping family matters private, the shame that would be caused by ruining the family's reputation, and the belief in the husband's right to discipline his wife. Participants in this conspiracy may include the victim and the abuser, their families, religious leaders, service providers, law enforcement, and possibly others (Ammar, 2000; Macey, 1999).

Women who choose to stay in an abusive relationship may struggle with many conflicting needs. Most of these women want the abuse to stop, while they also want to hold on to the marriage; they want their children to be safe, while they want their children to have a father (Nason-Clark, 2000). Other reasons for staying include the cultural stigma of divorce, the shame of being abused, self-blame for choosing the abusive spouse, feelings of failure if the marriage ends, lack of resources, and having nowhere else to go. There may be fears of losing the children through custody battles, removal by child protective services, or the abusive partner taking the children out of the country. There is also generally a belief that a two-parent home, even if it is violent, is better for the children than a single-parent home, even if it is peaceful (Dasgupta, 2000; Douki et al., 2003). When the abuse becomes unbearable, or in those cases where women refuse to accept any abuse at all, they may first try to seek help from relatives or family friends, then from the imam, and finally, as a last resort, from domestic violence agencies (Baobaid, 2002; Hassouneh-Phillips, 2001a).

Muslim victims of domestic violence may face multiple barriers to seeking help from domestic violence organizations or mental health services. Given the existing stereotypes about Muslims being violent, victims may fear making Muslims look bad by reinforcing stereotypes (Alkhateeb & Abugideiri, 2007; Eid, 2005). Other barriers include valuing the family's privacy, financial insecurity, fearing that their immigration status will be compromised or reported if they are undocumented, fear of being alone, unfamiliarity with the services available, mistrust of government services, racism and discrimination by service providers, negative beliefs about shelters, and language barriers (Abdul-Karim & Kiely-Froude, 2009; Abu Ras, 2007; Baobaid, 2002; Dasgupta, 2000; Halabu, 2006).

Family and Community Leadership Responses

Responses to domestic violence by community leadership can be quite varied and inconsistent due to insufficient training and a lack of a unified policy on how to deal with domestic violence, as well as the lack of an oversight body to regulate how Muslim leaders should intervene (Abdallah, 2007; Abugideiri, 2007; M. B. Alkhateeb, 2009; Eid, 2005; Halabu, 2006). Unhelpful responses from relatives or religious leaders range from revictimization by blaming the victim, denying or minimizing the abuse, or even relatives abusing the victim as a means to keep her in the marriage. Victims may be discouraged from utilizing government-sponsored programs (Ayyub, 2000) or seeking professional counseling, or religious leaders may insist on providing couples counseling without assessing the risks involved. Because religious leaders may prioritize reconciliation over safety (Nason-Clark, 2000), it is common for abused women to be urged to pray more, try harder to please their husbands, be more patient in the face of maltreatment, and forgive their husbands.

Those women who do choose divorce are likely to struggle not only with the stigma around divorce, but also with the real lack of support and resources within the Muslim community. The status earned by being married can be lost, and single women may be challenged to fit in and be accepted in social settings, in addition to being blamed for breaking up the family.

On the other hand, extended families often respond very positively by offering refuge and moral support, trying to intervene and confront the abuser, and providing financial resources and help with childcare (Halabu, 2006). There is a growing number of imams in the United States who are becoming educated on the issue of domestic violence and who intervene appropriately and effectively by recognizing the severity of the problem, prioritizing the safety and well-being of the victims, holding the abuser accountable, and taking any action that will interrupt the abuse, whether that means reporting it to the police, facilitating an Islamic divorce, or referring the victim to a domestic violence organization or shelter (Eid, 2005; Magid, 2007). In other countries, imams are taking a stand against domestic violence by speaking out during Friday sermons (Hamill, 2010) and by engaging in training programs to learn how to help victims of domestic violence (Karabat, 2010).

Clinical Interventions

It is critical to take the time to understand the client's perspective of the problem, the client's desired outcome, and how the client wants to be helped without imposing one's own agenda. Clinicians' self-awareness of biases is crucial to culturally competent treatment. Muslim clients are very sensitive to assumptions that Islam is inherently oppressive to women. Assuming that a victim of domestic violence is determined to seek a divorce (or that she will never leave) may negatively impact the treatment, preclude other options, and lead to premature termination of services. Assuming that a particular situation is abusive based on a projection of Western cultural norms may be detrimental. For example, a therapist should not assume that a recent immigrant Muslim client who has no information about the family finances is suffering from financial abuse. In contrast to her American counterpart, who may expect to be a full partner in financial earning and decision making, the Muslim client may not have needed that knowledge within her cultural context of being fully provided for, and may even prefer not to be burdened with this information.

In order to build and enhance the therapeutic alliance, clinicians should work hard to convey a nonjudgmental stance in which they are open to learning, be curious about what the client is hoping for from treatment, and actively search for resources from within the client's cultural and religious worldview that can be utilized in treatment.

Assessment Issues

Proper assessment is critical before any treatment planning can occur, and should consider the cultural and historical factors that have been discussed so far (see Table 16.1). In addition, it is important to consider that Muslim clients who agree with patriarchal social norms may not recognize they are in an abusive relationship (Ahmad et al., 2004), often seeking help for symptoms such as depression, anxiety, or marriage problems (Abugideiri, 2007). The significance of religion and spirituality should be assessed because Muslims impacted by abuse often find themselves reevaluating their religious beliefs as they work through the implications and consequences of the abuse. It may be tempting to assess the degree of religiosity by outward appearance, such as women wearing *hijab*, or men having a beard; however, it is more useful and informative to explore how Islam factors into the client's life, as well as the client's interpretation of religious beliefs (Abdul-Karim & Kiely-Froude, 2009). Muslims who may not be observing the ritual prayers or other areas of practice may still be concerned about observing Islamic marriage and divorce laws as they explore safety options.

Table 16.1 Factors to Consider during Assessment

Current and/or past abuse
    Specific abusive behaviors (hitting, isolation, threats, etc.)
    Level of anxiety or fear related to perpetrator
Preexisting trauma
    History of child abuse
    Other experiences of violence outside the home
    Living in war zones
        Torture and maltreatment in refugee camps
        Inner-city crimes
        Politically motivated torture
    Immigration-related
        Separation from significant family members (parent, spouse)
        Fear of deportation
        Safety threatened in process of leaving home country
History of oppression
    Colonization
    Slavery
    Discrimination
    Governmental persecution
Geopolitical circumstances (Ammar, 2000)
    Family members impacted by current wars in Muslim countries
    Frequent watching of news coverage depicting war casualties and destruction of country of origin
    Increased scrutiny of Muslims post 9/11; 2004 Madrid bombings; 2005 London bombings
Acculturation issues for immigrant Muslims
    Adjusting to individualistic culture
    Loss of socioeconomic status
    Lack of language and job skills
    Role reversal due to women's incomes
    Changes in gender roles
    Loss of extended family support
Cultural norms related to gender and violence
    Level of acceptance of domestic violence, and specifically male-perpetrated violence
    View of abuse by client, family, and community
    Sources of support within family and community
    Anticipated responses from family and community
Importance of religion and degree of practice
    Role of Islam in daily life, decision making, and current crisis
    Interpretation of Islamic teachings with regard to gender and violence

Treatment Approaches

An effective treatment approach will be congruent with Muslim clients' values, providing a safe space to address not only the clinical issues, but also the impact the experience of abuse may have had on the client's faith and spirituality. The objective for the majority of Muslim clients is to stop the abuse, and to preserve the marriage if at all possible (Abu Ras, 2007). Due to the collectivist, family-oriented values among most Muslims, interventions that are more family focused and systems oriented (Gil, 1996) may feel more congruent to the clients. Spiritually modified cognitive therapy (Hodge & Nadir, 2008) may be especially useful in helping clients distinguish between genuine theological beliefs and cognitive distortions that prevent healing and movement toward safety (Sweifach & Heft-LaPorte, 2007). The gender-inclusive approach (Hamel, 2005) may be more congruent with Muslims' cultural and religious values because it includes both partners, even if the sessions are not conjoint due to safety considerations. Advocates are encouraged to frame interventions as prioritizing safety and the health and well-being of all family members, rather than simply focusing on getting the woman out of the relationship.

Building on Cultural Values as a Resource

Extracting positive cultural values, and reframing others that may have been used negatively to contribute to domestic violence, can be an effective and culturally acceptable tool in preventing and treating domestic violence. The husband as head of the household is charged with protecting his family. The role of protector can be emphasized and explored with perpetrators to help them define how they would best like to protect their family, and what it means to be a protector. Appealing to the importance of family honor and reputation, abusive family members might be encouraged to consider how they would like to be known in their extended family and social circles: Do they treat all family members, including women, with dignity and respect, or do their female members live in fear and intimidation?

In considering the value placed on having intact families, education can be provided that the family unit is "broken" when abuse begins, not when the victim leaves. Utilizing family-focused interventions can emphasize the safety and well-being of each family member, including the abuser. Families need to be educated on the detrimental effects to children who witness abuse, the social and spiritual damage suffered by an abuser, as well as the short- and long-term consequences of abuse to the victim.

Although shame is often used as a social control mechanism to prevent victims from seeking help or leaving the marriage, this same mechanism can be redirected toward the perpetrator for protecting individuals under his or her care. By tapping into the collectivist mindset, immediate and extended family members, as well as community members and their leaders, can be reminded of their responsibility for the well-being of all individuals within the group.

Building on Islamic Values and Faith as Resources

Whether the clinician is providing treatment to the victim or to the abuser, religious teachings and values can be a source of strength and provide an incentive to change. Survivors often report that their relationship with God gave them strength at a time when they may have had no one else (Hassouneh-Phillips, 2003; Nason-Clark, 2000), and that their religious teachings empowered them to seek an end to the abuse (FaithTrust Institute & Gargiulo, 2007). Religion can also be used to challenge the abuser (Nason-Clark, 2000) and create an incentive to change one's behavior.

Muslim clients themselves may not be knowledgeable enough about Islamic teachings that can support them in their efforts to seek an end to domestic violence. For example, many women may not know that they have the right to initiate divorce, or they may believe an abuser who tells them that Islam gives husbands the right to beat their wives. Directing them to specific resources may help them (as well as the clinician) utilize more fully the resources that Islam has to offer.

BOX 16.2 DIVORCE IS *HALAL* (LAWFUL); ABUSE IS *HARAM* (PROHIBITED)

Latifah, a 30-year-old Arab mother of two children, was referred for therapy by her caseworker because she showed signs of depression and post-traumatic stress disorder. She had spent several sessions expressing her tremendous guilt about the divorce process, despite the fact that her husband was having an affair and had kicked her out of the house in the middle of a cold winter night. She had endured years of multiple forms of abuse, including severe beatings and being forced to engage in oral and anal sex.[1] The therapist had validated and empathized with her, explored the cultural conversations that reinforced this guilt, and addressed some of the cognitive distortions that she had been expressing such as, "I'm stupid," and "He was right, no one will ever want me." Then at one point she said, "Will

---

[1] In addition to the sexual abuse component of being forced to engage in this behavior, there is a spiritual dilemma that occurs due to Islam's prohibition against anal sex, which in many women's minds must be reconciled with her duty to comply with her husband's wishes.

> God ever forgive me?" With a slight tinge of impatience, the therapist remarked, "Forgive you for what? Divorce is *halal*; abuse is *haram.*" Latifah appeared stunned. "Really? Divorce is *halal*?" Now it was the therapist's turn to be stunned. After all these weeks, it had not occurred to the therapist that Latifah may not have known that Islam allows divorce, and that abuse and adultery are grounds for Islamic divorce. This piece of information was what Latifah had needed to overcome the spiritual struggle she had been undergoing, but she had never quite voiced it as such. Although she was not completely free of guilt, moving forward she would remind herself that God supported freedom from oppression and that divorce could be a peaceful and religiously sanctioned solution.

Knowing that God has witnessed all acts of abuse even when denied by the abuser or family members, and that the abuser will receive just punishment in the hereafter, even if it was not received in a court of law, can bring comfort to a victim and may even motivate a perpetrator to make some changes. Reminding victims of abuse that marriage is supposed to be grounded in mercy, love, and compassion helps to clarify that the abuser is the one who violated the marriage contract, not the victim by leaving or seeking help. It is important to challenge theological distortions, such as the belief that the abuse is a punishment for her past sins (Sweifach & Heft-LaPorte, 2007), or that she is a bad Muslim for filing a police report or seeking counseling.

Working Collaboratively

In order to provide effective treatment, clinicians must provide culturally appropriate services, or identify culturally appropriate referrals. Due to the complexity of the issue and the multiple layers of cultural and religious values, as well as the myriad obstacles to seeking help, clinicians may need to collaborate with multiple service providers who can address other facets of the problem. It is very helpful to identify and build relationships with Muslim community leaders, imams, and service providers in order to build credibility and trust, not only with the client, but with the Muslim community. Reaching out to get to know these potential allies can go a long way in providing the best possible care for clients, as well as in contributing to attitude changes that can ultimately reduce the risk of domestic violence and increase positive responses to help-seeking behaviors.

Conclusion

While this chapter has highlighted some of the significant layers that come into play when working with Muslims affected by domestic violence, clinicians should bear in mind that the complex nature of the phenomenon of domestic violence compounded by the diversity of Muslims in the West necessitates working carefully and patiently. Care should be taken to thoroughly understand relevant cultural and religious factors, and attention should be given to the client's description of the problem and treatment goals. Because the issue of domestic violence among Muslims can trigger biases and strong emotional responses among both the treatment provider and the client, it is important to conduct thorough assessments, obtain supervision and/or consultation when necessary, and work collaboratively with allies in the Muslim community who can provide much needed support and credibility to clinicians and their clients.

References

Abdallah, K. (2007). A peaceful idea, violent realities: A study on Muslim female domestic violence survivors. In M. B. Alkhateeb & S. E. Abugideiri (Eds.), *Change from within: Diverse perspectives on domestic violence in Muslim communities* (pp. 69–89). Great Falls, VA: Peaceful Families Project.

Abdul-Karim, S., & Kiely-Froude, C. (2009). Providing culturally conscious mental health treatment for African American Muslim women living with spousal abuse. *Journal of Muslim Mental Health, 4*, 175–186.

Abraham, M. (1999). Sexual abuse in South Asian immigrant marriages. *Violence Against Women, 5*, 591–618.

Abu Ras, W. (2007). Cultural beliefs and service utilization by battered Arab immigrant women. *Violence Against Women, 13*, 1002–1028.

Abugideiri, S. E. (2007). Domestic violence among Muslims seeking mental health counseling. In M. B. Alkhateeb & S. E. Abugideiri (Eds.), *Change from within: Diverse perspectives on domestic violence in Muslim communities* (pp. 91–115). Great Falls, VA: Peaceful Families Project.

Ahmad, F., Riaz, S., Barata, P., & Stewart, D. E. (2004). Patriarchal beliefs and perceptions of abuse among South Asian immigrant women. *Violence Against Women, 10*, 262–282.

Ali, A. Y. (1989). *The meaning of the Holy Qur'an* (New ed.). Beltsville, MD: Amana Publications.

Alkhateeb, M. B. (2009). *DV organizations serving Muslim women: Preliminary results of a 2009 quantitative survey.* Peaceful Families Project. Retrieved March 14, 2010, from http://www.peacefulfamilies.org/DVOrgsSurvey.pdf

Alkhateeb, M. B., & Abugideiri, S. E. (2007). Introduction. In M. B. Alkhateeb & S. E. Abugideiri (Eds.), *Change from within: Diverse perspectives on domestic violence in Muslim communities* (pp. 13–30). Great Falls, VA: Peaceful Families Project.

Alkhateeb, S. (1999). Ending domestic violence in Muslim families. *Journal of Religion and Abuse, 1*(4), 49–59.

Alwani, Z. (2007). The Qur'anic model for harmony in family relations. In M. B. Alkhateeb & S. E. Abugideiri (Eds.), *Change from within: Diverse perspectives on domestic violence in Muslim communities* (pp. 33–66). Great Falls, VA: Peaceful Families Project.

Alwani, Z., & Abugideiri, S. (2003). *What Islam says about domestic violence.* Herndon, VA: FAITH.

Ammar, N. H. (2000). Simplistic stereotyping and complex reality of Arab-American immigrant identity: Consequences and future strategies in policing wife battery. *Islam and Christian Muslim Relations, 11*, 51–71.

Ammar, N. H. (2007). Wife battery in Islam: A comprehensive understanding of interpretations. *Violence Against Women, 13*, 516–526.

Ayyub, R. (2000). Domestic violence in the South Asian Muslim immigrant population in the United States. *Journal of Social Distress and the Homeless, 9*, 237–248.

Baobaid, M. (2002). *Access to women abuse services by Arab-speaking Muslim women in London, Ontario. Background investigation and recommendations for further research and community outreach.* Centre for Research on Violence Against Women and Children. Retrieved March 13, 2010, from http://www.crvawc.ca/documents/Final-AccesstoWomenAbuseServicesbyArabSpeakingMuslimWomeninLondon_001.pdf

Chamie, J. (1986). Polygyny among Arabs. *Population Studies, 40*, 55–66.

Dasgupta, S. (2000). Charting the course: An overview of domestic violence in the South Asian community in the United States. *Journal of Social Distress and the Homeless, 9*, 173–185.

DeKeseredy, W. S., & Dragiewicz, M. (2007). Understanding the complexities of feminist perspectives on woman abuse: A commentary on Donald G. Dutton's rethinking domestic violence. *Violence Against Women, 13*, 874–884.

Douki, S., Nacef, F., Belhadj, A., Bouasker, A., & Ghachem, R. (2003). Violence against women in Arab and Islamic countries. *Archives of Women's Mental Health, 6*(3), 165–171.

Eid, T. Y. (2005). *Marriage, divorce, and child custody as experienced by American Muslims: Religious, social, and legal considerations.* Cambridge, MA: Harvard University. Unpublished doctoral dissertation.

Ellsberg, M., Jansen, H. A., Heise, L., Watts, C. H., & Garcia-Moreno, C. (2008). Intimate partner violence and women's physical and mental health in the WHO multi-country study on women's health and domestic violence: An observational study. *The Lancet, 371*, 1165–1172.

FaithTrust Institute (Producer), & Gargiulo, M. (Director). (2007). *Garments for one another: Ending domestic violence in Muslim families* [DVD].

Fortune, M. (1991). A commentary on religious issues in family violence. In Fortune, M., *Violence in the family: A workshop curriculum for clergy and other helpers* (pp. 137–151). Cleveland: Pilgrim Press.

Fortune, M. (2001). Religious issues and violence against women. In C. M. Renzetti, J. L. Edleson, & R. K. Bergen (Eds.), *Sourcebook on violence aginst women* (pp. 371–385). Thousand Oaks, CA: Sage.

Ghayyur, T. (2009). *Domestic violence survey analysis February-March 2009.* SoundVision. Retrieved August 10, 2010, from http://soundvision.com/info/domesticviolence/2009survey.asp

Gil, E. (1996). *Systemic treatment of families who abuse.* San Francisco, CA: Jossey-Bass.

Halabu, H. (2006). *Domestic violence in the Arab American community: Culturally relevant features and intervention considerations.* University of Michigan, Ann Arbor, Michigan. Unpublished doctoral dissertation.

Hamel, J. (2005). *Gender inclusive treatment of intimate partner abuse: A comprehensive approach.* New York, NY: Springer.

Hamill, J. (2010). Imams urged to condemn domestic abuse. *Herald Scotland.* Retrieved July 5, 2010 from http://www.heraldscotland.com/news/home-news/imams-urged-to-condemn-domestic-abuse-1.1036028

Hassouneh-Phillips, D. (2001a). American Muslim women's experiences of leaving abusive relationships. *Health Care for Women International, 22,* 415–432.

Hassouneh-Phillips, D. (2001b). Polygamy and wife abuse: A qualitative study of Muslim women in America. *Health Care for Women International, 22,* 735–748.

Hassouneh-Phillips, D. (2003). Strength and vulnerability: Spirituality in abused American Muslim women's lives. *Issues in Mental Health Nursing, 24,* 681–694.

Hodge, D. R., & Nadir, A. (2008). Moving toward culturally competent practice with Muslims: Modifying cognitive therapy with Islamic tenets. *Social Work, 53,* 31–41.

Ibrahim, N., & Abdalla, M. (2010). A critical examination of Qur'an 4:34 and its relevance to intimate partner violence in Muslim families. *Journal of Muslim Mental Health, 5*(3), 327–349.

Karabat, A. (2010, April 13). Imams to become women's rights activists across Turkey. *Today's Zaman.* Retrieved July 5, 2010 from http://www.todayszaman.com/tz-web/news-207267-101-imams-to-become-womens-rights-activists-across-turkey.html

Kasturirangan, A., Krishnan, S., & Riger, S. (2004). The impact of culture and minority status on women's experience of domestic violence. *Trauma, Violence, & Abuse, 5,* 318–332.

Krahé, B., Bieneck, S., & Möller, I. (2005). Understanding gender and intimate partner violence from an international perspective. *Sex Roles, 52,* 807–827.

Kulwicki, A. D., & Miller, J. (1999). Domestic violence in the Arab American population: Transforming environmental conditions through community education. *Issues in Mental Health Nursing, 20,* 199–215.

Macey, M. (1999). Religion, male violence, and the control of women: Pakistani Muslim men in Bradford, UK. *Gender and Development, 7*(1), 48–55.

Magid, M. (2007). Affecting change as an imam. In M. B. Alkhateeb & S. E. Abugideiri (Eds.), *Change from within: Diverse perspectives on domestic violence in Muslim communities* (pp. 187–202). Great Falls, VA: Peaceful Families Project.

Nason-Clark, N. (2000). Making the sacred safe: Woman abuse and communities of faith. *Sociology of Religion, 61,* 349–368.

Raj, A., & Silverman, J. G. (2002). Intimate partner violence against South Asian women in Greater Boston. *Journal of the American Medical Women's Association, 57*(2), 111–114.

Sokoloff, N. J., & Dupont, I. (2005). Domestic violence at the intersections of race, class, and gender: Challenges and contributions to understanding violence against marginalized women in diverse communities. *Violence Against Women, 11*, 38–64.

Sweifach, J., & Heft-LaPorte, H. (2007). A model for group work practice with Ultra-Orthodox Jewish victims of domestic violence: A qualitative study. *Social Work with Groups, 30*(3), 29–45.

Watlington, C. G., & Murphy, C. M. (2006). The roles of religion and spirituality among African American survivors of domestic violence. *Journal of Clinical Psychology, 62*, 837–857.

CHAPTER 17
Sexuality and Sexual Dysfunctions

AMAL KILLAWI

Sexual problems in a relationship can be challenging for any couple. One of the reasons couples may seek therapy is that one or both of the partners is experiencing a sexual dysfunction. A growing field, sex therapy is a specialized form of counseling that generally adheres to solution-focused and brief-treatment models and focuses on resolving sexual problems for both single and partnered individuals. This chapter is intended for sex therapists, marital counselors, and mental health providers from other disciplines who work with clients around problems of a sexual nature.

Religious beliefs and sexual values are considered some of the strongest and most important constructs held by individuals (Turner, Center, & Kiser, 2004). It is well known that sexual behavior is influenced by social and cultural factors (Kulhara & Avasthi, 1995), and that sexuality is defined within cultural and social settings (Bullough, 1976; Reiss, 1986). Religion and spirituality can be important sources of meaning and motivation (Turner et al., 2004) and have a powerful influence on attitudes about sexuality and sexual behavior. Religious beliefs can impact the etiology of sexual dysfunctions (Simpson & Ramberg, 1992) and influence their presentation, as well as client help-seeking behavior, and treatment compliance (de Silva & Rodrigo, 1995; Sungur, 1999). Yet, religion is often overlooked and not emphasized in sex therapy (Simpson & Ramberg, 1992). Mental health providers have paid less attention to the role of religious standards in the treatment of sexual dysfunctions (Ribner, 2003b). Currently, there exists a gap in the literature relating multicultural therapy to sex therapy (Peterson, Dobbins, Coleman, & Razzouk, 2007), and only recently have providers made an effort to merge spirituality and sexuality in counseling (Turner et al., 2004).

As mental health professionals increasingly find themselves serving culturally diverse clients from a variety of religious and spiritual backgrounds, they will very likely encounter clients from the Muslim faith. Muslims are not a monolithic group. They hold diverse personal and family values, and vary in their practice of Islam depending on their ethnicity, sectarian affiliation (e.g., Sunni, Shi'a, etc.), socioeconomic status, level of integration into society, and whether they are immigrants or native born. As in any faith group, the practice of Muslims may deviate from the guidelines set by the faith, and Muslims will vary in the way Islam plays a role in their lives.

Despite the heterogeneity that exists among Muslims, this chapter aims to provide an overview of sexuality from an Islamic perspective, discuss implications for clinical practice, and offer practical treatment recommendations. These guidelines are not meant to be conclusive and applicable to all Muslim clients. However, it is the author's hope that this information will assist mental health professionals in delivering quality services to a significant demographic of the world population.

Sexual Dysfunctions and Sex Therapy

The *Diagnostic and Statistical Manual of Mental Disorders* (DSM-IV-TR; American Psychiatric Association, 2000) classifies nine diagnostic categories of sexual dysfunction.[1] Further distinctions are made for etiology and treatment. The definition of a sexual dysfunction is influenced by social mores, values, and knowledge (Wincze & Carey, 2001). According to the DSM-IV-TR, one of the criteria for a sexual dysfunction diagnosis is that "the disturbance causes marked distress or interpersonal difficulty." It is important to note here that some individuals may have what is classified as a "dysfunction," but the symptoms are not a cause of distress or dissatisfaction for them or their partners. This could be due to mutual acceptance; for instance, both partners may not find it problematic that the husband ejaculates quickly after vaginal penetration. It can also be due to lack of education or cultural beliefs about the right to sexual satisfaction. For example, in many cultures, sex for women is not expected to be pleasurable, but rather considered an obligation toward the husband. Alternatively, some people may experience problems and dissatisfaction with their sexual functioning, but still not meet the criteria for a sexual dysfunction. An example of this is age-related changes that may result in

---

[1] The DSM V, to be released in 2013, plans to combine arousal and desire disorders into one category based on the Basson (2001) model of female sexual response, which demonstrates that arousal and desire occur simultaneously.

vaginal dryness in women and the need for increased stimulation before an erection for men.

A variety of factors can contribute to sexual difficulties. In order to establish causality and arrive at a comprehensive case formulation, it is important for providers to conduct a careful and thorough evaluation during the assessment process and to provide referrals for a medical assessment as needed. When developing a treatment plan, Wincze and Carey (2001) urge providers to customize treatments utilizing the biopsychosocial approach. This means that providers should recognize the "psychological, biological, pharmacological, relational, and contextual contributors to sexual problems" (Leiblum, 2007, p. 8) and address multiple etiologies with various treatment options. Therapists are encouraged to use an integrative treatment approach that utilizes a variety of cognitive-behavioral and systematic interventions, such as sexual education, sensate focus, communication training, and couple counseling, along with pharmacological, medical, and psychological interventions as needed (Leiblum & Wiegel, 2002; Wincze & Carey, 2001).

Cultural Competence in Sex Therapy

As sexual dysfunctions are multifaceted and cannot be attributed to one cause, competent clinical practice requires clinicians to value complexity and view their clients holistically. Providers must acknowledge the reality of cultural and religious influences on clients (Peterson et al., 2007) and be willing to challenge clinical bias about other cultures and faiths. When working with sexual values different from their own, clinicians should acknowledge cultural and religious biases and avoid "cultural ethnocentrism" (Ribner & Kleinplatz, 2007) and stereotyping, which can jeopardize the effectiveness of treatment.

Professionals practicing sex therapy should be respectful and nonjudgmental (Simpson & Ramberg, 1992), and should adopt a "curious stance of genuine not-knowing" (Anderson & Goolishian, 1992). Providers should strive to acquire education about the different values, traditions, and beliefs held by various ethnic and religious groups, and to understand these groups' sexual values in their respective contexts (Ribner & Kleinplatz, 2007). It is also equally important to demonstrate sensitivity to the uniqueness of each client (Carolan, Bagherinia, Juhari, Himelright, & Mouton-Sanders, 2000). Peterson and colleagues (2007) review a "three-step guide" for cultural competency: Providers should (a) acknowledge and express respect for the cultural differences between them and clients, (b) ask clients about the influences of their cultural beliefs on their concept of health and illness and preference for treatment interventions, and (c) share their professional expertise, while also inviting clients to share about their own cultural and individual values.

Accepting clients' cultural and religious values as a behavioral construct can significantly define the therapeutic framework during treatment (Burt & Rudolph, 2000; Simpson & Ramberg, 1992). Providers should integrate the clients' religious beliefs and attitudes about sexuality into the therapeutic process (Simpson & Ramberg, 1992). Opposing cultural and religious mandates or denying their validity will undermine any efforts to build therapeutic trust with clients (Ribner, 2003a). Thus, in order to minimize resistance and maximize potential for change, it is important for providers to work accordingly with client belief systems and engage in creative modifications of treatment processes as needed (Ribner, 2003b).

Sexual Values in Islam

> Values surrounding sexuality are based on the recognition that there is Something Beyond. Life here is meaningful, when lived in accordance with Divine Revelation and Guidance found in the Qur'an and the Hadith, where people fulfill the trust bestowed on them. (Compton, 1989, p. 80)

By definition, a Muslim is one who accepts and submits to God. Muslims are primarily guided by two sources: first and foremost by the Qur'an, Islam's holy scripture considered to be the highest form of religious law, and second by the Prophetic traditions or *ahadith*,[2] a compilation of Prophet Muhammad's (PBUH)[3] teachings and normative example or *Sunnah*. Additionally, Muslims may refer to accounts of how the companions and followers of the Prophet (PBUH) implemented his teachings. The traditional texts are the sources of *Sharia*, also known as the "instructions which regulate everyday activity of life to be adhered to" by practicing Muslims (Serour, 1996, p. 102). *Sharia* provides the framework for a healthy and God-conscious lifestyle.[4] Understanding the role of these sources is important because of the implications they may have on treatment interventions, particularly those that are perceived to be against religious norms, as addressed later in the chapter.

---

[2] Plural term of *hadith*, which is a saying or narration of the Prophet Muhammad's (PBUH) speech, deed, or spoken or tacit approval or disapproval of an issue.

[3] Out of reverence for the Prophet Muhammad (PBUH), Muslims follow each reference to his name with this acronym, which stands for "May God's peace be upon him."

[4] Muslims do not have a religious hierarchy. The Qur'an is considered the highest authoritative source. If there are multiple interpretations of a Qur'anic verse, Muslims refer to the *Sunnah* of the Prophet for the appropriate application or understanding. In case an issue is not addressed in either, Muslims may consult an Islamic scholar who will then use analogical reasoning and draw on relevant principles in the Qur'an and the *Sunnah* to come to a conclusion (Al-Hibri & El Habti, 2006, pp. 153–154).

As Islam is considered a way of life, God touches on every aspect of the human experience, including sexuality. Islam has a rich discourse around sex and sexuality, and sexual references in the Qur'an and Prophetic traditions are positive. Sex is considered a gift from God and a glimpse of the pleasures of Heaven (Badri, 1979). Some classical Islamic scholars have noted that orgasm is the closest one can come to experiencing Heaven (Farah, 1984). Islam considers sexual activity to be a necessary and natural part of life, reserved exclusively for the marital relationship. Muslims are encouraged to enjoy sex within the framework of marriage (Al-Sawaf & Al-Issa, 2000).

These beliefs are in direct contrast to the cultural taboos about sex present in many Muslim communities today. Historically, sex was not viewed as conflicting with the Islamic faith, but rather "encouraged as a natural means towards the happiness of the individual, the stability of the home, and . . . the achievement of the union symbolic of the unity of the Divine" (Walton, 1963, p. 41). Classical scholars within the Islamic tradition dedicated entire chapters to enhancing the sexual relationship,[5] and many books were written explicitly describing sexual behavior and technique. Perhaps the most famous is Al-Ghazali's *Book on the Etiquette of Marriage*, part of his larger work, *The Revival of the Religious Sciences*, written between 1096 and 1106. Al-Ghazali outlines the etiquette of sexual relations, emphasizing the importance of women's sexual satisfaction, and offering husbands specific recommendations such as that "sex should begin with gentle words and kissing . . . and (that) he should caress the breasts and nipples, and every part of the body" (Khan, 2006, p. 422). Farah (1984) writes that "upon reading his instructions, it is difficult to believe that it was written in the eleventh century and not by a present-day psychologist" (p. 32). Another popular manual is *The Perfumed Garden*, written by Al-Nefzawi in the 16th century. Al-Nefzawi discusses sexual technique and coital positions, recognizing differences in the sexual responses of men and women, and encouraging foreplay and mutual satisfaction (Al-Sawaf & Al-Issa, 2000). It is important to note that many of the Islamic references address their instructions to men because they are often the initiators of sexual relations, and women are more likely to be sexually neglected or uncomfortable discussing their pleasure (Kotb, 2004).

Marriage and Family Practices

The Qur'an emphasizes the common origin and equal value of men and women (Ansari, 2002) and states, "It is He Who created you from a single person, and made his mate of like nature, in order that he might dwell with her (in love)" (7:189). Created from a "single soul," men and women have

---
[5] Refer to Al-Kawthari (2008, p. 3) for a partial list.

the same essence and enjoy mutual rights and responsibilities (Al-Hibri & El Habti, 2006). In marriage, their roles are complementary and equal in value. The marital relationship is described as a covenant with God, a relationship that provides security and tranquility and is based on love, mercy, and affection, as evidenced by the following verse:

> And among His signs is this, that He created for you mates from among yourselves, that you may dwell in peace and tranquility with them, and He has put love and mercy between your (hearts): Verily in that are signs for those who reflect." (Qur'an 30:21)

The Prophet Muhammad (PBUH) taught Muslims that "the most perfect of believers in faith is the one who has the best morals, and the best of you are the kindest of you to their wives" (*Sunan al-Tirmidhi*, as cited in Al-Hibri & El Habti, 2006, p. 193). The Qur'an tells Muslims that "they (spouses) are your garments and ye are their garments" (2:187). Both partners must strive to the best of their ability to sustain each other emotionally, spiritually, intellectually, and sexually, and thus be garments for one another, offering each other mutual protection, comfort, support, service, and companionship (Farah, 1984).

Muslims are highly encouraged to marry, as marriage lays the foundation for society and family life, and one of its major objectives is to satisfy sexual needs. *Nikah*, or intercourse, is the Arabic word for marriage (Al-Jibali, 2000), and most classical Islamic law texts state that marriage is a contract that permits sexual contact between a man and a woman (S. Webb, personal communication, September 26, 2010). Even though marriage may be postponed, celibacy and asceticism are discouraged (Al-Jibali, 2000). Single Muslims are expected to remain abstinent from sex[6] and strive to marry.[7]

Marriage practices vary and are influenced by cultural norms, religious practice, and family traditions (Altareb, 2008). Although some Muslims may date, as is commonly practiced in Western cultures, it is not religiously permitted. The Islamic marriage process is purposeful and aims to help single individuals make objective life decisions without the complexity of

---

[6] As evidenced by the verse, "But let them who find not (the means for) marriage abstain (from sexual relations) until Allah enriches them from His bounty" (Qur'an, 24:33). This applies to both men and women, as "Muslims who follow the Spirit of Islam, would claim a single sexual standard for all (single) men and women.... The sexual urge is recognized as natural, and all-consuming at certain stages of life, so there is a constant struggle between passion and good judgment" (Compton, 1989, p. 82).

[7] As narrated in a *hadith*, "Oh young people. Whoever among you can marry, should marry, because it helps him lower his gaze and guard his modesty (i.e., his private parts from committing illegal sexual intercourse) and whoever is not able to marry, should fast, as fasting diminishes his sexual desire" (*Sahih al-Bukhari*, Volume 7, Book 62, Number 4).

emotional and sexual relationships (Altareb, 2008). The methods for choosing one's spouse can range from families arranging chaperoned meetings to introductions facilitated by friends, religious leaders, or even online social networks. Compatibility may be sought based on similarities in age, education, ethnic background, religious sect, and religious practice (Abdul-Rauf, 2007). Consent is required by both parties in order for the marriage to be valid. After officiating a marriage contract, a public celebration is typically held, and the couple is free to consummate the marriage (Altareb, 2008).

Having children is encouraged, as they are considered to be a blessing from God. Muslim couples may utilize various birth control methods, depending on the religious interpretations they follow. Abortion is permitted in cases where the health of the mother or the child is in danger, or if the pregnancy resulted from rape or incest, but it cannot be used as a form of birth control. Couples experiencing infertility may utilize various treatments; however, treatment cannot include a third party's "genetic or conceptional contribution" (Serour, 1996, p. 104), such as egg or sperm donation, or surrogate mothering, because they "intrude into the (couple's) marital functions of sex and procreation" (Serour, 1996, p. 106). After birth, Muslim boys are circumcised, as they are in the Jewish tradition. Female circumcision, also known as female genital mutilation, is not an Islamic practice, and this is quite evident when reviewing reports from different countries where cultural norms encourage such behavior among people of different faiths.

Most Muslim marriages are monogamous. Although polygamy is permitted conditionally, it is considered to be an exception rather than the rule (Ansari, 2002) and must be practiced with justice and fairness.[8] Gay relationships are prohibited in Islam for both men and women. However, Islam makes a distinction between feelings and actions (Altareb, 2008). It is not considered sinful to identify as gay and acknowledge same-sex attraction, but it is prohibited to engage in gay sexual activity. Some Muslims may struggle to reconcile their religious, cultural, and sexual identities. Clinicians working with Muslims around sexual orientation issues should practice compassion, empathy, and sensitivity.

Sex as Worship and a Right for Both Spouses

The Islamic view of sexuality is based on the ideal of establishing equilibrium between spirituality and the fulfillment of earthly desires and needs. When the sexual act occurs within legitimate bonds (marriage), pleasure becomes a recognized right for both spouses and does not generate any guilt (Al-Hibri & El Habti, 2006, p. 206).

---

[8] The Qur'an says, "... if you fear that you shall not be able to deal justly (with them), then only one" (4:3) and, "You are never able to be fair and just as between women, even if it is your ardent desire" (4:129).

For Muslim couples, marriage is a means to provide sexual satisfaction according to the limits set by God. Sex can serve multiple purposes within marriage: providing enjoyment and sexual gratification; preserving chastity and protecting individuals from fornication and lustful gazes at others; and facilitating procreation and contributing to offspring (Al-Kawthari, 2008). Sex is also meant to enhance the physical and emotional bond between the couple, increasing intimacy and strengthening their relationship. Muslim religiosity does not mean inhibition of sexuality (Al-Sawaf & Al-Issa, 2000). For Muslims living a God-centered life, even sexual relations should be practiced with transformative objectives. The spiritual relationship between husband and wife is the basis of sexual relations; thus, sex with one's spouse becomes a form of worship and *sadaqa* (charity)[9] that merits God's pleasure and reward if performed with God's consciousness and an awareness of His objectives.[10] The goal is shared emotional and sensual satisfaction of the couple, with special consideration given to women as evidenced by the Qur'anic verse, "Women shall have rights similar to the rights upon them; according to what is equitable and just" (2:228) and the following Prophetic saying:

> When one of you has sexual intercourse with his wife, he must always be conscious of her needs. If he finishes before her, he then must not rush her and must wait for her until she is satisfied, because that frustrates her and prevents her from enjoying her sexuality. (Ibn Qudamah, as cited in Al-Hibri & El Habti, 2006, p. 211)

Each partner must strive to provide sexual fulfillment for the other, but men must pay particular attention to the sexual satisfaction of their wives, given the difference in arousal patterns. Al-Ghazali advises husbands to be patient with their wives and to seek "congruence in attaining . . . climax" for that is "more gratifying to her" (Farah, 1984, p. 107).[11]

---

[9] It is narrated that the Prophet (PBUH) said, ". . . and in the sexual act of each of you there is sadaqah (charity). [The Companions said], O Messenger of Allah! One of us fulfills his sexual desire and he is given a reward for that? And he said, Do you not see that were he to act upon it unlawfully, he would be sinning? Likewise, if he acts upon it lawfully, he will be rewarded" (Sahih Muslim, as cited in Al-Kawthari, 2008, p. 10).

[10] "Islam considers this (sexual) act as one of the five basic elements of Faith, as important as belief, worship, fasting and pilgrimage! . . . Al-Ghazali . . . said, . . . if one even cohabits with one's own wife—not for the . . . carnal pleasure, but for perform(ing) . . . the duty imposed by God, then that is an act of piety and devotion" (Hamidullah, 1969, section 108).

[11] Al-Ghazali writes, "Once the husband has attained his fulfillment, let him tarry until his wife also attains hers. Her orgasm may be delayed, thus exciting her desire; to withdraw quickly is harmful to the woman. Difference in the nature of [their] reaching a climax causes discord whenever the husband ejaculates first. Congruence in attaining a climax is more gratifying to her because the man is not preoccupied with his own pleasure, but rather with hers; for it is likely that the woman might be shy" (Farah, 1984, p. 107).

Spouses are to beautify themselves for each other and be sexually available to one another. As part of marital obligations, both men and women are expected to engage in sexual relations, and to deprive the other of sexual fulfillment without a valid reason is considered a sin. Some couples may mistakenly believe that only the husband has the right to sexual fulfillment, when in fact sexual relations are the right of both partners. Given the variation in libido between individuals, ultimately it is up to the couple to mutually agree on the frequency with which they will engage in sexual activity. Islam stresses on moderation and finding a middle course (Al-Kawthari, 2008). Sexual dysfunction and/or lack of sexual relations can be a prerequisite for divorce for both men and women.

Sex Play

Many Islamic references highlight the importance of sex play in a couple's relationship. Couples are free to engage in various forms of sex play and to decide on the level of coverage they observe during sexual relations, including direct observation of each other's genitals. Sex is to involve mutual consent and be free of harm. Cultural factors will determine the couple's level of comfort and choice of sexual activity; additionally, they may be guided by their subscription to certain Islamic legal opinions that limit the permissibility of some types of sex play. A general principle of Islamic jurisprudence is that in matters of daily life, everything is *halal* (permissible) except for what is expressively forbidden (*haram*) in the religious text. For example, the majority of Islamic jurists consider anal sex to be an abhorrence based on various *ahadith* of the Prophet (although it is permitted by some Shi'a scholars).

Couples are encouraged to be creative in their lovemaking positions and engage in foreplay, as clarified by the Qur'an using the simile of a farmer planting his seeds in a field:

> Your wives are your tilth; go, then, unto your tilth as you may desire, but first provide something for your souls, and remain conscious of God, and know that you are destined to meet Him. And give glad tidings unto those who believe. (2:223)[12]

This is also supported by the Prophetic tradition advising husbands that they should not fall upon their wives like animals, and instead should

---

[12] Another Islamic scholar, Abul-Ala Mawdudi, adds, "The farmer sows the seed in order to reap the harvest, but he does not sow it out of season or cultivate it in a manner which will injure or exhaust the soil. He is wise and considerate, and does not run riot" (Rahman, 1981, p. 285).

first allow for a messenger (i.e., kisses and romantic words) between them (Al-Kawthari, 2008; Farah, 1984).

Sex toys are permitted, but their use will depend on the individual preferences of each couple. The general rule is that the spouse should generate stimulation (Al-Kawthari, 2008). Muslim couples are expected to limit their fantasies to each other and refrain from looking elsewhere for pleasure. Thus, any material that displays naked bodies or sexual content, including books, magazines, educational material, videos, and pictures, is prohibited, based on the rules of modesty and the belief that adultery can be committed in other ways, even without direct participation in sexual activity. Additionally, any sexual activity that involves others outside of the marital relationship, for example, adding partners or exchanging partners, is prohibited. The principle of marriage is for each spouse to derive pleasure exclusively from the other; their relationship is to remain private to protect its sacredness.

Historically, individual masturbation has been strongly discouraged and constituted by most Islamic scholars as a transgression of God's boundaries for sex. Other scholars allowed it with some conditions: that individuals are unmarried and fear that they will have sex if they do not masturbate, and that it is releasing sexual tension rather than fulfilling sexual desire (Kotb, 2004). Kotb (2004) argues that because masturbation is not clearly and absolutely forbidden like sex outside of marriage, the law of necessity allows for some flexibility. Contemporary scholars may allow for masturbation in the face of serious challenges, such as fear of engaging in sex outside of a marital relationship or as a requirement for the treatment of a sexual dysfunction, provided that there is evidence of its effectiveness (S. Webb, personal communication, September 26, 2010).

Muslim couples are to abstain from sexual activity during certain times.[13] For example, during *Ramadan*, the month of fasting, any type of sexual activity is prohibited between sunrise and sunset to practice self-restraint and spiritual development. During menstruation and postnatal bleeding, it is forbidden for Muslim couples to engage in sexual intercourse (coitus) so as to not cause discomfort for the wife.[14] However, couples are free to negotiate other forms of sexual activity during this time. Couples that perform

---

[13] Although there are no prescribed times for sexual activity, the Qur'an notes three occasions when children should make an extra effort to seek their parents' permission before entering their bedroom: in the early morning, afternoon, and late night, because these are times when parents may be more likely to engage in sexual activity.

[14] This is based on the following Qur'anic verse: "They question you concerning menstruation. Say it is a harm (a damage) so refrain from women during menstruation and do not approach them until they are purified. Once they purify themselves, then enjoy them from where God has instructed you. Truly God loves the repenters and those who care for purity" (2:222).

the five daily prayers, as is required of Muslims, may prefer not to have sexual relations between prayers, because the couple must be mindful of performing the *ghusl*[15] (ritual washing) in time for the next prayer.

Modesty and Sex Education

Although there is an abundance of positive traditional Islamic knowledge around issues of sexuality, the reality is that sex continues to be a taboo subject among Muslims, mainly due to the intersection of various cultural attitudes and practices. Many Muslims adhere to religious mandates that define and influence gender interactions and intimate relationships. Islamic tradition preaches modesty and makes a distinction between public and private space. Men and women are both instructed to observe modest dress and behavior. Levels of modesty differ based on context,[16] and modesty is expected even among members of the same sex. Sexuality is not to be flaunted. The sexual relationship is considered a special and private matter, reserved exclusively for one's spouse, and thus not to be discussed with others. Similar to the Jewish tradition (Ribner & Kleinplatz, 2007), Islam's emphasis on privacy of the body and sex is not due to shamefulness, but is rather considered a form of protection from casual observation to be revealed only during the right time and to the right person. Like their Jewish brethren, Muslims are not inclined to "display open that which is cherished most" (Ribner & Kleinplatz, 2007, p. 47).

For these reasons, sex tends to be reserved for discussion within the family and within a religious context. Sex education, if there is any, does not occur at a specific age. During the study of the Qur'an and Prophetic traditions, one may be exposed to sexual information when learning about the various religious obligations and rituals that govern Muslim life. Some Muslims may have attended school-based education programs; others may have obtained information from their peers, books, the media, and online sources. However, Muslim parents may not provide their children with comprehensive sexual education, mainly because their own cultural and traditional upbringing lacked appropriate sexual health information

---

[15] Required to fulfill various rituals and prayers, *ghusl* is the bathing and purification of the body and is mandatory after sexual intercourse, any sexual discharge, and completion of the menstruation cycle.

[16] In public, women are to cover their bodies except for their face and hands; some opinions allow for the feet to be uncovered. Men are to cover from the navel to the knees, with some opinions also including the chest and back. Among members of their sex, men and women must cover from the navel to the knees. In the private home environment among close male relatives, women may uncover, but still adhere to a greater level of modesty than they might among other women. Between spouses, the rules of modesty no longer apply, and couples are free to dress as they like.

(Khan, 2006). Additionally, in Western environments characterized by sexualized media and sexually active peers, Muslim families may find it challenging to provide sex education that is in line with Islamic values. Even within a religious context, many Muslim intellectuals, educators, religious leaders, and parents are uncomfortable discussing sexual issues publicly (Ahsan, 2007). Compared to the historical plethora of Muslim writings about sex and sexuality, in today's time, only a few books have been authored by Muslims (Ahsan, 2007). It should be noted, however, that there has been some progress. Muslims are increasingly discussing sex, and a number of people are working around sexual health issues as educators and counselors within their communities.

Sexual Dysfunctions among Muslims

Research in the general population shows sexual dysfunctions to be prevalent, but estimates vary across studies. Community samples have provided estimates ranging from 10% to 52% of men and 25% to 63% of women (Feldman, Goldstein, Hatzichristou, Krane, & McKinlay, 1994; Frank, Anderson, & Rubenstein, 1978; Rosen, Taylor, Leiblum, & Bachman, 1993; Spector & Carey, 1990). A U.S. study found that sexual dysfunctions were present in 43% of women and 31% of men (Laumann, Paik, & Rosen, 1999). In a review of the international literature, Simons and Carey (2001) used community samples to estimate the following prevalence rates: male orgasmic disorder (3%), male hypoactive sexual desire disorder (3%), erectile disorder (5%), premature ejaculation (5%), and female orgasmic disorder (10%). More specifically, the chief complaints are premature ejaculation for men (21%) and low sexual desire for women (22%) (Laumann et al., 1999).

Little research exists on rates of sexual behavior and sexual problems among Muslims. Most of the available information originates from mental health clinics in the Middle East dominated by Western treatment methods (Al-Sawaf & Al-Issa, 2000). In a one-year study in a hospital outpatient clinic in Saudi Arabia, out of a sample of 38 men, 25 men (66%) were seen for erectile dysfunction and 13 men (34%) were seen for "ejaculation disorder" with weak or partial erection. Only five women were seen during this time: three women for dyspareunia, and two women for vaginismus. No women were seen for desire or orgasmic disorders (Al-Sawaf & Al-Issa, 2000). Turkish studies have found vaginismus to be the most commonly diagnosed sexual dysfunction among women (Oniz, Keskinoglu, & Bezircioglu, 2007; Yasan & Gürgen, 2009), and premature ejaculation the most commonly diagnosed among men (Yasan & Gürgen, 2009).

There is much we don't know about the sexual dysfunction rates of Muslims living in Western countries. The information we do have is usually derived from clinical observation rather than empirical research.

Two British studies found that men from Muslim backgrounds present more frequently with premature ejaculation (Richardson & Goldmeier, 2005; Steggall, Pryce, & Fowler, 2006), while another concluded that they may be more at risk for this sexual dysfunction (Richardson, Wood, & Goldmeier, 2006). Based on personal correspondence with providers and religious leaders in the West, as well as an informal survey of online help forums, it is reasonable to assume that Muslims in the West may be experiencing similar rates of sexual dysfunctions. Many providers and religious leaders have also observed a growing number of Muslims seeking help for affairs, sexual addictions, pornography, and other Islamically unlawful means of sexual gratification.

Implications for Practice and Treatment Recommendations

It is important for therapists to recognize that the culture and faith traditions of clients influence their presentation of sexual problems, how they manage them, and the types of treatments they seek (de Silva & Rodrigo, 1995; Sungur, 1999). Cultural and religious beliefs may either generate resistance to the therapy or provide strong motivation for change (Sungur, 1999); thus individuals may be hesitant to seek treatment or fully utilize the benefit of counseling. Sungur (1999) provides a helpful framework for conceptualizing how various cultural and religious factors can manifest in sex therapy. For the purposes of this chapter, they have been modified and are as follows:

- Definition of the problem and motivation for treatment
- Problem attribution and expectations for treatment
- Choice of helping agencies
- Provider preferences and dynamics in therapy
- Acceptance of and compliance with intervention techniques

In this section, practical treatment guidelines for working with Muslim clients are also presented.

Definition of the Problem and Motivation for Treatment

Social mores, values, and knowledge (Wincze & Carey, 2001) can impact the definition and experience of sexual dysfunctions, more specifically, what people consider to be problematic sexual functioning, how they experience their symptoms, and how they respond to them. Because symptoms can be culturally determined, Western diagnostic labels may not always be applicable and may even be inappropriate sometimes (Kleinman, 1987). Muslim clients may present with concerns different from their Western counterparts or with culturally specific sexual dysfunctions. For example, in a country such as Saudi

Arabia whose culture equates masculinity with sexual potency and fertility and emphasizes female virginity, Al-Sawaf and Al-Issa (2000) note the prevalence of performance anxiety and concern about "sexual prowess" among men, and complaints about physical performance and avoidance of sex among women. In a Turkish study, Yasan and Gürgen (2009) found that none of the women in their sample complained about orgasmic difficulties.

Cultural beliefs, expectations, and individual experiences can contribute to certain types of sexual problems. Some newlyweds may experience anxiety shifting from abstinence to sexual exploration after marriage. Prior to the wedding night, couples may not have had any physical or sexual contact with the other sex and little sexual education. Similar to the experience of many Orthodox Jewish couples (Ribner, 2003a), the expectation of consummation combined with limited sexual experience and knowledge can contribute to the development of sexual problems soon after the wedding. Couples may experience general awkwardness, discomfort, pain, and unfamiliarity with the body, such as the inability to identify genitalia or locate the vaginal opening. More specifically, men may experience premature ejaculation or erectile dysfunction due to expectations that they should always be able to perform, and women may be at risk of developing vaginismus due to cultural beliefs restricting the insertion of any object into the vagina (i.e., tampons or pap smears), as well as the exaggerated belief in pain upon rupture of the hymen. Cultural traditions such as displaying the blood-stained linen the day after the wedding,[17] can also generate anxiety for couples. It is also worthy to note that arranged marriages, specifically those without consent, can contribute to sexual problems, especially if there is limited attraction between the couples (Al-Sawaf & Al-Issa, 2000; Yasan & Akdeniz, 2009; Yasan & Gürgen, 2009).

Clients may seek treatment after triggers, such as an impending divorce, marital conflict, or miscarriage. Clinicians would do well to first address the trigger problem in treatment[18] (Sungur, 1998). However, cultural and religious factors can also influence motivation for treatment. Al-Sawaf and Al-Issa (2000) observed that women in Saudi Arabia sought treatment only when prompted by the husband and if there were concerns about infertility. Yasan and Gürgen (2009) found that the greatest motivation for sex therapy in Turkey was the "desire to maintain the marriage and to have children" (p. 71). More specifically, women's priority

---

[17] Limited to certain regions of the Muslim world, this practice is strictly a cultural one and is against the Islamic norms of modesty and privacy.

[18] Although the goal of sex therapy is symptom resolution, clinicians may have to explore and focus on underlying causes if there is no improvement. Sungur (1999) argues that marital therapy does not have to remain separate from sex therapy, and that both can be provided to stabilize and enhance the relationship.

was to have children, and men's priority was their own pleasure (Yasan & Gürgen, 2009). Yasan and Gürgen (2009) also hypothesized that as long as Turkish couples are having intercourse, they may not seek therapy for other sexual problems.

Depending on their cultural background and level of religious practice, Muslim couples in the West may present similarly, but other concerns may prompt them to seek sex therapy as well. Based on the clinical experience of many providers, a common complaint from men is that their wives are not responsive or lack interest in sexual relations, particularly after childbirth. Providers also report working with women who are uncertain about the cultural implications of initiating sexual activity. Women may also present with feelings of shame and guilt related to the husband's request during sexual relations for religiously prohibited behaviors such as anal sex and viewing pornographic content. At times, interfaith couples and individuals married to recent immigrants may present with problems related to sexual incongruence and conflicting expectations. Individuals may present seeking to resolve sexual trauma, deal with gay feelings, or address a spouse's compulsive/addictive sexual behavior. In some communities, sexual dysfunctions can make individuals susceptible to social stigma and loss of social status as a result of failing to fulfill the expectations of marriage (Yasan, Essizoglu, & Yildirim, 2009). Some providers have observed couples seeking help after numerous years, as a "last resort" before divorce.

Problem Attribution and Expectations for Treatment

As is the case of many culture-bound syndromes, problems may be attributed to a variety of factors (de Silva & Rodrigo, 1995), such as possession by evil spirits, the evil eye, or sorcery (Al-Sawaf & Al-Issa, 2000). Due to a lack of sexual education, some couples may believe their problem to be only a physical one, and as a result only accept physical treatment (Sungur, 1999). For example, they may seek medications or a hymenectomy (removal of the hymen) for dysfunctions like vaginismus or dyspareunia, instead of behavioral treatments, such as sensate focus or dilator therapy. Thus, before beginning treatment, it is important for clinicians and clients to have a mutual understanding of the problem (Sungur, 1999) and its causes, and then proceed to negotiate mutually acceptable treatment options.

During the assessment process, it is good practice to begin with general demographic questions before obtaining a psychosocial and psychosexual history and inquiring about the presenting problem (Wincze & Carey, 2001). Clinicians should explore clients' religious and cultural beliefs regarding sex, as well as their attitudes about health, marriage, and gender roles. It is also important to take a religious history to assess how devout the couple is, their level of practice, and whether they perceive a connection between their problems and sinful behavior or laxity in faith (Chaleby, 1992; Hedayat-Diba, 2000). Caution should be observed when administering assessment measures, as the normative data may not be representative of Muslims and thus may not account for cultural and religious differences.

Choice of Helping Agencies

It is important to consider how couples are being referred to treatment (Nasserzadeh, 2008). Professional mental health treatment is often a last resort for Muslims. This is due to the stigma and shame associated with mental illness, as well as the communal culture that emphasizes problem solving within the family and community. In general, before seeking professional help, Muslims may first seek guidance from their family, friends, community leaders, and/or religious leaders. However, for sexual difficulties, couples may choose to hide the nature of their problems from their family and community and resort to medical and mental health professionals instead. Prior to seeking sex therapy, individuals may have tried folk remedies (Sungur, 1999), consulted with traditional healers and religious leaders, and visited multiple doctors such as primary care physicians and psychiatrists. For example, Yasan and Gürgen (2009) found that many clients did not know where to seek help, and that four out of five cases had consulted a physician first. Similarly, in a sample of Saudi Arabian clients, the majority of the male patients and all of the female patients were referred to treatment from medical clinics, with only five patients consulting the outpatient clinic directly (Al-Sawaf & Al-Issa, 2000). In addition, 80% of the patients with erectile disorder, as well as the two women with vaginismus, sought help from a traditional healer (Al-Sawaf & Al-Issa, 2000).

Couples counseling may also be pursued first before sex therapy; however, other couples may not even consider therapy due to unfamiliarity with counseling as a health-seeking option. Additionally, the limited number of providers familiar with Islam and Muslim cultures may discourage Muslim couples from seeking treatment. There may also be shame and embarrassment associated with discussing sex and sexual dysfunctions. As such, sexual problems may be discovered within the context of couples counseling or other mental health treatment, and may not present until much later in the counseling process. Still, as documented in British, Saudi Arabian, and Turkish studies (Al-Sawaf & Al-Issa, 2000; Richardson & Goldmeier, 2005; Steggall et al., 2006; Yasan & Gürgen, 2009), some Muslims do approach sexual dysfunction clinics directly seeking help. Couples may choose non-Muslim providers over Muslim providers out of embarrassment, greater comfort discussing sexual issues with a non-Muslim, and concerns of confidentiality with Muslim providers being from the same community as the client.

Provider Preferences and Dynamics in Therapy

During counseling, providers should acknowledge the potential discomfort in discussing sexual issues and should inquire if the client feels that the therapist is a good fit (Wincze & Carey, 2001). Due to Islamic guidelines about gender relations, and discomfort in discussing sexual issues, Muslim clients may prefer a provider of the same gender. If a couple seeks treatment together and there is a male-female therapist team, the presence of a male therapist can be uncomfortable for some women, and some men may consider it culturally unacceptable for their wives to be sharing their most intimate moments with a "strange" man (Al-Sawaf & Al-Issa, 2000). Thus, a couple may prefer a female therapist.

During therapy, clinicians should be considerate of the language they use with Muslim clients. Due to cultural and religious norms around modesty and sexual privacy, some clients may be uncomfortable with explicit language, and may instead use certain connotations to refer to sexual organs and sexual activity. Some may find it challenging to hold an explicit sexual conversation and may be hesitant to disclose details about their sexual encounters.[19] Muslim couples are religiously discouraged to divulge this aspect of their life to anyone. However, when there are sexual problems, it is considered acceptable to share with professionals. As such, clinicians should demonstrate patience and sensitivity, encouraging clients to use words they are comfortable with and to share as much information as is necessary for effective assessment and treatment. It is important to note that a couple's level of sharing will depend on their cultural and social backgrounds, and therefore some clients may be more comfortable talking about sex than others. Clinicians should also be aware of the power dynamics (Nasserzadeh, 2007) and diversity in communication patterns between couples, which may influence their sexual communication and willingness to accept certain treatment protocols.

Although couple therapy may be strongly preferred according to Western treatment methods, dual therapy may not always be a viable option for Muslim couples. Depending on their cultural and personal value systems, some individuals may be reluctant to engage in therapy because they may find it challenging, embarrassing, and inappropriate to reveal their most intimate moments and discuss their sexual difficulties in front of their spouse or with a stranger. In such cases, therapists can encourage presenting partners to bring their spouses to the sessions to ensure implementation of the treatment plan (Sungur, 1999). If that is not possible,

---

[19] They may cite the following Prophetic tradition: "The most wicked among the people in the sight of God on the Day of Judgment is the man who goes to his wife and she comes to him, they have intercourse, and then he divulges her secrets by describing what they did in their intimacy" (Sahih Muslim, as cited in Al-Hibri & El Habti, 2006, p. 210).

"remote control therapy" may be used (Sungur, 1999). Therapists can provide clients with culturally and religiously appropriate reading material and instructions and encourage them to share this information with their spouses, thus engaging them in the treatment process (de Silva & Rodrigo, 1995). Individual sessions may be especially important and recommended for clients working to resolve sexual abuse or trauma.

Occasionally, single clients may present for therapy, for example seeking help for a sexual dysfunction that contributed to a divorce or due to a sexual aversion preventing them from getting married. Working with single Muslim clients poses its own ethical challenges, and given clients' level of religious practice, therapists may find it helpful to work in conjunction with religious leaders to address the permissibility of sex therapy techniques without a partner.

Acceptance of and Compliance with Intervention Techniques

Prior to providing treatment interventions, clinicians should begin by exploring client inhibitions and preferences (Nasserzadeh, 2007). Clinicians that are able to establish a trusting therapeutic relationship can improve treatment compliance (Sungur, 2007). According to Nasserzadeh (2009), sometimes what matters most is not the type of techniques used with Muslim couples, but rather how these techniques are introduced and used within treatment. Challenges to treatment compliance can be attributed to religious reasons, cultural discomfort, and living arrangements.

When resistance is based on legitimate religious beliefs, it is important for clinicians to understand and work within the perceived religious guidelines of clients. Depending on their preferences, clients may research religious guidelines alone, directly consult with Islamic scholars, or connect the counselor with a religious leader, such as an imam. Some clients will not know that Islamic law can be flexible in cases of necessity, and what is forbidden can become permitted depending on urgency, need, and availability of options (Nasserzadeh, 2009). Consultation with a religious scholar can be helpful in determining if a given situation constitutes an exception and has grounds for flexibility. Additionally, Islam teaches that behaviors are based on intentions; treating sexual dysfunctions with the intention to strengthen and preserve the marriage is an honorable goal in the eyes of God. Utilizing the principle of necessity and reframing Islamic beliefs can help in decreasing client anxiety about engaging in religiously prohibited behavior. It is important to note here that because religious leaders may refer Muslim couples to counseling, therapists should consider the important role these leaders can play in the treatment of sexual dysfunctions. Religious leaders can work in concordance with couples and their therapists by encouraging referrals to professional help, providing religious consult about permissibility of treatment options, and suggesting treatment modifications to conform with Islamic law.

Some Muslim couples may refuse certain intervention techniques or be noncompliant with homework instructions because they are uncomfortable with the exercises prescribed in sex therapy (Sungur, 1999). To practice culturally sensitive sex therapy and accommodate client norms and beliefs, clinicians are expected to utilize a variety of intervention techniques and be creative in their modification (Ribner, 2004). Sometimes an intervention may be religiously prohibited or culturally unacceptable, so clinicians will have to use alternative interventions and be creative in modifying existing interventions, as well as adjust their expectations for treatment (Ribner, 2004). For example, in the treatment of vaginismus, some couples may find individual masturbation and dilator insertion to be objectionable. Thus, clinicians may have to modify dilator therapy accordingly by prescribing partner masturbation and instructing the husband to insert the dilators or his fingers instead. In the treatment of many sexual dysfunctions, such as hypoactive sexual desire or orgasmic disorders, clients are often prescribed individual masturbation and fantasy training along with erotic exposure, and are instructed to masturbate while fantasizing about various sexual encounters and viewing material that displays naked bodies and sexual activity. From the perspective of sexual ethics in Islam mentioned earlier in the chapter, such activity is prohibited and akin to adultery. However, traditional treatment can be modified, and clients may be more willing to accept partner masturbation instead, as well as fantasy training and erotica focused exclusively on the partner.

Therapists should also ensure that they utilize material that is culturally appropriate, linguistically appropriate, and religiously sensitive (Nasserzadeh, 2009). Instructional videos and photographs that display naked bodies and sexual activity would be unacceptable for couples abiding by Islamic sexual ethics. Instead, depending on the acceptance of clients, therapists can use anatomical drawings, models of the body, and verbal or written instructions. During sex therapy, clinicians may find themselves working with multiple behavioral, cognitive, and medical interventions, and at times, it can be challenging to honor client preferences if they involve a request for unusual or nonempirically supported interventions. For instance, contrary to the more commonly prescribed dilator therapy, Al-Sawaf and Al-Issa (2000) successfully treated a case of vaginismus in a Saudi Arabian couple by placing the woman on medication for depression and anxiety, providing her with sexual health education, engaging her in relaxation training, and then surgically removing her hymen.

Gaining familiarity with religious restrictions allows clinicians to make a distinction between normative responses and the use of religious beliefs as a tool to resist treatment. For example, in working with a man with erectile dysfunction who objected to the wife-on-top position, Al-Sawaf and Al-Issa (2000) noted a Qur'anic verse (2:223) to clarify that all sexual positions are acceptable in Islam. Referring to the religious obligation to care for one's health and sexually satisfy one's spouse, as mentioned earlier in the chapter, can be helpful in encouraging an unwilling partner to consider participating in treatment. Clinicians can also help decrease feelings of guilt and shame associated with sexual difficulties by reminding clients of the Islamic belief that illness can be God's test for the faithful and that they will be rewarded for their struggles and hard work. In addition, clients who feel ashamed of their sexual desires or urges can be reminded that they are religiously permitted to engage in a variety of sexual activity with their partners for sexual satisfaction. Educating clients about Islam's positive perspective on sex and reminding them of its acceptance as part of human nature can help in promoting treatment processes (Al-Sawaf & Al-Issa, 2000). Sungur (1994) reports that a significant number of couples presenting for therapy had their problems addressed simply by providing sexual education without additional interventions.

Treatment noncompliance can sometimes be simply due to living arrangements. In some Muslim cultures, married couples may be expected to live with their extended family and may have little privacy to complete their homework assignments. In Turkey, a private ward was established in the hospital to accommodate such couples in sex therapy (Sungur, 1999). Thus, during the clinical interview, it is necessary to obtain information about living arrangements that can impact potential treatment interventions.

Technology and Sex Therapy

Technological advances can provide viable alternatives for Muslim clients preferring greater anonymity and privacy in the treatment of their sexual problems. Clinicians can explore the possibility of providing phone and online counseling, and an increasing number of clinicians are incorporating these technological tools in their practice. Although research on the efficacy of online therapy is limited, a pilot study by Hall (2004) demonstrated that it may be preferable for some clients, making it a potentially attractive option for Muslim clients who want to avoid the embarrassment of in-person sessions. Additionally, clinicians should familiarize themselves with the online sources accessed by some couples before they present for professional treatment. Online support groups, for example, can bring people together with a common purpose, providing self-help, social support, and psychoeducation (Perron & Powell, 2009). Enabling couples to privately and anonymously communicate their experiences and concerns, online support groups can be especially useful for individuals from communities in which immense stigma is still attached to seeking professional mental health services.

Case Illustration

Aisha and Omar are a young Yemeni couple who sought treatment with a female therapist for Aisha's depressive symptoms due to a referral by her physician. Born and raised in the United States, Omar was still a student when he was introduced to Aisha during his visit to extended relatives in Yemen. After the wedding, Aisha came to the United States with her husband, where he manages a business and she attends a community college. The couple had been married for one year and maintained traditional and conservative cultural and religious beliefs. During the intake session, Aisha was silent and teary-eyed as her husband described her depressive symptoms and the resulting tension in their marriage. In discussing medication options, including the possibility of sexual side effects, Aisha and Omar became embarrassed, but Omar noted that it wouldn't matter anyway because they had been experiencing sexual problems for the past year. The therapist asked for permission to discuss their sexual relationship. Further assessment revealed a diagnosis of vaginismus for Aisha, and that the decrease in her mood was associated with the sexual dysfunction and being away from her family. The therapist thanked the couple for sharing and validated and normalized their concerns. Reminding them of Islam's encouragement to seek help, the therapist suggested sex therapy and explained to the couple what it would entail. After answering their questions and assuring them of confidentiality, Aisha and Omar agreed to therapy and planned to meet individually with the therapist before returning for a joint session.

In her individual session with the therapist, Aisha spoke about her fear of penetration, explaining that she was able to experience sexual arousal but was having difficulty continuing with intercourse. Aisha's sex education was limited to the brief wedding night talk by a relative, who shared incorrect and exaggerated information. During his individual session, Omar acknowledged Aisha's pain, but expressed his frustration at being unable to have sex with his wife. With gentle probing by the therapist, Omar revealed that he also felt guilty about masturbating when his wife could not sexually satisfy him. After the individual sessions, Aisha was referred back to her physician to rule out any medical problem, and therapy continued with joint sessions.

The therapist explored with the couple their concerns and feelings about sexuality, encouraging them to think about Islamic teachings regarding marriage and sex. Aisha and Omar were taught effective communication skills and were encouraged to be more open with each other. With their permission, the therapist shared with the couple simple drawings of human anatomy and verbally explained the dynamics of intercourse including sexual arousal and response and different sexual techniques. When discussing treatment options, Aisha and Omar revealed that they were not comfortable with dilator therapy, as they were unsure about its religious permissibility. Additionally, Aisha was afraid to use them alone and had no experience with her body. After consulting with a local imam who explained to them the Islamic principle of necessity allowing for dilator therapy for the benefit of their marriage, the couple was able to positively reframe their understanding of sex therapy. Thus, they eventually agreed to dilator therapy provided that Aisha insert the dilators without masturbation, and that if she were to include Omar in the exercises, he would stimulate her himself. The therapist instructed Aisha in Kegel exercises and relaxation techniques, and prescribed the couple sensate focus exercises. She also reminded them about Islam's permissibility of creative sex play, thus decreasing performance anxiety about intercourse. After completing these treatment prescriptions in the privacy of their home, the couple was encouraged to attempt intercourse. A weeks later, Aisha called to report to the therapist that they were able to have intercourse for the first time, and that she had noticed an improvement in her mood.

Conclusion

It is well known that minority groups tend to underutilize mental health services, and when they do seek treatment, they often terminate early on in the process (Margolese, 1998). A key factor in the outcome of therapeutic work with Muslims is professionals' knowledge about and attitude toward Islam and Muslims (Nasserzadeh, 2007). In one study, it was found that over 85% of the Muslim respondents believed that it was important for the counselor to have an understanding of Islamic values (Kelly, Aridi, & Bakhtiar, 1996). Thus, in order to address the mental health needs of Muslims and better engage them in mental health services, it is vital for providers to familiarize themselves with their Muslim clients' religious beliefs, customs, and traditions (Hedayat-Diba, 2000; Rehman & Dziegielewski, 2003).

Sexual dysfunctions can cause pain and despair for many couples. Clinicians can play a crucial role in assessing and relieving the concerns of couples experiencing sexual problems, but they have the obligation to do so while respecting client cultural and religious beliefs. Clinicians should apply the principles of cultural competency and multicultural therapy when addressing sexual health issues (Peterson et al., 2007). Cultural and religious factors can influence whether Muslim individuals will seek help for their sexual dysfunction, and can either generate resistance to therapy or provide strong motivation for change (Sungur, 1999). Several treatment approaches, such as masturbation or fantasy training, may conflict with some of the cultural or religious beliefs of Muslim clients. Clinicians should also be cautious in defining what constitutes success. It is important to remember that client expectations for treatment may not always align with what is understood in the field, and clinicians should be willing to adjust their expectations.

Islam's openness toward sex and sexual health, as well as its emphasis on mutual pleasure and spousal enjoyment, can be a powerful promoter of change. Clinicians will find that most Muslim couples will be open to satisfying each other and resolving their sexual difficulties. However, some challenges remain. Culturally sensitive resources are limited, and treatment processes may take longer. Additionally, collaboration is urgently needed between providers of sexual health and Islamic scholars to further explore and address sexual health issues. Providers who are sensitive to their clients' religious and cultural beliefs, aware of their personal biases, and creative in adapting treatment interventions will increase the likelihood of successful treatment outcomes and be able to provide more culturally competent care.

Acknowledgments

I am grateful to the following people for their constructive feedback and assistance with this chapter: Abdullah Hasan, MD; Sarah Nasserzadeh, PhD; Imam Suhaib Webb; Nadia Bazzy, MA; Imen Alem; and the anonymous providers who shared their clinical insight.

References

Abdul-Rauf, M. (2007). *The Islamic view of women and the family*. Alexandria, VA: Al Saadawi Publications.

Ahsan, M. (2007). Review of "Sex and sexuality in Islam." *Culture, Health & Sexuality, 9*(5), 551–552.

Al-Hibri, A., & El Habti, R. (2006). Islam. In D. S. Browning, M. C. Green & J. Witte Jr. (Eds.), *Sex, marriage, and family in world religions* (pp. 150–225). New York, NY: Columbia University Press.

Al-Jibali, M. (2000). *The Muslim family—The quest for love and mercy: Regulation for marriage and wedding in Islam*. Arlington, TX: Al-Kitab and As-Sunnah Publishing.

Al-Kawthari, M. (2008). *Islamic guide to sexual relations*. Tooting, London: Huma Press.

Al-Sawaf, M., & Al-Issa, I. (2000). Sex and sexual dysfunction in an Arab–Islamic society. In I. Al-Issa (Ed.), *Al-Junūn: Mental illness in the Islamic world* (pp. 295–311). Madison, CT: International Universities Press.

Altareb, B. (2008). The practice of marriage and family counseling and Islam. In J. D. Onedera (Ed.), *The role of religion in marriage and family counseling* (pp. 89–104). New York, NY: Routledge/Taylor & Francis Group.

American Psychiatric Association. (2000). *Diagnostic and statistical manual of mental disorders* (Revised 4th ed). Washington, DC: Author.

Anderson, H., & Goolishian, H. (1992). The client is the expert: A not-knowing approach to therapy. In S. McNamee & K. Bergen (Eds.), *Therapy as social construction* (pp. 25–39). Newbury Park, CA: Sage.

Ansari, Z. (2002). Islamic psychology. In R. P. Olson (Ed.), *Religious theories of personality and psychotherapy: East meets west* (pp. 325–357). New York, NY: Haworth Press.

Badri, M. B. (1979). *The dilemma of Muslim psychologists.* London: MWH.

Basson, R. (2001). Female sexual response: The role of drugs in the management of sexual dysfunction. *Obstetrics and Gynecology, 98,* 350–353.

Bullough, V. (1976). *Sexual variance in society and history.* Chicago, IL: University of Chicago Press.

Burt, V. K., & Rudolph, M. (2000). Treating an orthodox Jewish woman with obsessive compulsive disorder: Maintaining reproductive and psychologic stability in the context of normative religious rituals. *American Journal of Psychiatry, 157,* 620–624.

Carolan, M., Bagherinia, G., Juhari, R., Himelright, J., & Mouton-Sanders, M. (2000). Contemporary Muslim families: Research and practice. *Contemporary Family Therapy, 22,* 67–79.

Chaleby, K. (1992). Psychotherapy with Arab patients: Towards a culturally oriented technique. *Arab Journal of Psychiatry, 3,* 16–27.

Compton, A. Y. (1989). Multicultural perspectives on sex education. *Sexual & Marital Therapy, 4*(1), 75–85.

de Silva, P., & Rodrigo, E. K. (1995). Sex therapy in Sri Lanka—Development, problems and prospects. *International Review of Psychiatry, 7,* 241–247.

Farah, M. (1984). *Marriage and sexuality in Islam: A translation of al-Ghazali's book on the etiquette of marriage from the ihya'.* Salt Lake City, UT: University of Utah Press.

Feldman, H. A., Goldstein, I., Hatzichristou, D. G., Krane, R. J., & McKinlay, J. B. (1994). Impotence and its medical and psychosocial correlates: Results of the Massachusetts male aging study. *Journal of Urology, 151,* 54–61.

Frank, E., Anderson, C., & Rubenstein, D. (1978). Frequency of sexual dysfunction in "normal" couples. *New England Journal of Medicine, 299,* 111–115.

Hall, P. (2004). Online psychosexual therapy: A summary of pilot study findings. *Sexual and Relationship Therapy, 19,* 167–178.

Hamidullah, M. (1969). *Introduction to Islam.* Pakistan: Darul Ishaat. Retrieved from http://muslim-canada.org/hamidullah_all.html

Hedayat-Diba, Z. (2000). Psychotherapy with Muslims. In P. S. Richards & A. E. Bergin (Eds.), *Handbook of psychotherapy and religious diversity* (pp. 289–314).Washington, DC: American Psychological Association.

Kelly, E. W., Aridi, A., & Bakhtiar, L. (1996). Muslims in the United States: An exploratory study of universal and mental health values. *Counseling and Values, 40,* 206–218.

Khan, M. A. (2006). *Sex and sexuality in Islam.* Lahore, Pakistan: Nashriyat.

Kleinman, A. (1987). Anthropology and psychiatry: The role of culture in cross-cultural research on illness. *British Journal of Psychiatry, 151*, 447–454.

Kotb, H. (2004). *Sexuality in Islam*. Doctoral dissertation. Retrieved from http://www2.hu-berlin.de/sexology/GESUND/ARCHIV/kotb2.htm

Kulhara, P., & Avasthi, A. (1995). Sexual dysfunction on the Indian subcontinent. *International Review of Psychiatry, 7*(2), 231–240.

Laumann, E. O., Paik, A., & Rosen, R. C. (1999). Sexual dysfunction in the United States: Prevalence and predictors. *Journal of the American Medical Association, 281*(6), 537–544.

Leiblum, S. R. (2007). Sex therapy today: Current issues and future perspectives. In S. R. Leiblum (Ed.), *Principles and practice of sex therapy* (4th ed., pp. 3–22). New York, NY: Guilford Press.

Leiblum, S. R., & Wiegel, M. (2002). Psychotherapeutic interventions for treating female sexual dysfunction. *World Journal of Urology, 20*, 127–136.

Margolese, H. C. (1998). Engaging in psychotherapy with the Orthodox Jew: A critical review. *American Journal of Psychotherapy, 52*, 37–53.

Nasserzadeh, S. (2007). *Counseling the Muslim couple—Using religious values rather than fighting them*. Symposium presentation at the 18th World Congress for Sexual Health, Sydney, Australia.

Nasserzadeh, S. (2008, June). *Are we sensitive enough?* Keynote address at the British Association for Sex and Relationship Therapy Annual Conference (BASRT), Coventry, UK.

Nasserzadeh, S. (2009, June). *Sexual and relationship therapy in the context of the world's major religions*. Symposium presentation at the 19th World Congress for Sexual Health, Gutenberg, Sweden.

Oniz, A., Keskinoglu, P., & Bezircioglu, I. (2007). The prevalence and causes of sexual problems among premenopausal Turkish women. *Journal of Sexual Medicine, 4*, 1575–1581.

Perron, B., & Powell, T. J. (2009). Online groups and social work practice. In A. Gitterman & R. Salmon (Eds.), *The encyclopedia of social work with groups*. New York, NY: Routledge.

Peterson, F. L. Jr., Dobbins, J., Coleman, F., & Razzouk, J. (2007). Culturally competent sex therapy. In J. W. Bley (Ed.), *Innovations in clinical practice: Focus on sexual health* (pp. 245–260). Sarasota, FL: Professional Resource Press/Professional Resource Exchange.

Rahman, A. (1981). *Qur'anic sciences*. London: Muslim Schools Trust.

Rehman, T. F., & Dziegielewski, S. F. (2003). Women who choose Islam. *International Journal of Mental Health, 32*, 31–49.

Reiss, I. L. (1986). A sociological journey into sexuality. *Journal of Marriage and Family, 48*(2), 233–243.

Ribner, D. S. (2003a). Determinants of the intimate lives of Haredi (ultra-orthodox) Jewish couples. *Sexual and Relationship Therapy, 18*(1), 53–62.

Ribner, D. S. (2003b). Modifying sensate focus for use with Haredi (ultra-orthodox) Jewish couples. *Journal of Sex & Marital Therapy, 29*(2), 165–171.

Ribner, D. S. (2004). Ejaculatory restrictions as a factor in the treatment of Haredi (ultraorthodox) Jewish couples. *Archives of Sexual Behavior, 33*(3), 303–308.

Ribner, D. S., & Kleinplatz, P. J. (2007). The hole in the sheet and other myths about sexuality and Judaism. *Sexual and Relationship Therapy, 22*(4), 445–456.

Richardson, D., & Goldmeier, D. (2005). Premature ejaculation—Does country of origin tell us anything about etiology? *Journal of Sexual Medicine, 2*, 508–512.

Richardson, D., Wood, K., & Goldmeier, D. (2006). A qualitative pilot study of Islamic men with lifelong premature (rapid) ejaculation. *Journal of Sexual Medicine, 3*, 337–343.

Rosen, R. C., Taylor, J. F., Leiblum, S. R., & Bachman, G. A. (1993). Prevalence of sexual dysfunction in women: Results of a survey of 329 women in an outpatient gynecological clinic. *Journal of Sex and Marital Therapy, 19*, 171–188.

Serour, G. I. (1996). Traditional sexual practices in the Islamic world and their evolution. *The Evolution of the Meaning of Sexual Intercourse in the Human, 10*, 101–110.

Simons, J. S., & Carey, M. P. (2001). Prevalence of the sexual dysfunctions: Results from a decade of research. *Archives of Sexual Behavior, 30*, 177–219.

Simpson, W. S., & Ramberg, J. A. (1992). The influence of religion on sexuality: Implications for sex therapy. *Bulletin of the Menninger Clinic, 56*(4), 511–523.

Spector, I. P., & Carey, M. P. (1990). Incidence and prevalence of the sexual dysfunctions: A critical review of the empirical literature. *Archives of Sexual Behavior, 19*, 389–408.

Steggall, M. J., Pryce, A., & Fowler, C. G. (2006). Is ethnicity and religion an aetiological factor in men with rapid ejaculation? *Sexual and Relationship Therapy, 21*(4), 429–437.

Sungur, M. (2007). *Does being Muslim make any difference in practice of sex therapy: Experiences from a secular Muslim country (Turkey)*. Symposium presentation at the 18th World Congress for Sexual Health, Sydney, Australia

Sungur, M. Z. (1994). Evaluation of couples referred to sexual dysfunction unit and prognostic factors in sexual and marital therapy. *Sexual and Marital Therapy, 9*, 251–265.

Sungur, M. Z. (1998). Difficulties encountered during the assessment and treatment of sexual dysfunction—A Turkish perspective. *Sexual and Marital Therapy, 13*, 71–81.

Sungur, M. Z. (1999). Cultural factors in sex therapy: The Turkish experience. *Sexual and Marital Therapy, 14*(2), 165–171.

Turner, T. E., Center, H., & Kiser, J. D. (2004). Uniting spirituality and sexual counseling. *The Family Journal, 12*(4), 419–422.

Walton, A. (1963). Introduction. In S. Nefzawi (author), *The perfumed garden* (R. Burton, Trans.). London: Neville Spearman.

Wincze, J. P., & Carey, M. P. (2001). *Sexual dysfunction: A guide for assessment and treatment* (2nd ed.). New York, NY: The Guilford Press.

Yasan, A., & Akdeniz, N. (2009). Treatment of lifelong vaginismus in traditional Islamic couples: A prospective study. *Journal of Sexual Medicine, 6*(4), 1054–1061.

Yasan, A., Essizoglu, A., & Yildirim, E. A. (2009). Inappropriate treatment of a woman with vaginismus and social and psychiatric consequences in a traditional culture. *Sexual and Relationship Therapy, 24*(3/4), 286–291.

Yasan, A., & Gürgen, F. (2009). Marital satisfaction, sexual problems, and the possible difficulties on sex therapy in traditional Islamic culture. *Journal of Sex & Marital Therapy, 35*(1), 68–75.

CHAPTER 18
Substance Abuse

LYNNE ALI-NORTHCOTT

Substance use among Muslims in Western countries like the United Kingdom was virtually undocumented before and during the 1980s. Since then, the number of Western Muslims using drugs and alcohol has steadily increased, as indicated by ethnicity records of those accessing treatment (Fountain, 2009b). As a result, treatment centers, researchers, and practitioners are increasingly realizing the need for greater cultural awareness training for workers, as well as new initiatives needed to engage and retain Muslim clients in treatment (Arfken, Berry & Owens, 2009). It is time practitioners went beyond the wide generalization of incorporating "spirituality" into treatment, and instead focus on the specific aspects of Islam that are unique to the individual's makeup and deep rooted in their beliefs and practices. In doing so, clinicians will be able to better meet the needs of Muslim clients.

This chapter focuses mainly on the process of addiction treatment for Muslims in the United Kingdom, with some references to the United States. The chapter focuses on behaviors associated with substance use and the psychological processes of addiction and recovery. It first reviews a historical account of the Islamic prohibition of intoxicants and then outlines some of the issues related to Western Muslims who use substances. A discussion regarding how religio-cultural norms and values can both impede and facilitate recovery from substances is presented. The chapter also stresses the importance of incorporating spirituality into the treatment journey, more specifically highlighting the various concepts and rituals of Islam that can benefit clients seeking treatment for substance misuse. The chapter does not differentiate between specific substances; rather, it is a guide for all substances that intoxicate and have the potential to become addictive, such as alcohol, cocaine, cannabis, and heroin. Considerations for the different kinds of treatment settings are presented before demonstrating the synopsis of the chapter with a client case study. As a practitioner I follow an abstinence-based approach to recovery, and therefore the chapter is written with this assumption. The terms substance "users" or "misusers" are used interchangeably throughout the chapter; however, as the chapter later illustrates, in Islam there is no concept of social using, and therefore for most Muslims, any *use* is considered *abuse*. To illustrate some of the concepts, I present throughout the chapter quotations and a case study of Muslim addicts in the United Kingdom; however, identifying information has been removed to protect their identities.

What Does Islam Say about Substances?

The Arabic word for intoxicant mentioned in the Qur'an is *khamr* and derives from the root word *khamara*, which literally means to cover, veil, and hide as well as to possess, seize, or overcome (Wehr, 1980). Therefore, *khamr* refers to any substance that covers, overcomes, or befogs the mind and the intellect (Mikhalak & Trocki, 2007); decreases the ability to think and feel rationally; negatively impacts decision making; and lowers inhibitions. Box 18.1 demonstrates the criteria often used to determine those substances that are considered forbidden. At the same time, those substances when found in products, such as cooking sauces with white wine or chocolates containing alcohol, are also prohibited. This is further emphasized by the saying of the Prophet Muhammad, "Whatever intoxicates in large quantities, then a small quantity of it is also forbidden" (Sunan Abu Dawud, No. 3673, al-Tirmidhi, al-Nasa'i). Therefore, substances such as alcohol, cocaine, cannabis, and so on are forbidden in Islam, whether it is consumed in small or large quantities.

> **BOX 18.1   CRITERIA FOR ESTABLISHING FORBIDDEN SUBSTANCES**
>
> 1. Harmful to health
> 2. Harmful to the health of others
> 3. Wasteful of wealth
> 4. Sedates
> 5. Takes one out of his or her senses
> 6. Distorts rational thinking
> 7. Intoxicates and clouds the mind
> 8. Distorts physical motor skills

A Historical Review of the Prohibition of Substances in Islam

Prior to the introduction of Islam to Mecca in Saudi Arabia, there was a popular culture of socializing through the drinking of alcohol. In the initial years of Islam, early Muslims were not required to give up drinking alcohol. The first Qur'anic verse that was revealed regarding alcohol is as follows: ". . . concerning alcoholic drink and gambling . . . In them is great sin, and some benefits for men, but the sin of them is greater than their benefit" (2:219). Thus God revealed His dislike of alcohol and other intoxicants, and although God did not outlaw them at this stage, many Muslims became abstinent immediately while some did not. Others reduced or curtailed their drinking because they understood that Allah disliked it, they began to develop feelings of guilt, and they were concerned that they might be sinning (Badri, 1976). This demonstrates that Muslims began to put forward the pleasure of God over any enjoyment they may have personally gained from drinking alcohol. This paved the way for further revelations regarding inebriation.

Thereafter, Muslims were discouraged from approaching prayer while in the state of intoxication. This was the command in the second verse that was revealed: "O you who believe! Do not go near prayer when you are intoxicated until you know (well) what you say . . ." (Qur'an 4:43). This verse further emphasized God's dislike of substances that intoxicate, and facilitated an increased number of Muslims becoming teetotalers, because they understood that anything that prevented them from prayer could not be beneficial. Finally, the last verse concerning intoxicants was revealed and this completely outlawed the use of substances, as follows: "O you who believe! Intoxicants and gambling . . . are an abomination of Shaitaan's handiwork, so avoid strictly all that in order that you may be successful" (Qur'an 5:90).

Islamic scholars teach that with the emergence of Islam, faith in—and love of—God was firmly established in the hearts of the early Muslims, which enabled them to abstain from alcohol. By the time the prohibition occurred the early Muslims were more able to accept this because they had become spiritually strong. This demonstrates that Islam recognizes that becoming abstinent from intoxicants is not always easy, and that increased faith can promote gradual recovery from substances.

Why Were Substances Prohibited?

Using substances is considered to be a major sin in Islam. The verse 2:219 mentioned previously recognizes that intoxicants have some purposes for humankind, yet at the same time the verse reminds the reader that the harm outweighs benefits derived from those qualities. For example, it is reported that drinking red wine in moderation may prevent heart disease (Agewall, Wright, Doughty, Whalley, Duxbury, & Sharpe, 1999). However, Islam recognizes that the use of substances like alcohol can negatively impact society at large, causing more harm than any benefit derived from them. As well as the medical problems associated with alcohol and drugs, intoxicants are often the root of social problems such as family breakdowns, domestic violence, and a massive financial cost to the country due to crime and occupational problems (Fisher & Harrison, 2009). Therefore, Islam takes a preventative approach so that such problems can be avoided, and a complete prohibition of substances is used to avoid negative social impacts.

Not only does Islam completely outlaw the imbibing of intoxicants, it also forbids a person from all dealings concerned with the production, distribution, and selling of them. This is illustrated in the following saying of the Prophet Muhammad:

> God's curse falls on ten groups of people who deal with alcohol. The one who distils it, the one for whom it has been distilled, the one who drinks it, the one who transports it, the one to whom it has been brought, the one who serves it, the one who sells it, the one who utilizes money from it, the one who buys it and the one who buys it for someone else. (Sunan Ibn-I-Majah, Volume 3, Book of Intoxicants, Chapter 30, Hadith No. 3380)

Although this saying is specific to alcohol, the same would apply to intoxicants in general. In Muslim lands where Islamic law is implemented there are grave penalties, in some cases fatal, for those who are found with it in their possession, even if they have not actually imbibed it themselves. Perhaps this is why so many Arab Muslims are now seeking treatment for substance misuse in Western countries. Islam does not always take such a punishing approach to those who are lost in their own addictions. The Prophet Muhammad realized that not all of his followers were able to become abstinent from alcohol immediately after the prohibition was revealed in the Qur'an. He preferred to guide them toward repentance rather than punish them.

Islamic scholars suggest that a contributing factor that causes an individual to turn to substances may be a diminished sense of faith in God (see Michalak, Trocki, & Katz, 2009) and an inability to control one's desires, stemming from a sickness of the heart (Imani, 1992). They believe that a heart void of the remembrance of God is a sick heart and can lead to a diminished sense of spirituality and faith, which can lead to a number of sinful activities.

Substance Use among Muslims Living in the West

It is impossible to isolate the exact number of Muslims who use or misuse substances in Western countries, mainly due to lack of data and also how well hidden the problem is among Muslim communities. In the United Kingdom, the National Treatment Agency only began recording clients' religion in 2009 and has yet to publish its findings. Even if the exact number of Muslims accessing treatment were recorded, this would merely be the tip of the iceberg because many may never seek treatment due to the taboo of addiction. Muslims are moreover generally more wary of approaching Western services, as they are afraid it could compromise their culture or religion (Arfken et al., 2009). Many Muslims try to overcome their problems through the family, community, or in their family's country of origin, as shown in Box 18.2. It is hard to determine the exact number of Muslims who do *not* come forward for help, and also those who become substance-free without any need to contact agencies.

> **BOX 18.2   COMMON REACTIONS OF MUSLIM CAREGIVERS**
>
> When Western caregivers discover that a loved one has substance misuse problems they usually urge him or her to seek treatment in the relevant agencies. However, in my experience, Muslim caregivers will often seek help from Western treatment services after they have exhausted everything else. One of the common reactions is to make *du'aa* (supplication to God). Many Muslim caregivers believe that if they remain patient and just pray to God, eventually their loved one will stop using substances. Another nonaction approach is to ignore the problem and stay in denial. As discussed earlier, Muslims often believe that they can resolve the problem within their own home, and there have been many cases of drug and alcohol users being locked up in a room. Their caregivers lack understanding about the process of addiction and see it as merely a physical problem, and that once detoxified their loved one will be cured. Another problematic response for caregivers is to arrange a marriage for the substance user, thinking that by forcing responsibility upon the user it will cause him or her to become abstinent. Unfortunately, in most of these cases the substance use continues and results in damaged marriages. Usually the penultimate reaction is to send their loved one to a clinic in their country of origin, believing that it will better meet their loved one's religio-cultural needs than any Western service can. Unfortunately, in many cases caregivers are naive about what can actually happen in such clinics. Jamal was forced to attend a residential unit by his family in Bangladesh and explains what happened to him.
>
> > Most of the time I was completely out of it on sedatives. Sometimes they would wake me to throw cold water over me

> and tell me how much of a pig I was. I was beaten and tied to a ceiling fan. When I told my parents what was happening they said that the doctors told them I would say such things just so that I could leave and take drugs again. When it was time to go they said I had been uncooperative and needed further treatment just so that my parents would give them more money to keep me in longer.

Finally, when caregivers realize that all else has failed, they make a decision to contact a Western service. This delay can be avoided if Western services are able to build bridges between themselves and the Muslim community, and gain cultural understanding and competence to retain Muslims in treatment. Western Muslims need to come to realize that treatment in their *resident* country has to be the first port of call and not the last. It is the responsibility of practitioners and service managers to find ways of building relationships with Muslim caregivers in order to gain their trust and find ways of meeting the cultural and religious needs of their loved ones.

Interestingly, out of those who do seek treatment at agencies, the drug of choice for Muslims in the United Kingdom appears to be heroin (Fountain, 2009b), while in America Muslim youth reporting substance use most often reported cannabis use (Ahmed, Arfken, & Abu-Ras, 2010). Muslim heroin use in the United Kingdom rarely escalates to intravenous use, as it is seen as unclean and a "white man's" method of using, in comparison to other cultural groups (Fountain, 2009b). In contrast, however, in some Arab countries such as United Arab Emirates injecting is more common and Muslims have been found to inject substances that include opiates, such as cough mixtures (Tahboub-Shulte, Ali, & Khafaji, 2009). It is possible that this is done due to the scarcity of heroin availability. This is important for Western professionals to be aware of, as there are large numbers of international Muslims seeking private treatment for their substance use in Western countries. Foreign Muslims accessing treatment in the West will perhaps have even more diverse needs than those of Western Muslims, and further research is needed to determine what those needs are and how clinicians can meet them.

How Does Culture Influence Substance Use and Vice Versa?

It is no revelation that minority and marginalized groups, such as ethnic minorities, are more likely to indulge in problematic substance misuse, mostly due to economic and educational disadvantages. It is also important to consider how the stress of migration, adjustment to new communities, and discrimination can also heighten the chances of minority groups turning to substance use to cope (Arfken, Kubiak, & Koch, 2007). As with most substance abusers, the most common cause of experimentation is due to peer-led exposure to substances. It is an innate human quality to want to belong to a group, as group affiliation provides social, psychological, and physical well-being (Fiske, 2004). In situations where peers are engaging in risky behaviors, such as substance use, this has the potential to lead toward individual use. Adolescents who use drugs often initially begin as a means to connect with and be accepted by peers already using drugs. It is under these circumstances that experimentation with substances can lead to addiction and dependency (Orford, 2001). There can be a tendency for people to conform to new behaviors, even though it may contradict their morality and personal values. And it is through this conformity that a new set of norms and values may be established among peers and by which addiction may develop. Muslims living in the West may feel the desire to fit in with the wider social sphere, thus experiencing a cultural conflict, and may pull away from the culture of their parents. A second-generation British Pakistani named Syed, who has been struggling with heroin addiction, explains why he first began taking drugs.

> I felt like a misfit. I didn't feel like I belonged to my parents' Pakistani traditions, nor was I accepted by the white kids at school. Drug culture gave me a sense of belonging, albeit quite false, and I had a commonality with the other South Asian boys who were all going through the same identity crisis that I was. When we later entered the club scene, drugs and music promoted a sense of togetherness that broke down all cultural barriers, and the white kids accepted us into their group.

The guidance once promoted by their culture and religion may become lost as young Muslims seek their place within the Western context. Sometimes the desire to fit in and belong can be at the very root of their addiction. However, first experiences using substances does not always occur during adolescence with everyone. In my experience working in the field of substance treatment, I have noticed that immigrants of a more mature age may start experimenting with drugs and alcohol even though they may have never tried it in their country of origin. Ultimately, however, connectedness among individuals using drugs tends to decline as the addiction intensifies. Very often they begin to find an increasing lack of connectedness within their social group and isolation emerges (Parrott, Morinana, Moss, & Scholey, 2004). Thus, individuals find themselves cut off from their own culture, the family, and the local community. It is not surprising that a reaction would be to seek further solace in their substance misuse.

The general public views addiction as a moral problem (Parrott et al., 2004), stereotyping and excluding addicts (Twenge, Catanese, & Baummeister, 2002). Similar stigmatization occurs within Muslim communities, in both Western and Arab countries (Maalouf & Arfken, 2009). As a result of their use, addicts may feel excluded from the wider society, which may lead them to experience feelings of shame and guilt, which may in turn lead them toward greater substance misuse (Parrott et al., 2004). Substance misuse is well hidden in many Muslim communities, and family members often stay in denial due to cultural taboos of substance use. This may prevent clients from seeking treatment earlier than their Western counterparts (Arfken et al., 2009), thus Muslims may take longer to recover. The cultural implications of the number of Muslims seeking help for substance use is demonstrated in Box 18.3.

> **BOX 18.3 CULTURAL ISSUES SURROUNDING MUSLIM DRUG USERS IN THE UNITED KINGDOM**
>
> Following are some of the key research findings of a nationwide study of ethnicity and drug treatment in U.K. treatment centers (Fountain, 2009a, 2009b):
>
> - Among all religions, groups, and institutions, mosques were the least likely to accept that a problem with drugs exists in their communities.
> - Family and community is an integral part of a Muslim's culture, and therefore treatment centers need to focus on building relationships with local Muslim leaders and community members in order to build confidence and understanding of the treatment process.
> - Involving families in the treatment of the client helps retain clients in treatment and aids in achieving successful long-term recovery.
> - South Asian families (many of whom are Muslim) are the least likely to contact U.K. drug services.
> - South Asian families are most likely to try and deal with the drug problem of their loved ones through their own family or community leaders without seeking support from Western services.

So far this chapter has presented how culture can influence or exacerbate an addiction. On the other hand, cultural values can also have a positive impact on how communities view substance use. Studies have shown that when Muslim drug users try to make changes to their lifestyle by seeking help from services and/or religious leaders, the Muslim neighborhood readily welcomes them back into the community (Arfken et al., 2009). Muslim clients who find a sense of acceptance from institutions, such as the family and mosques, may find it easier to come out of the isolation into which the substance misuse ultimately led them. Given that Muslims are encouraged to prefer mercy over punishment, when the community sees individuals return to their faith, the community may encourage them and welcome them, which can help prevent relapse.

The Importance of Enhancing Spirituality in Addiction Services

The preceding provides a brief look at how cultural values can increase opportunities for Muslim substance users to gain abstinence. When Muslim clients take the step to come into treatment, it is important for clinicians to understand how issues of culture can also benefit the recovery journey. Treatment goals need to focus on the individual as a whole, and be tailor-made to suit specific needs unique to each client. Alongside the inclusion of goals around physical, psychological, and social needs, no thorough treatment/care plan can afford to exclude an exploration of spirituality, regardless of the ethnicity, culture, or religious orientation of the client. In the West, psychotherapeutic theorists have advanced in their thinking since the days of Freud, who was among the first to claim that religion has the potential to be a negative force in an individual's development (Fukuyama & Sevig, 1999). Spirituality can be a protective mechanism against relapse and a template for conducting everyday life in all areas such as family, work, parenting, and relationships (Tonigan, Toscova, & Connors, 2005).

In addiction counseling, clients may often claim to feel spiritually dead. In early recovery, clients may recognize lack of spirituality as a sense of emptiness (Narcotics Anonymous, 1998). Thus, it may be beneficial for the therapist to explore this spiritual void with the client and aid him or her in finding new ways of filling this void.

In my experience, Muslims greatly welcome the exploration of spirituality in their treatment journey, and it allows them the opportunity to be open with their therapist regarding their religious and cultural needs. Recovering Muslim substance users have found that the rediscovery of their faith has been the very catalyst needed to become abstinent from their drug of choice. By gaining a greater understanding and education around Islamic principles, the therapist will be more able to support Muslim clients' spiritual exploration.

When exploring spirituality in the early stages of the treatment process, the practitioner should be relaxed, informal, and begin with a few open-ended questions to give the client permission to consider how their spirituality or religion can help them in their recovery (Miller, 1999). The following questions may be helpful: "What is your experience of being Muslim and using substances?" "What aspects of your faith might be useful in helping you in your recovery?" In addition, questions such as, "Is there anything you feel is relevant for me to understand about what Islam means to you and how we might channel this into your treatment program?" may assist the practitioner in tailoring the treatment to the client's needs. The more explicit practitioners are when asking clients about their beliefs and values the better the treatment outcome (Tonigan et al., 2005). Practitioners can ask clients how they would like to explore their spiritual growth in order to create a sense of well-being and meet their religio-cultural needs.

Some treatment centers think that the best way to meet religio-cultural needs is to pair up Muslim clients with Muslim counselors; however, this is not always effective (Arfken et al., 2009). Some clients may feel ashamed to admit that they are not ready to practice elements of Islam or are reluctant to admit their "sins." It would be preferable for practitioners to ask clients if they have a preference for a Muslim counselor (where available), rather than assume they would like someone from their own religio-social background. Having said this, culturally sensitive treatment services by both Muslim and non-Muslim practitioners are seen as the way forward in working with Muslim clients, so that their many cultural needs can be met. Some examples of religio-cultural sensitivity may include the provision of *halal* food, a place to pray, family interventions in different languages, understanding around family commitments, and perhaps time away from the program during Ramadan and religious festival holidays called *Eid*.[1] Further explorations of these issues are discussed in the following.

Islamic Concepts That May Be Considered in the Treatment Process

Muslims prefer to define Islam as a "way of life," not a "religion." This means that daily life should entail a consciousness of God in all actions. Islamic scholars advise vigilance in all life roles, such as the way we interact with loved ones, friends, and strangers, as well as how we behave in our private sphere, in order to encourage lifelong abstinence (Michalak et al., 2009). The following are some of the Islamic concepts that Muslim clients might be able to capitalize on in their recovery, and it is worthwhile for professionals working alongside them to be aware of these concepts.

---

[1] There are two *Eids* in the Islamic year. The first is known as *Eid ul Fitr* and signifies the end of Ramadan. The second *Eid* is known as *Eid ul Adha* and coincides with the annual pilgrimage to Mecca, known as Hajj.

Increasing God-Consciousness (Taqwa)

A sense of shame may be deeply internalized in Muslim clients for their substance use. Clients may go to great lengths to hide their addiction from their family and community. However, Muslims may also have a constant uncomfortable feeling of knowing that they are sinning before God. Helping the client to attain a deeper consciousness of God (*taqwa*) can be a motivating factor in relapse prevention. It may be helpful for clients to focus on God not only as being All-Punishing, but as All-Forgiving and Merciful too. A *hadith*, or saying by the Prophet Muhammad, explains that before God created mankind He wrote down the decree of all that was to come in the future and then He said, "My Mercy prevails over My Wrath" (as cited in ul-Hasan, 1996).

Intention (Niyah)

Most counselors will assert that recovering substance misusers must not enter into recovery for anyone but themselves, not even for the sake of their loved ones. Some counselors may even say that the individual should not enter treatment even for the sake of God. Should practitioners suggest this to a Muslim, it may cause friction between them and the client in the therapeutic relationship. An integral part of Islam is to direct all words and actions toward the pleasure of God. Therefore, challenging the intention (*niyah*) of giving up for God may be sacrilegious in many Muslim clients' eyes. In cognitive psychology, intention is vital in creating a new set of automatic behaviors (Bargh, 1997). When clients keep the focus on making their efforts for the sake of God, it creates an increased awareness of accountability of one's actions before God and can be a means of relapse prevention. This may also help to keep the client in the maintenance stage of recovery (Al-Krenawi & Graham, 1997). Knowing that they are working toward abstinence by seeking the pleasure of God gives some Muslim clients the sense that they have God's help on their side. They may have hope in His reward for their efforts, which gives them the motivation to keep trying, even when they might relapse.

Increasing Faith (Iman)

Iman is the Arabic word for "sincere faith" and is balanced by having love, fear, and hope in God. Love of God increases the desire to please Him; fear of His Punishment causes a person to stay away from sin; and hope in His reward provides the motivation to keep striving. To illustrate this, Delroy, an ex-crack user of Caribbean heritage who became Muslim during his early stage of treatment, explains: "If it wasn't for my hope that Allah would guide me and keep me on the straight path I know I would have relapsed. My faith gave me something to cling to when my cravings became overwhelming." Hope in the Mercy of God and that He will give help enables some Muslims in recovery to remain strong and hopeful when staying abstinent becomes a struggle. Fearing God can also prevent clients from engaging in negative behaviors, as Ali, a recovering alcoholic of Moroccan ethnicity, relates: "Whenever I had the urge to relapse I thought of the Hell Fire and that was enough to keep me in recovery." Practitioners can explore with clients ways of increasing *iman*, perhaps using some of the rituals of Islam discussed later in the chapter.

Family Interdependence

In my experience working with Muslim caregivers, when clients enter recovery, their family begins to expect more from their loved ones, thinking they are indefinitely cured and that their ordeal is finally over. This experience may be more common among Muslim clients from South Asian and Arab cultures, in which young adults are expected to play key roles in the family, such as running errands, keeping chores, helping with childcare, and so on. Family pressures can become a barrier to the treatment process (Shaikh & Reading, 1999). The practitioner may consider exploring how the client can balance family life and his or her own recovery, while balancing obedience to one's parents, an obligation highlighted in the Qur'an that Muslims can often take very seriously, albeit some begrudgingly.

Social network theories stress the importance of a newly recovering client having in place a positive group of core caregivers who share treatment goals and aid in preventing relapse (Copello, Orford, Hodgeson, Tober, & Barrett, 2002). When Muslim families are part of the treatment process the chances of the program being successful for the client are increased manifold (Al-Krenawi & Graham, 1997). Educating Muslim families about treatment, including them in group sessions, and involving them in the care plan could prove vital to ensuring ongoing recovery for the client and help family members understand that recovery is a lifelong commitment.

There may initially be a lack of participation from family members when they first begin to engage with services. However, this should not be confused with a lack of interest or concern. It is possible that family members may feel uncomfortable meeting therapists or other families due to the stigma attached to having a substance misuser in the family. Clinicians might therefore find it useful to locate translators or provide literature about substances and recovery in various languages. In my experience, culturally sensitive caregiver groups have shown to be a beneficial way of providing Muslim families with appropriate guidance to support clients and help them stay in the treatment process.

Brotherhood/Sisterhood (Ukhuwa)

A common dilemma newly recovering clients often face is how to move away from negative peers and find new friends. Clients often use loneliness and boredom as a justification for why they relapse. Congregational prayer, educational opportunities, and social events can offer Muslims avenues to find positive peers and hobbies within an Islamic environment where abstinence from substances is the social norm. Yasmine, a recovering cocaine user of European ethnicity who became Muslim in her early recovery, experienced this process:

> When I stopped using drugs I walked into the local mosque one day and sat down and joined a sisters' [religious study] circle where I could learn about Islam. Without my sisters in Islam I would never have been able to forget my old using friends and stay clean.

Having a sense of belonging is a core social motive that enables individuals to further their personal development and promote ongoing change (Fiske, 2004). Practitioners should help their Muslim clients explore pathways for social reintegration (Tahboub-Schulte et al., 2009) and consider building links with mosques and Islamic education centers so that the practitioner can be aware of courses, events, and sporting activities run by Muslims in their locality.

Satan (Shaitan)

In Western treatment centers statements like, "My *addict* convinced me to relapse," or "my *addict* justified why it was okay for me to use," are common. Many Western clients separate their logical, recovering, personality with the irrational, addicted side of their thinking and tend to blame their addicted "self" for their substance use. Muslims may engage in a similar approach, using Satan (*Shaitan* in Arabic) to symbolize the influence on the addicted self.

The Qur'an asserts that intoxicants are the "handiwork of Satan, hindering mankind from the remembrance of God and from prayer" (Qur'an 90:05). The Qur'an frequently reminds humans how *Shaitan* is an open enemy to mankind attempting to lead mankind astray through satanic whispers and suggestions to perform deeds that are displeasing to God, for example, "Satan makes them promises, and creates in them false desires; but Satan's promises are nothing but deception" (Qur'an 4:120). It is because of this understanding that *Shaitan* may play a prominent feature in a Muslim's recovery. Substance misusers may feel that the cause of their slips and relapses is due to succumbing to satanic whispers. I have heard innumerable numbers of Muslim clients express a belief that it was *Shaitan* who lured them back to their substance misuse, or even that black magic had been performed on them. Clinicians who do not believe in satanic whispers or black magic may assert that it is merely the clients' internal voice. However, it will not be beneficial to the therapeutic relationship to disparage the client's beliefs. Instead, counselors need to work within the client's worldview. However, clients should stop using *Shaitan* as a justification for why they are using substances and realize that they can develop strategies to counteract this unseen force, including prayer, recitation of Qur'anic verses, supplications, glorification of God, being in a state of cleanliness, and other Islamic rituals.

Counselors may find it useful to educate clients around conditioned psychological processes and how those processes are also responsible for relapses. They should also explore culturally sensitive relapse prevention techniques (see Islamic Rituals section) alongside universal ones. By engaging in new behaviors, the client can counteract the conditioned responses to nonconscious triggers, as well as take responsibility for not following the suggestions of the *Shaitan*. The practitioner can perhaps discuss with clients the following Qur'anic verse: "Those who fear God and observe His commandments, when a passing stroke from Shaitan troubles them, they immediately remember (God), and lo! They are all aware" (Quran 7:201).

Afterlife (Akhirah)

Muslims believe that the purpose of life is to submit to and worship God, and that their actions will be judged by Him after their death. The *akhira* refers to life after death, including the Day of Judgment and subsequently Heaven and Hell, and is an important concept in Islam. In recovery, Muslims may begin to take stock of their actions during their life and reflect on how this might influence their status in the Hereafter. For example, Muslim therapists in Palestine have encouraged clients to explore the life they might face after death. They have utilized death anxiety as a therapeutic tool in order to cultivate motivation to abstain from substances (Al-Krenawi & Graham, 1997). In theory, Muslims are reminded of death and the afterlife five times a day during prayer, as they address God as the Master of the Day of Judgment, so a conversation around their Hereafter might ensue in a useful discussion.

Accountability (Muhassaba)

Muhassaba means to bring oneself to account completely—realistically including one's strengths and flaws. Self-awareness is paramount in Islam, and that is why daily reflection is encouraged. Further emphasis is placed on the *akhira*, as Muslims are encouraged to assess themselves before death, when they will be judged by God. This is illustrated in the Qur'anic verse, "O you who believe! Fear God and observe your duty to Him. And let every soul consider what it has prepared for the morrow" (59:18). Performing daily inventories, as encouraged in the Twelve Steps, is therefore a useful tool for self-analysis. *Muhassaba* is about looking at what one needs to change about oneself and trying to be proactive about improving one's behaviors.

It is important for Muslims in recovery to stop and think about their actions in order to prevent them from engaging in automatic behaviors associated with their substance use, and in order to advance toward recovery. Practitioners may consider exploring with their clients in what positive behavior they think they can regularly engage. Replacing old behaviors with new, positive ones is the best way to ensure successful recovery from substances (Al-Krenawi & Graham, 1997), as emphasized by the following saying of the Prophet Muhammad: "Fear Allah wherever you are, and follow up a bad deed with a good one and it will wipe it out, and behave well towards people" (as cited in Ibrahim, 1997, Hadith no. 18). *Muhassaba* is particularly useful for clients who relapse because it helps them to assess what went wrong and how they can behave differently to prevent themselves from falling back into the cycle of addiction.

Islamic Rituals Useful in Facilitating Successful Recovery

In addition to Islamic concepts that can be considered by clinicians, there are also rituals that can be integrated into effective recovery. The following are some of those acts of worship specific to Islam that can be incorporated into the care plan.

Ritualistic or Congregational Prayer (Salah)

Prayer in Islam is a combination of invoking God, praising Him, and asking for help and guidance alongside prescribed bodily movements such as standing, bowing, and prostrating to God. Muslims are required to pray five times per day at prescribed times. This ritualistic prayer, or *salah*, is often found to be a time of reflection and calm in a day that might be full of tensions and cravings. Studies have shown that prayer and meditation reduces anxiety and depression (Al-Krenawi & Graham, 1997), thus preventing a client from relapsing. It is believed to be one way of cleansing negative emotions such as anger. Often when clients are struggling to cling to their abstinence, Western clinicians encourage them to work their program one day at a time. Phrases used by Twelve Step programs such as, "Keep it in the day," help take the pressure off when clients ask themselves questions like, "Can I really stay clean forever?" Muslims who establish the daily ritual prayers are mindful of their timetable, setting their daily routines around the timings of prayer, thus enabling them to work their recovery program from one prayer to the next. Prayers can be very helpful in establishing a new routine in recovery and offering a new mindset that can prevent the recovering individual from slipping back into old behaviors.

Some Muslims have a misunderstanding and lack of knowledge about their faith and believe they cannot approach their prayer until the drug has completely left their system, and for some this might include methadone. They may believe that praying five times a day will help them stay clean and sober, but at the same time feel that they cannot *start* praying *until* they are clean and sober. However, as reviewed by Michalak and colleagues (2009), Islamic scholars encourage Muslims to turn back to God at the nearest opportunity. The Qur'an states not to approach prayer in the state of intoxication, but does not require the substance to be entirely out of the body before one can pray. Clinicians can suggest that clients offer prayers unless psychologically or physically impaired due to intoxication.

Supplication (Du'aa)

Du'aa is most commonly understood as the act of asking God for help and guidance. Addiction is very internal and isolating, and as a result, contemporary theorists are increasingly directing clients toward prayer and meditation as a means of filling the spiritual void that addiction leaves behind. Muslims may have a deep sense of knowing that God is the only One who can truly help them (Imani, 1992). Through the very act of asking for help and guidance from God, recovering Muslims can learn to reach out beyond their own selves (Finley, 2004). Muslims believe that through the power of *du'aa* even the most seemingly impossible goals can become achievable. In addition, the knowledge that God is listening to them may offer recovering addicts a sense of no longer being completely alone.

Fasting

Fasting is the act of abstaining from food, drink, and sexual activity during the daylight hours. It is obligatory for Muslims to fast throughout the Holy month of Ramadan. Ramadan is a helpful behavioral milieu for giving up substances because so many changes in routine take place (Ali-Northcott, 2008). While working with Muslim clients, I have seen many heavily dependent heroin addicts manage to abstain, in some cases, throughout the entire 30 days of Ramadan and report minimal cravings during the fasting period. This may have been possible due to many new behaviors being put into practice, such as a change of peer group, engaging in prayers, and reading the Qur'an. This demonstrates that the implementation of some of the rituals and practices mentioned in this section of the chapter may offer success in aiding abstinence.

Treatment centers and clinicians might find benefit from promoting their services in the period leading up to Ramadan, as this is a time when Muslims may be more socially cued and determined to make changes. A study suggests that there is a positive correlation between the "religiosity" of Muslims and the ability to refrain from nicotine during Ramadan (Hameed, Jalil, Noreen, Mughal, & Rauf, 2002). In a study in which Muslim smokers were primed with Ramadan-related stimuli, their cravings for nicotine were significantly decreased both at an implicit and explicit level

(Ali-Northcott, 2008). Further research is needed to test if the same is true of other substance addictions.

Muslims can fast outside of Ramadan as well. It was a habit of the Prophet Muhammad to fast on Mondays and Thursdays. Some Muslims believe that fasting increases their faith and consciousness of God and enables them to abstain from substances, as explained by Hassan, a British-born Pakistani:

> When I was in my early days of recovery, I fasted a lot. The very thought of putting a crack pipe to my lips after I had been fasting repulsed me whenever I got thoughts of using. I have no doubt that fasting helped me stay clean.

Repentance (Tawba)

Seeking forgiveness from God directly (*tawba*) with no intercessors needed is a fundamental practice in Islam. Repentance can help clients put the past behind them and focus on ongoing change. Clients can work toward ongoing self-development and spiritual and psychological change by asking God to remove negative flaws in their character (Gorski, 1992) and forgive them for their mistakes. Seeking forgiveness from God and those who have been harmed by the addiction offers clients a sense of relief and aids in the process of a fresh start and a clean slate. Negatively dwelling on past mistakes can often cause feelings of self-pity that usually feed the addiction. I have regularly heard clients express that they feel overburdened with sins; they fear that they have transgressed so much that God will never accept them. Contemporary therapists must help clients to accept the reality of the past, to understand that they cannot change their negative actions yet they have the capacity to take responsibility for them (Sanderson & Linehan, 2005). The Qur'an can help recovering Muslims counter negative thoughts with the frequent reminders that God is All-Forgiving and forgives all sins, even if these sins reach the sky. For example, the Qur'an states, "Say: O my Servants who have transgressed against their souls! Despair not of the Mercy of Allah: for Allah forgives all sins: for He is Oft-Forgiving, Most Merciful" (Qur'an 39:53). When clients learn of verses such as this, it can often increase their motivation and hope that they can have a clean slate before the eyes of God.

Recitation/Memorization of Qur'anic Verses

As a counselor, Muslim clients have frequently told me that reciting the Qur'an has provided them with many benefits including occupation of their time, serving as a distraction when cravings occur, providing them with a sense of well-being and harmony, and enabling them to reflect on the messages in the Qur'an that relate to their own lives (and their hopes and fears for their afterlives). Muslims may believe that the Qur'an is a cure for the sickness of the heart, and recitation of it or listening to a CD can bring about a sense of peace and relaxation. Runa, a Bangladeshi ex-crack user, explains how recitation of the Qur'an benefited her recovery:

> During my using days I would drop the kids off to school and already be planning how to buy my drugs. When I started to give up, I began reciting Qur'an with the kids all the way to school. It helped me stop thinking about drugs and by the time I got there I didn't even want to use drugs at all.

The rituals described are just some of the many variations of Islamic worship that can be considered in treatment recovery. Some centers, catering to Muslim clients, have created a program that integrates Islamic worship within the program. A residential treatment center in South Africa, Crescent of Hope, is one such example. Recitation of the Qur'an, private contemplation, spiritual walks, congregational prayers, and even sleeping routines all aid in establishing something that can be continued once the patient has left the treatment center. The center's typical timetable includes these activities and works them around the five daily congregational prayers.

Religio-Cultural Considerations for the Treatment Settings

How easily the above-mentioned Islamic concepts and rituals can be integrated into treatment journeys can vary according to the treatment setting. This section presents some considerations that can aid in retaining Muslims in the treatment setting. The chronological order of a treatment journey differs immensely for different clients and different regions. In most cases, public funding in the United Kingdom is not usually granted for residential rehabilitation until the client has spent at least 12 weeks in day care and proved his or her level of motivation to stop using substances. However, those who can privately fund their recovery program will usually go straight into residential care. In the case of alcohol and opiate use, individuals will commonly have to experience detoxification prior to entering residential treatment. It is with this in mind that the structure of this section has been presented and discusses how the different kinds of settings can best accommodate Muslim clients and meet their religious and cultural needs.

Day Program

In the day care setting, clients tend to recognize one another from the local area. The Muslim community is typically tightly knit, but even more so among those who are using substances, as they tend to form their own subgroups. This tends to be the case more so in cities with large Muslim communities. In my experience working with both Muslim and non-Muslim clients, shame appears to be more deeply internalized in Muslims, and it can often be a barrier for them against expressing their thoughts and feelings freely in group settings. Practitioners would do well to discuss this openly and create a group confidentiality contract that will enable clients to feel safer around self-expression. It is also important to be aware that it can take more time for Muslim clients to build enough trust to explore their thoughts and feelings openly with practitioners and their peer group.

Muslim clients often need more gentle probing to open up about difficult issues. Within the context of the day care center clinicians should be aware that clients might leave the building at the end of the day holding some difficult emotions. Relapses can sometimes occur when clients open up about deep issues. This does not mean that day care clients should be prevented from opening up; rather, clinicians can explore with clients how to keep themselves safe using adequate support networks outside of the day care program or finding ways to manage emotions alone, such as through thought diaries.

Practitioners in day programs will also need to understand that the needs of Muslims can change drastically during the Holy month of Ramadan. Taking medication during daylight hours nullifies the ritual fast. Therefore, practitioners may need to help clients on maintenance prescriptions, such as methadone, naltrexone, and Subutex, to arrange with prescribing agencies to pick up their prescriptions at different times to allow clients to fast. Allowances may also be required so that clients can leave the program on the *Eid* holidays.

Residential Setting and Detoxification Units

Muslim clients may not be used to being away from their family for extended periods of time. This section considers some of the ways residential units can achieve maximum retention and successful outcomes for Muslim clients. Most Western residential programs run for approximately 12 weeks, some up to six months or a year. In order to be able to retain Muslim clients for the full duration of their treatment, it is vital for the residential unit to meet the needs of its Muslim clients. This may include providing *halal* food[2] and a place for them to pray during the prescribed prayer times. Some clients may wish to attend the local mosque on Fridays for congregational prayers, which residential centers should consider accommodating. Congregational prayers may be important in their recovery and spiritual

---

[2] *Halal* food refers to that which is lawful in a Muslim's diet. For example, Muslims are forbidden from eating pork and its by-products. Meat must also be slaughtered in accordance with Islamic law and is usually purchased from specialist butchers.

growth, because it entails establishing a new routine and helps to prepare the individual for reintegration into the community. Residential centers can assist clients in obtaining a copy of a local prayer timetable from the Internet, and work out suitable times with their clients so that daily prayers can be worked around counseling or peer group sessions.

In addition, the residential center should try to meet the emotional needs of clients. It is important to remember that Muslim clients often come from close families and can feel isolated in treatment, because they are not used to being away from their close relatives for so long. Regular visitations could help keep clients in treatment longer, as supported by a quotation from Faruq, a Bangladeshi heroin user, who said,

> When I was in detox I was not allowed any visitors at all. I was lonely, in pain, and feeling miserable. I missed my wife and kids so much that as soon as the withdrawals became just bearable enough, I discharged myself and missed out on my place in secondary care.

Unfortunately, because Faruq left treatment before the prescribed time, he was automatically denied the opportunity to join the aftercare programs provided by the detoxification center.

As discussed earlier, the emotional and cultural needs of Muslim clients play a big part in how comfortable individuals feel in their environment. They can also impact the way clients may feel in relation to their peer groups. For example, group-counseling sessions encourage clients to be open about much of their private thoughts and experiences. It is important for practitioners to understand that Muslims may feel uncomfortable exploring subjects such as sexual relations, especially when members of the opposite gender are present. Islam forbids Muslims from talking about their personal sexual experiences with anyone, with the exception of professionals addressing a specific problem. Addiction recovery units that have client groups that include clients who are seeking help for sex addiction are becoming more common in private residential units in the United Kingdom, and perhaps practitioners need to think carefully before referring Muslim clients to these settings. Treatment centers focusing exclusively on substance addiction are most likely the better option for Muslim clients. There are also issues of Muslims not wishing to reveal past negative behaviors to the group. This may be based on Islamic beliefs that discourage them from openly revealing sinful behaviors. Practitioners might want to speak to Muslim clients about this rather than dismiss the clients as being unresponsive and unwilling to engage. Another consideration to take into account is that gender-specific treatment centers or same-sex gender groups may be preferred by Muslim clients, especially women. Muslim clients may feel uncomfortable in treatment centers, such as those that adopt a Twelve-Step model, when the mixed-gender group hold hands at the end of the session and say a prayer together. This is due to their religious understanding or culturally based discomfort around touching nonfamily members of the opposite sex. It may also be useful to consider preferences of gender when allocating the focal clinician to a Muslim. Being alone in a closed room with someone of the opposite sex who is not closely related by blood is regarded as prohibited in Islam. There is greater likelihood of clients feeling free to express their emotions when the professional working alongside them is of the same gender.

Aftercare

Once clients complete their journey in most residential units, and some day programs, aftercare treatment is highly recommended to increase the chance of long-term recovery. Recovering substance abusers need to establish a routine that is realistic to their social, religious, and cultural environment, so that it can be maintained upon leaving the treatment setting. Discharge plans must not be composed merely at the end of the program, but throughout the treatment journey. By the time clients reach the aftercare stage of their treatment, they ought to be drug-free because of the new behaviors they have implemented in their new lifestyle.

The role of the clinician at this stage is to help clients focus on what is working for them in their program and what they could do differently. The clinician needs to be ready to support the client should relapse occur. In my experience, when Muslim clients relapse, they often feel a lot of guilt, especially those who have been consciously trying to increase their faith. In these situations, it is important to remind them of God's Mercy and Forgiveness, and to remember that some of the earlier followers of Islam were unable to give up substances immediately, as discussed earlier in this chapter. Clients must also understand that relapses are a natural part of recovery, and there is a lot to be learned from them. The clinician can help clients explore ways to avoid another relapse by using a technique called "rewinding the tape." Clients retrace the events that led up to the relapse, gaining some insight into how they could have acted differently.

The Twelve-Step Orientation

Fellowships such as Alcoholics Anonymous and Narcotics Anonymous have become increasingly popular in Western countries, and as a result there has been a growth in treatment centers that integrate the Twelve-Step model. It is a model that is largely based on the theory that people are addicted due to a biological predestination rather than environmental factors alone. Therefore, addiction is seen as a disease. It claims to be a program that all recovering addicts can embrace wholeheartedly, regardless of religious or cultural orientation. The concept of turning to a Higher

Power, whether it is Jesus, Jehovah, a Group of Drunks (GOD) (Gorski, 1992), one's deceased grandmother, or an inanimate object, is deemed to be so universal that any recovering addict can incorporate the steps into his or her life. However, some Muslims report feeling as though they were compromising aspects of their Islam when attending fellowship meetings or placed in treatment centers that adopt the Twelve-Step program. Jameel, a Bangladeshi former heroin user, explains:

> The counselors told me that my belief in Allah as my Higher Power was not working for me and that I should be more open-minded towards choosing another God. We battled over this until it caused me to leave the rehab.

Another conflict for Muslims is that according to the Twelve Steps, making amends is discouraged until the ninth step. Sometimes clients take their steps very slowly and can come to this step at a late stage of recovery. Practitioners need to be aware that when Muslims delay the making of amends it can cause cultural conflicts within the family. In Islam, making amends in relationships is seen as a matter of great urgency as there is an emphasis on doing so in case a person dies before they have the opportunity to settle disputes. This is shown by the Prophetic saying, "Whoever has wronged his brother with regard to his honor or something, let him ask him for forgiveness before the time when there will be neither dinar nor dirham"[3] (Sahih al-Bukhari, hadith no. 541, Vol. 008, Book 076).

In some ways the model is acceptable to the Islamic faith and many Muslims have found sobriety through the Twelve Steps. However, for other Muslims, the notion that addicts are born with a predestined disease is interpreted as going against their religious beliefs, as it suggests that God has in some way forced addiction on that person. Rather, Muslims may believe that people are responsible for their own behaviors and have the ability to change their fate by being conscious of bettering themselves. They may also believe that wherever there is an ailment, God has provided a cure.

Another consideration for clinicians following a Twelve-Step model is that therapy is a vehicle for establishing a new way of life, and Muslims may find aspects of the Twelve Steps unrealistic to integrate into their new lifestyle. An example of this is demonstrated by the following quotation from Syed, who was mentioned earlier in the chapter. He said,

> In my discharge plan I agreed to attend thirty Narcotics Anonymous meetings in thirty days, like everyone else did when they were getting

---

[3] Dinars and Dirhams make up the Arab currency, and this Prophetic saying implies that one should hasten toward resolving conflicts before either death or the Day of Judgment arrives.

ready to leave the rehab. But I knew full well I never would because I didn't see the point when I could go to the mosque every day instead.

Having spoken to many Muslims who have been through residential programs that adopt the Twelve Steps, I have found that where lifestyle suggestions have been made Muslims will tend to find avenues from their religion or culture to replace them. Examples may include attending prayers instead of the meetings, praying to God instead of writing a "gratitude list," or contemplating and performing *muhassaba* instead of writing daily inventories.

Millati Islami

An alternative for American Muslims seeking a fellowship like the Twelve Steps, without compromising their Islam, is Millati Islami (MI). Millati Islami means "Path to Peace" and was established in the United States for Muslim recovering addicts (Imani, 1992). At first glance, one might think that there is very little difference between this model and the traditional Twelve Steps; however, a deeper look at the model proves it to be quite unique. According to this model, addiction is seen as a disease but not in the way we have come to understand it in the West. It is seen as a disease of the heart, a spiritual void, where the owner of that heart has become distant from the love and remembrance of God. It is the reestablishment of faith and love of God that will help to change behaviors and motivate followers to become abstinent from substances (Imani, 1992).

The Millati Islami steps offer ways of understanding and bettering oneself and one's relationships with others just like the Twelve-Step model; however, the main focus is that the intentions of following each step are orientated toward attaining the pleasure of God. This model does not label the follower as an addict for life, as the traditional Twelve Steps does; rather, it is the submission to the Will of God that frees one from one's addiction. There is an emphasis on how Islamic beliefs and practices, such as recitation of the Qur'an, can be the cure for the sick heart. Before recovery, one's social life and friends would have revolved around using substances, which cements the emergence of addiction (DiClemente, 2003). Fellowships in general can compensate for unsupportive social networks that can be a threat to recovery (Tonigan et al., 2005) and can provide a source of relapse prevention that is around the clock. This prevents the "dry drunk" stage (Lefever, 2003) and is thus perhaps an important part of a Muslim's recovery. Maryum, an American fellowship member of MI shares her experience:

> Being in this community offers me hope and allows me to understand that Muslims are not perfect. However, we strive to be pleasing to Allah. The literature reinforces the evidence that using drugs is

not permissible or pleasing to Allah. It also provides me information on how to not use mind- or mood-altering substances. One of the most profound things for me in the MI literature is that "we recover from *salat* to *salat* [prayer to prayer]." I am more aware of Allah in the MI meetings than the other Twelve Step fellowship that I attend.

This chapter presented the varying considerations for the different treatment settings and will now demonstrate how these issues may be incorporated into a client's treatment journey. The brief case study that follows highlights how Delroy became abstinent from crack cocaine using Islamic values and practices.

A Case Study: Delroy

Delroy is of Jamaican origin and had spent his life abusing drugs since his early teens. By the time he entered his 50s he had been on crack for more than 20 years and felt as though there was nothing for him to live for. Having accessed a day program that offers culturally sensitive services in East London, United Kingdom, Delroy became exposed to Muslims in recovery that made up a large part of his client peer group. On his 55th birthday, during Ramadan, Delroy became a Muslim and has since found that Islam has helped him to develop a recovery program that has enabled him to stay free from drugs. Delroy has found that the rituals such as prayer give him focus in his life to get through each day. He says:

> The thing about Islam, taking drugs and drinking are all wrong, and I started to find faith that Islam would help me to give them up. Through my prayer I get answers from Allah and courage to do the things that are right. If I thought of ever doing wrong, I think of Allah and do the right thing because I fear Him.

Delroy coupled Islamic practices (like prayer, attending Islamic lectures, fasting, and reading the Qur'an) with the treatment he was getting from his day care program. His new-found religion gave him an opportunity to replace his old behaviors. For example, Delroy was well known in his drug-using community and initially found it difficult to overcome the temptation to use drugs with old peers whenever his path would meet theirs. He found that by attending the mosque he would always have a number of Muslim "brothers" ready to socialize with him. He also started attending a religious study circle for new Muslims every weekend, thus creating some structure in his life and providing a way of utilizing his time effectively. His cognitive-behavioral counseling (CBT) enabled him to retrain his thoughts and behaviors and challenge some of his old thinking habits that had kept him in his drug use for so long, namely his sense of hopelessness. Moreover, he found that Islam complemented his turning over of a new leaf, by encouraging him to become a more honest person. Islam also helped him focus on being more self-aware and improving his character. Delroy found that his faith gave him something to reach out to and increase his hope in himself. Through practicing Islam and continuing with his aftercare, Delroy has remained drug free for two years, is now employed as a drug outreach worker, and is also training to become a substance misuse practitioner so that he can help others who have been through similar journeys.

Conclusion

For a person who has been compulsively engaging in one set of behaviors to stop, it is vital for him or her to find a new set of behaviors in which to engage. It is essential for the newly recovering client to find something to be passionate about and establish a routine that can be realistically maintained as a "positive addiction," meaning one that does not have negative consequences (Glasser, 1985). By exploring the concepts and rituals mentioned in this chapter, clients may find a way of life that enables them to establish a structure for their lives that can facilitate their recovery from substances. When Muslim clients embrace Islam as a way of life, they are putting into practice a whole repertoire of alternative behaviors that can be completed regularly and automatically. As a result, thoughts of using substances may be expelled, drug-related stimuli may no longer trigger them to use, and cravings may subside (Ali-Northcott, 2008). Clients who embrace Islam as part of their recovery program may find the discipline in the reconditioning of their minds and behavior through Islamic practices and concepts. This is supported by Yasmine, who was quoted earlier in this chapter, who said,

> Islam gave me focus to change my behaviors. By being conscious of Allah in my daily tasks I increased my fear of Him and was able to retrain my thoughts by occupying myself in directing all my deeds for Allah's Pleasure.

In general, it is vital that recovering clients make a commitment to sustain their new behavior consistently. When clients begin to drop aspects of their routine, without replacing them with something positive, they leave themselves vulnerable to relapse. The way of life in Islam is not just about the rituals and practices, such as those mentioned throughout this chapter. Any action that does not invoke the displeasure of God is deemed as worship. Islam does not ban fun and it is important for Muslim clients in recovery to find new ways of finding enjoyment and natural ways of evoking gratification. Activities such as attending gym and other exercise classes, socializing, or other hobbies are just some examples that can be classed as worship if the intention is to please God. If the clinician can explore the religio-cultural considerations that have been presented throughout this chapter, this may make the way for a successful treatment journey. The role of the clinician is to help clients explore what makes them a complete person, to aid them in establishing a way of life that will promote well-being and contentment, as well as maintain a routine that will help secure their recovery from substances.

The very meaning of the word "Islam" is "submission" to God's pleasure, and through that submission and commitment one can maintain a successful recovery and a fruitful way of life, as complemented by the Qur'anic verse, "Indeed in the remembrance of God to hearts find contentment" (13:28).

Acknowledgments

I would like to extend my gratitude to my clients for their insightful contributions to this chapter and the fellowship member who enlightened me about Millati Islami. I would also like to thank my colleagues at Nafas, as well as Elaine Dixon and Mohammad Elsamra for their valuable feedback, and our editors for their continual support and mentoring.

References

Agewall, S., Wright, S., Doughty, R., Whalley, E., Duxbury, M., & Sharpe, E. (1999). Does a glass of red wine improve endothelial function? *Oxford Journals, 1*, 74–78.

Ahmed, S., Arfken, C., & Abu-Ras, W. (2010). *Risk-taking behaviors of U.S. Muslim college students*. Presented at the 13th Biennial Meeting of the Society for Research on Adolescence, March 11, Philadelphia, PA.

Ali-Northcott, L. (2008). *The effect of Ramadan on Muslim tobacco smokers, how does Ramadan reduce cravings?* London South Bank University, UK. Unpublished doctoral dissertation.

Al-Krenawi, A., & Graham, J. R. (1997). Alcohol and drug abuse from an Islamic perspective: Implications for intervention. *Transcultural Pyschiatry, 34*, 377–391.

Arfken, C. L., Berry, A., & Owens, D. (2009). Pathways for Arab Americans to substance abuse treatment in Southeastern Michigan. *Journal of Muslim Mental Health, 31*(4), 31–46.

Arfken, C. L., Kubiak, S., & Koch, A. (2007). Arab Americans in publicly financed substance abuse treatment. *Ethnicity and Disease, 17*, 72–76.

Badri, M. B. (1976). *Islam and alcoholism*. Plainfield, IN: American Trust Publications.

Bargh, J. (1997). The automaticity of everyday life. In R. S. Wyer (Ed.), *Advances in social cognition, Volume X* (pp. 1–59). Mahwah, NJ: Lawrence Erlbaum Associates.

Copello, A., Orford, J., Hodgeson, R., Tober, G., & Barrett, C. (2002). Social behavior and network therapy, basic principles and early experiences. *Addictive Behaviors, 27*, 345–366.
DiClemente, C. C. (2003). *Addiction and change: How addictions develop and addicted people recover.* New York, NY: Guilford Press.
Finley, R. (2004). *Integrating the Twelve Steps into addiction therapy: A resource collection and guide for promoting recovery.* Hoboken, NJ: Wiley.
Fisher, G. L., & Harrison, T. C. (2009). *Substance abuse: Information for school counselors, social workers, therapists, and counselors.* Boston, MA: Pearson.
Fiske, S. (2004). *Social beings: A core motives approach to social psychology.* New York, NY: Wiley.
Fountain, J. (2009a). *Issues surrounding drug use and drug services among Black African communities in England.* Retrieved March 2010 from http://www.nta.nhs.uk/publications/documents/2_black_african_final.pdf
Fountain, J. (2009b). *Issues surrounding drug use and drug services among the South Asian communities in England.* Retrieved March 2010 from http://www.nta.nhs.uk/publications/documents/1_south_asian_final.pdf
Fukuyama, M. A., & Sevig, T. D. (1999). *Integrating spirituality into multicultural counseling.* Thousand Oaks, CA: Sage.
Glasser, W. (1985). *Positive addiction.* New York, NY: Harper & Row.
Gorski, T. (1992). *Understanding the Twelve Steps.* New York, NY: Fireside.
Hameed, A., Jalil, M. A., Noreen, R., Mughal, I., & Rauf, S. (2002). Role of Islam in prevention of smoking. *Journal of Ayub Medical College Abbottabad, 14*(1), 23–25.
Ibrahim, E. (1997). *Translation of Al-Nawawi's Forty Hadith.* Cambridge, UK: Islamic Texts Society.
Imani, Z. (1992). *Millati Islami The Path of Peace: Islamic Treatment for Addiction.* Baltimore, MD: New Light Publishing.
Lefever, R., (2003*). Break free from addiction using the Twelve-Step Program.* London: Carlton Books.
Maalouf, M., & Arfken, C. I. (2009). Assessing the problem of substance abuse in the Arab world. *Journal of Muslim Mental Health, 4,* 5–8.
Michalak, L., & Trocki, K. (2007). Alcohol and Islam: An overview. *Contemporary Drug Problems, 33,* 523–562.
Michalak, L., Trocki K., & Katz, K. (2009). "I am a Muslim and my dad is an alcoholic—What should I do?" Internet-based advice for Muslims about alcohol. *Journal of Muslim Mental Health, 4,* 47–66.
Miller, W. (1999). *Integrating spirituality into treatment.* Washington, DC: American Psychological Association.
Narcotics Anonymous. (1998). *It works how and why: The Twelve Steps and Twelve Traditions of Narcotics Anonymous.* Los Angeles, CA: Narcotics Anonymous World Services.
Orford, J. (2001). *Excessive appetites: A psychological view of addictions* (2nd ed.). Chichester, UK: Wiley.
Parrott, A., Morinana, A., Moss, M., & Scholey, A. (2004). *Understanding drugs and behavior.* Chichester, UK: Wiley.
Sanderson, C., & Linehan, M. (2005). Acceptance and forgiveness. In W. Miller (Ed.), *Integrating spirituality into treatment: Resources for practitioners* (pp. 199–216). Washington, DC: American Psychological Association.

Shaikh, Z., & Reading, J. (1999). *Between two cultures, effective counselling for Asian people with mental health and addiction problems.* Middlesex, UK: EACH.

Tahboub-Schulte, S., Ali, A. Y., & Khafaji, T. (2009). Cultural formation treating substance dependency in the UAE: A case study. *Journal of Muslim Mental Health, 4,* 67–75.

Tonigan, S., Toscova, R., & Connors, G. (2005). Spirituality and the 12-step programs: A guide for clinicians. In W. Miller (Ed.), *Integrating spirituality into treatment.* Washington, DC: American Psychological Association, pp. 111–131.

Twenge, J. M., Catanese, K. R., & Baummeister, R. F. (2002). Social exclusion causes self-defeating behavior. *Journal of Personality and Social Psychology, 83*(3), 605–615.

Ul-Hasan, S. M. (1996). *Translation of 110 Hadith Qudsi.* Riyadh, SA: Darussalam.

Wehr, H. (1980). *A dictionary of modern written Arabic–Arabic–English.* Lebanon: Librarie du Liban.

Index

A

Addiction treatment, *see* Substance abuse
Adolescents and emerging adults, 251–280
   behavioral manifestations in faith, 263
   bias, educational assessment, 264
   communication style, 263
   convert parents, 261
   cultural brokers, 262
   development, 252–260
      biological changes, 252–253
      case study, 258–260
      criminal activity, 258
      identity, 253–254
      risky behaviors, 255–260
      self-injurious behaviors, 256–257
      spiritual development, 254–255
      substance use, 257–258
   exosystem, 272–276
      case study, 275–276
      creative arts, 272–273
      impact of media, 274
      Internet, 273–274
      racism and discrimination, 274–275
   family tensions, 261
   functional Islamic literacy, 255
   harmful behaviors, 258
   human ecological theory, 251
   Islamophobia, 270
   macrosystem, 276–277
      global events, 276
      political environment, 276–277
   mesosystem interaction, 269–272
      acculturation, 270
      case study, 271–272
      family-school collaboration, 269–270
      socioeconomic status, 270–271
   microsystem, 260–269
      case study, 268–269
      community settings, 265–269
      community youth organizations, 267–269
      educational institutions, 264–265
      family setting, 260–262
      gender interaction, 263–264
      Muslim and ethnic community, 266–267
      neighborhood and geographic location, 265–266
      peer influence, 262–264
   Muslim Youth Helpline, 256
   negative stereotype, 254
   non-religious programs, 267
   peer norms of smoking behavior, 257
   socioeconomic status, 270
   teacher bias, 264
   teacher expectations, low, 264
   trauma symptoms, 261
   wearing of *hijab*, 252

384 • Index

Alcohol, interview discussion about, 60, *see also* Substance abuse
Assessment, *see* Psychological testing and assessment

B

BDI, *see* Beck Depression Inventory
Beck Depression Inventory (BDI), 80
Bias
  clinician awareness of, 9, 320
  educational assessment, 264
  identification of, 309
  negative experiences associated with, 218
  popular media, 90
  practitioner
    countertransference and, 4
    home-based social services, 210
  susceptibility to effects, 71
  teacher, 264
"Blaming" self, 151

C

Case study
  adolescents and emerging adults
    development, 258–260
    exosystem interactions, 275–276
    mesosystem interaction, 271–272
    microsystem settings, 268–269
  cognitive-behavioral model, 101–103
  converts to Islam, 230–231
  humanistic-experiential model, 109–111
  individual psychotherapy/counseling, 95–96
  Muslim couple and family relational issues
    child-rearing practices, 128–130
    gendered relationships, 125–126
    problem solving and communication, 130–131
  patient–provider relationship and communication
    diagnosis and psychoeducation, 187–188
    informed consent and patient confidentiality, 189
    involuntary commitment, 185–186
  psychoanalytic/psychodynamic model, 95–96
  refugees, 282, 300–302
  sexuality and sexual dysfunctions, 349–350
  substance abuse, 378–379
  tasawwuf-based model, 150–151
  university counseling centers, 214–216
CBT, *see* Cognitive-behavioral therapy
Children, *see also* Adolescents and emerging adults
  custody battles, 318
  ethnic identity, 127
  family socioeconomic status, 270
  identity issues, 9, 12
  impact of misconceptions on, 9
  mini-narrative, 129
  refugee, 289–290, 296
  sexual education, 339
  stressor, 261
  translating for parents, 208
Cognitive-behavioral model, 96–101, *see also* Psychotherapy/counseling
  case study, 101–103
  intervention, 98–101
  theory, 96–98
Cognitive-behavioral therapy (CBT), 108, 142
  adapted models, 143
  automatic thoughts modified during, 97–98
  case study, 101–103, 378
  effectiveness, 96
  emphasis, 97
  intervention requirement, 101
  Islamic teaching incorporated into, 142–143
  logical analysis, 98
  Muslim understanding of, 97
  religious patients, 113
Cognitive functioning, assessment, 77–79
Community
  responses to domestic violence, 319
  youth organizations, 267–269
Community-based prevention and intervention, 161–180

challenges to making
  recommendations, 162–163
cultural characteristics influencing
  help-seeking, 164–166
  beneficial community qualities,
    164–165
  qualities presenting barriers to
    treatment, 165–166
disclosure, 161
elders, references to, 164
faith community nursing, 168
future directions, 174–176
holistic view of individual, 168
imam responsibilities, 167
media campaigns, 171
Muslim culture and mental health
  service scale, 178–180
obstacles to mental health treatment,
  162
parish nursing, 168
prototype of community outreach
  program, 174
recommendations, 166–173
  conferences and professional
    training, 170–171
  creation of community advisory
    panel, 172
  cultural competence training,
    169–170
  databases identifying culturally
    competent mental health
    providers, 173
  imams, 166–167
  integrating mental health
    treatment with mosque
    services, 167–169
  Internet, 169
  Islamic schools, 168
  mental health providers, 169
  mental health screenings, 171
  mosques and community
    education, 167
  nurturing relationships between
    Muslims and non-Muslim
    mental health providers,
    172–173
  outreach to Muslim community,
    171
  prevention and intervention
    strategies targeting Muslim
    community, 166–169
  prevention and intervention
    strategies targeting
    non-Muslim community,
    169–171
  schools, 169
  strengthening of ties between
    Muslim community and
    non-Muslim mental health
    providers, 171–173
  theoretical framework, 163–164
Conceptualizations of mental health,
  illness, and healing, 15–31
  case study, 27–28
  causes of mental illness, 17–22
    biological, psychological, and
      environmental theories, 17–18
    clinical implications related to
      supernatural beliefs, 21
    cultural variations in
      explanations of mental illness,
      21–22
    evil eye, 20
    magic, 19
    possession by jinn, 20–21
    spiritual disease, 18
    supernatural explanations, 19
    whispering, 19
  obedience to Allah, 24
  prevention, healing, and treatment,
    24–27
    clinical applications of Islamic
      concepts, 26–27
    importance of prevention, 25
    patience and reliance upon Allah,
      25–26
    treatment with *ruqyah*, 27
  punishment, mental illness as, 24
  purpose of mental illness, 23–24
    expiation for sins/increase in
      rewards, 23
    punishment/reminder from
      Allah, 23–24
    spiritual growth and purification,
      24
    test and trial from Allah, 23
  soul substance, 22
  theistic psychotherapy, 26
  view of physical and mental health,
    16
Confidentiality
  adolescents, 262

breached, 36, 249
discussion of with client, 52
ethics, 208
evaluation, 35
group contract, 373
home-based social services, 207–208
patient, 7, 188–190
refugee concern with, 293
Converts to Islam, 229–250
  case study, 230–231
  conversion process, 231–234
    conversion, 233–234
    exploratory phase, 232–233
  corporal punishment, 231
  counseling Muslim converts, 244–249
    assessment, 244–247
    gathering history, 246
    help-seeking approaches, 246–247
    mental health attribution, 246
    potential convert assessment questions, 245
    religious consultants and resources, 248
    transference and countertransference, 248–249
    treatment, 247–248
  declaration (*shahadah*), 229
  discrimination, 244
  ethnic groups, 237
  facilitated marriage, 229
  factors impacting clinical presentation, 234–244
    environmental context, 241–244
    ethnic or racial background, 237
    family life cycle, 237–241
    family of origin, 237–239
    friends, 242
    individual factors, 234–237
    Islamic beliefs and practices, 235–236
    marriage, 239–240
    marriage search, 239
    mental health, 234–235
    Muslim community, 242–243
    parenting, 240–241
    sociopolitical context, 243–244
  family history, 232
  halal meat, 236
  help-seeking approaches, 247
  initial years of conversion, 233
  interest (*riba*), 236
  loneliness, 242
  marriage issues, 240
  name change, 238
  people of the book, 240
  self-medication, 234
  within-group differences, 230
  worldview, 243
Coping, *see* Traditional mental health coping and help-seeking
Counseling, *see* Psychotherapy/counseling
Cultural ethnocentrism, 331
Cultural formulation, *see* Mental health interview and cultural formulation

D

DBT, *see* Dialectical behavioral therapy
Diagnostic and Statistical Manual of Mental Disorders IV–Text Revision Cultural Formulation (DSM-IV TR), 51, 330
Dialectical behavioral therapy (DBT), 302
Discrimination
  acculturative stress, 55
  adolescents and emerging adults, 274–275
  converts experiencing, 239, 244
  criminal activity and, 258
  documented reports of, 286
  European vs. American, 9
  implicit forms of, 274
  importance of community amid, 164
  job, 220
  minority groups and, 265
  post-9/11, 44, 107, 185
  protection from, 215, 288
  refugee, 284
  religious, 53
  socioeconomic status and, 270
  stereotyping and, 10
Divorce, 315
  bias, 200
  case study, 95
  families, 199
  guilt about, 323–324
  Islamic views on, 5, 44
  last resort, 343

prerequisite for, 337
pronouncements of, 315
request for, 272
sexual dysfunction contributing to, 346
shame of, 317
stigma, 121
threat of, 42
Domestic violence, 309–328
abused verse from Qur'an, 311
acculturation-related stressors, 313
alternate terms for, 309
basis of marriage, 310
building credibility, 324
child custody battles, 318
clinical interventions, 320–324
assessment issues, 320
building on cultural values as resource, 322–323
building on Islamic values and faith as resources, 323–324
divorce, 323–324
factors to consider during assessment, 321
nonjudgmental stance, 320
treatment approaches, 322
working collaboratively, 324
divorce, shame of, 317
domestic violence in Muslim community, 312–318
contributing cultural values, 314–315
culture-specific manifestations of domestic violence, 315–316
exacerbating factors, 313–314
prevalence, 312–313
role of religion, 316–318
extended families, 319
factors to consider during assessment, 321
female reverts, 314
identity, 315
Islamic paradigm, 310–312
nonjudgmental stance, 320
polygyny, 316
pronouncements of divorce, 315
punishment, abuser receiving, 324
shame, 322
stereotypes, 309
victim and community responses to domestic violence, 318–319

family and community leadership responses, 319
victim responses, 318–319
Draw a Person test, 79
Drugs, *see also* Substance abuse
addict, 231
analogy, 6
case study, 268
consumption rates, 263
interview discussion about, 60
life-saving, 192
prevention, 25
self-medication, 234
DSM-IV TR, *see* Diagnostic and Statistical Manual of Mental Disorders IV–Text Revision Cultural Formulation

E

Early marriages, 127
Educational assessment, 264
Emotion-focused therapies, 108
Employer lack of understanding, 286
Evidence-based techniques, 140
Exosystem interaction (adolescents), 272–276
case study, 275–276
creative arts, 272–273
impact of media, 274
Internet, 273–274
racism and discrimination, 274–275
Expiation for sins, 23

F

Faith community nursing, 168
Family
communication style, 130
dynamics, refugees, 287–291
harmony, restoration of, 219
hospital communication with, 184–185
life cycle, conversion to Islam and, 241
Muslim identity and, 164
practices, sexuality and, 333–335
responses to domestic violence, 319
-school collaboration, 269–270
socioeconomic status, 270
violence, *see* Domestic violence

Family systems therapy and postmodern
   approaches, 119–134
  clinical implications, 131–132
  dynamics of family relationships in
     Islam, 120–121
   family in Islam, 120–121
   institution of marriage, 121
  early marriages, 127
  false stereotypes, 120
  family systems theory, 122–123
  imbalance, 127
  mini-narratives, 124
  mitigated punishment, 130
  Muslim couple and family relational
     issues, 125–131
   case study, 125–126, 128–130,
      130–131
   child-rearing practices, 126–128
   gendered relationships, 125–126
   problem solving and
      communication, 130–131
  physical punishment, 127
  postmodernist perspectives, 123–124
  premarital sex, 127
  relationship between spouses, 121
Fasting
  case study, 214
  definition, 194, 370
  during Ramadan, 5, 66, 338
  inpatient psychiatric units, 194–195
  psychiatric inpatients, 195
  puberty and, 252
  substance abuse recovery and, 371
  whole-body ritual washing and, 192
Feedback
  advice to therapists, 94
  checking perceptions through, 156
  countertransference, 96
  psychological testing and assessment,
     81–83
Freudian slip, 91

G

Gender interaction (adolescents),
   263–264
Global events, 276
Guilt
  acculturative stress, 55
  blaming self, 151, 152
  case study, 230

child's, 216
client relapse, 375
clinician, 63
collective, 96
counselor interpretations provoking,
   94
divorce, 323–324
explanation, 16
family, 40
help-seeking, 200
refugee youth, 261, 290
sexual activity, 61, 74
socioeconomic circumstances, 64
superego, 92

H

Hamilton Depression Rating Scale
   (HDRS), 80
HDRS, see Hamilton Depression Rating
   Scale
Healing, see Conceptualizations of
   mental health, illness, and
   healing
Help-seeking, see Traditional
   mental health coping and
   help-seeking
  approaches, Muslim converts,
   246–247
  behavior, university counseling
   centers, 220
  cultural characteristics influencing
   help-seeking, 164–166
Home-based social services, 197–211
  assessment, 199
  best practice, 197
  "blaming of the religion," 200
  data gathering, 199
  demographics, 198–199
  ethical considerations, 207–210
   challenges to maintaining
      boundaries, 209
   confidentiality, 207–208
   language concerns, 208–209
   practitioner bias or lack of
      cultural awareness, 210
   profanity, 209
  evaluation, 200
  family system configurations, 198
  home-based service provision,
   199–204

assessment, 203
conceptual differences in time,
    200–201
data gathering, 202–203
hospitality, 202
intervention, 203–204
rapport building, 200–202
social etiquette when entering the
    home, 201–202
termination, 204
interfaith marriage, 198
intervention, 199
need for translator, 208, 209
nonrelated persons, references to,
    198
personal questions, 209
profanity, 209
rapport building, 199
religious, cultural, and social
    considerations, 204–207
    decision making, 206–207
    family dynamics, 206
    modesty, 205–206
    prayer, 204–205
termination, 200
women's head covering, 205
Hooka, 60
Human ecological theory, 251
Humanistic-experiential model, 103–
    111, *see also* Psychotherapy/
    counseling
    case study, 109–111
    intervention, 107–109
    theory, 103–107

I

Identity
    adolescents and emerging adults,
        253–254
    crisis, children, 12
    family and, 164
    intersecting, 217
    issues, adolescents struggling with, 9
    stigmatized, 220
    terminology defining, 53
Illness, *see* Conceptualizations of mental
    health, illness, and healing
Individual psychotherapy/counseling,
    see Psychotherapy/counseling
Inpatient psychiatric units, 183–196

congregational Friday prayer
    (*jumu'a*), 193, 194
dietary requirements, 191–192
fasting, 194–195
hygiene, 192–193
language barriers, 186
modesty/privacy, 190–191
Muslim population in United States,
    183
patient–provider relationship and
    communication, 184–190
    case study, 185–186
    diagnosis and psychoeducation,
        187–188
    informed consent and patient
        confidentiality, 188–190
    interpreters, 186–187
    involuntary commitment, 185
    understanding Muslim families,
        184–185
prayer, 193–194
problem as punishment, 187
religious needs reported, 184
ritualized prayer (*salah*), 193
ritual washing prior to prayer (*wudu*),
    192
supplication (*dua'a*), 193
threats of deportation, 188
whole-body ritual washing (*ghusl*),
    192
Intellectual functioning, nonverbal tests
    of, 78
Interview, *see* Mental health interview
    and cultural formulation
Intimate partner abuse, *see* Domestic
    violence
Islam, Muslim definition of, 364
Islamic-based interventions, 135–160
    "being in the world, but not of it"
        (*tasawwuf*), 153
    "blaming" self (*nafs al-lawwamma*),
        151
    cognitive therapy incorporating
        Islamic teachings, 142–143
    contemporary context, 139–141
    direction or orientation of prayer,
        150
    doctor (*hakim*), 144
    evidence-based techniques, 140
    facing *qibla*, 150
    hallucinations, 138

historic place of Islamic counseling and psychotherapy, 137–139
humility, 156
interplay of self and soul, 150
intuition, 154
models, 141–142, 145–146
nafsiyyat (Islamic science of self), 136–137
names of God, 150
openness to revealed knowledge, 139
paradox, 151, 153
prophetic medicine (*tibb an-nabawi*), 143
spiritual emptiness, 140
tarbiyyah and orientation, 150
tasawwuf-based model, 144–147, 148–157
   case study, 150–151
   concepts and processes in Islamic counseling, 150–154
   critical process of *tarbiyah*, 149–150
   inculcating virtues, 156–157
   Islamic counseling training, 154–156
   levels of self in Qur'an, 152
   reflective exercise, 155
   therapeutic relationship, approach to, 147–148
tibb-based model, 143–144
Islam, Muslims, and mental health, 3–14
   basic tenets of Islam, 4–5
   contemporary issues facing Muslims in the West, 9–12
      Islamophobia, 10
      jihad and terrorism, 11–12
      women in Islam, 10–11
   contributions to psychology, 8
   criminal punishments, 6
   demographics of Muslims living in Western countries, 8–9
   Divine Laws (*shariah*), 6
   fasting (*sawm*), 5
   greater jihad, 11
   historical perspective, 7
   identity issues, 9
   Islamophobia, 10
   laws of human conduct, 6
   Muslims in post-9/11 world, 12
   Oneness of God (*tawhid*), 4
   pilgrimage (*hajj*), 5
   sources of Muslim legal code, 5–7
   suicide bombings, 11
   vague claims, 12
Islamophobia, 10, 270

J

Jinn possession, 20, 22

L

Language
   acquisition, 285–286
   assessment and, 72–74
   barriers, inpatient psychiatric units, 186
   children translating for parents, 208
   concerns, home-based social services, 208–209
   differences, 77

M

Marriage
   arranged, 342, 359
   basis of, 310
   biracial, 96
   chastity until, 61
   contract, 121, 334
   conversion and, 239
   cultural beliefs surrounding, 166
   deterioration of, 150
   early, 127
   facilitated, 229
   family practices and, 333–335
   family relationships and, 121
   interfaith, 198
   Islamic premises, 120
   newlyweds, 342
   perfect, 95
   polygamy, 11
   principle, 338
   purposes of sex in, 336
   relationship between spouses, 121
   search, 239
   sexuality and, 333–335
   status of women in, 11
Mental health, *see* Conceptualizations of mental health, illness, and healing; Islam, Muslims, and mental health, 3–14

Mental health interview and cultural formulation, 51–69
  components of cultural formulation, 52
  confidentiality, 52
  corporal punishment, 58
  countertransference theme, 63
  cultural components of psychosocial environment, 57–60
    community-based psychosocial factors, 59
    concept of self in collective culture, 59–60
    family psychosocial factors, 57–59
  cultural formulation, overall assessment, and management options, 65–66
  cultural identity, 53
  culturally informed mental health interview, 52–57
    acculturative stress assessment, 55–56
    cultural identity of individual, 52–53
    explanatory model of individual's illness, 56–57
    immigration history, 54–55
    religiosity assessment, 53–54
  difficult topics of discussion, 60–61
    sexual activity, 61
    suicide, 61
    tobacco, drugs, and alcohol, 60–61
  disease manifestations (cultural elements), 64–65
  dreams, 65
  evil eye (*jinn*), 56
  individual–clinician relationship (cultural elements), 61–64
    countertransference, 63, 64
    intercultural considerations, 62
    transference, 62–63, 63–64
  Ramadan fast, 59
  representative Muslim, 63
  transition object, 59
  translator, 52
  water-pipe smoking, 60
Microsystem interaction (adolescents), 260–269
  case study, 268–269
  community settings, 265–269
    community youth organizations, 267–269
    educational institutions, 264–265
    family setting, 260–262
    gender interaction, 263–264
    Muslim and ethnic community, 266–267
    neighborhood and geographic location, 265–266
    peer influence, 262–264
Minnesota Multiphasic Personality Inventory-2 (MMPI-2), 79
MMPI-2, *see* Minnesota Multiphasic Personality Inventory-2
Muhammad, *see* Prophet Muhammad
Muslim Youth Helpline (MYH), 256
MYH, *see* Muslim Youth Helpline

N

Name change, 238
Names of God, 150
Newlyweds, 342
Nonjudgmental stance, 320
Non-religious programs, 267
Nonverbal tests of intellectual functioning, 78

O

Obedience to Allah, 24
Obedience to parents, 366
Observational learning, 97
Obstacles to mental health treatment, 162
Oneness of God (*tawhid*), 4
Openness to revealed knowledge, 139
Overdose, 300

P

Parents
  arguments, 42
  authoritarian, 184
  children translating for, 208
  concerned, 28, 219
  convert, 241
  discovery of son's drugs, 268
  discussing sexual issues, 340
  ethnic identity, 127
  immigrant, 53, 253

lack of involvement, 286
obedience to, 366
protective, 39
psychoeducation, 257
recent-convert, 241
refugee, 286, 290–291
role reversal, 55
strategies, 291
tumultuous relationship, 275
Parish nursing, 168
Patient confidentiality, 7, 188–190
Peak experience, 105
Peer-counseling service, 256
Peer influence, 262–264
Political environment, 276–277
Prayer
   congregational Friday prayer
      (*jumu'a*), 193
   home-based social services, 204–205
   inpatient psychiatric units, 193–194
   ritualized prayer (*salah*), 193
   supplication (*dua'a*), 193
Prophet Muhammad
   abstinence from alcohol, 358
   anger, 99
   biological, psychological, and
      environmental attributions to
      disease, 17
   blessings people lose, 16
   cleanliness, 192
   community-oriented practices, 59
   dietary requirements, 191
   expiation for sins, 23
   fasting, 371
   greater jihad, 11
   last prophet, 4
   life of, 311
   migration of, 297
   modeling of positive behaviors, 97
   modesty, 190
   perfection, 98
   Prophetic traditions (*ahadith*), 332
   Qur'an and, 6
   recovery from substances, 369
   saying by (*hadith*), 203, 248, 365
   sense of altruism, 104
   teaching of Islam, 7
Psychiatric units, *see* Inpatient
      psychiatric units
Psychodynamic models, *see*
      Psychotherapy/counseling

Psychological testing and assessment,
      71–85
   apathy, 82
   bias effects, 71
   case study, 82
   conducting assessment, 75–80
      cognitive functioning, 77–79
      emotional functioning, 80
      personality functioning, 79–80
      selection of assessment tools,
         76–77
      testing environment, 75–76
      timing and scheduling, 76
   depression scale, 79
   factors to consider, 72–75
      expectations and goals of
         assessment, 75
      language, 72–74
      presenting problem, 74–75
   language differences, 77
   letter-sequencing test, 77
   mischaracterization of Muslim
      clients, 71
   mood disturbance, 82
   nonverbal tests of intellectual
      functioning, 78
   over-reliance on nonverbal measures,
      77
   post-assessment, 81–83
      providing feedback, 81–83
      reporting and interpretation of
         findings, 81
   self-report questionnaires, 80
Psychotherapy
   contemporary context, 139–141
   historic place of, 137–139
   refugees, 292–300
      case formulation, 295–296
      case study, 300–302
      clinical introduction, 293
      cultural differences, 298–299
      intake screening, 292–293
      obtaining history, 294–295
      psychological safety, 296–297
      rapport building, 294
      religious resources, 297
      sexual trauma, 299
      therapeutic interventions, 296
      transference and
         countertransference, 299–300
   theistic, 26

Psychotherapy/counseling (individual), 87–117
  acknowledging resentment, 94
  additional and alternative models, 111–112
  altruism, 104
  biracial marriage, 96
  cognitive-behavioral model, 96–101
    case study, 101–103
    intervention, 98–101
    theory, 96–98
  consequences to behaviors, 97
  countertransference, 96
  dreams, 95
  emotion-focused therapies, 108
  Freudian slip, 91
  homework, 101
  humanistic-experiential model, 103–111
    case study, 109–111
    intervention, 107–109
    theory, 103–107
  logical analysis, 98
  natural inclination (*fitrah*), 105
  observational learning, 97
  peak experience, 105
  popular media, biases of, 90–91
  psychoanalytic/psychodynamic model, 91–96
    case study, 95–96
    intervention, 93–95
    theory, 91–93
  reliance on Allah (*tawakkul*), 100
  religio-cultural considerations, 88–91
  research evidence, 112–113
  sacrilegious notion, 96
  self-actualization, 104
  self-regard, 105
  unconditional positive regard, 105
Punishment
  abuser receiving, 324
  corporal, 58, 231, 291
  criminal, 6
  mental illness as, 24
  mercy over, 363
  mitigated, 130
  physical, 127
  problem as, 187

Q

Qur'an
  abused verse from, 311
  environmental factors, 17
  levels of self in, 152
  memorization of verses, 371–372
  verse regarding alcohol, 357

R

Rapport
  building, 35, 200, 294
  clinician–client, 61, 120, 187, 294
  hospitality and, 202
  insufficient time to build, 200
  practitioner bias and, 210
Rational Emotive Behavioral Therapy (REBT), 142
REBT, *see* Rational Emotive Behavioral Therapy
Refugees, 281–305
  adaptation stress, 291
  attempted suicide, 300
  case study, 282
  children's psychological symptoms, 290
  confidentiality, 293
  corporal punishment, 291
  defense mechanisms, 297
  dialectical behavioral therapy, 302
  employer lack of understanding, 286
  family dynamics, 287–291
    children, 289–290
    men, 288
    parenting, 290–291
    women, 289
  interpersonal backlash, 284
  mental health interventions, 291–302
    case formulation, 295–296
    case study, 300
    clinical introduction, 293
    community outreach, 291–292
    cultural differences in communication, 298
    cultural differences in time, 298–299
    intake screening, 292–293
    obtaining history, 294–295
    psychological safety, 296–297
    psychotherapy, 292–300

rapport building, 294
religious resources, 297
sexual trauma, 299
therapeutic interventions, 296
transference and countertransference, 299–300
migratory process, 282–287
  acculturation, 287
  asylum-seeking stage, 283–284
  education and language acquisition, 285–286
  financial stability and reemployment, 286
  health care, 284–285
  housing, 284
  premigratory stage, 282–283
  resettlement stage, 284–287
  social support, 286–287
resettlement agencies, 285
social support groups, 291
trauma, exposure to, 283
violence within refugee camps, 284
Remote control therapy, 346
Research evidence (psychotherapy/counseling), 112–113

S

Self
  Islamic science of (*nafsiyyat*), 136–137
  levels of in Qur'an, 152
Self-actualization, 93, 104, 139
Self-regard, 105
Sexuality and sexual dysfunctions, 329–354
  abortion, 335
  case study, 349–350
  contrasting beliefs, 333
  cultural competence in sex therapy, 331–332
  cultural ethnocentrism, 331
  dilator therapy, 350
  familiarity with religious restrictions, 347
  fantasy training, 347
  female circumcision, 335
  hymenectomy, 343
  implications for practice and treatment recommendations, 341–349
  acceptance of and compliance with intervention techniques, 346–348
  choice of helping agencies, 344
  definition of problem and motivation for treatment, 341–343
  problem attribution and expectations for treatment, 343–344
  provider preferences and dynamics in therapy, 345–346
  technology and sex therapy, 348–349
  infertility, 335
  instructional materials, 347
  instructions regulating everyday activity of life (*Sharia*), 332
  marriage and family practices, 333–335
  marriage objective, 334
  masturbation, 338
  modesty and sex education, 339–340
  mutual acceptance of partners, 330
  necessity, Islamic principle of, 350
  newlyweds, 342
  "not-knowing," 331
  opposing cultural and religious mandates, 332
  polygamy, 335
  remote control therapy, 346
  sex play, 337–339
  sexual dysfunction among Muslims, 340–341
  sexual dysfunctions and sex therapy, 330–331
  sexual values in Islam, 332–333
  sex as worship and right for both spouses, 335–337
  socioeconomic status, 330
  specific disorders, 340
Sexual trauma, refugees, 299
Sheesha, 60
Social justice
  advocacy, 220–222
  training, 216
Socioeconomic status, 270–271
Spousal abuse, *see* Domestic violence
Spouse, *see* Marriage

Substance abuse, 355–382
  arranged marriage for substance user, 359
  case study, 378–379
  common reactions of Muslim caregivers, 359–360
  conformity, 361
  criteria for establishing forbidden substances, 356
  cultural issues surrounding Muslim drug users in United Kingdom, 362
  detoxification, 372
  emergence of addiction, 377
  family education about treatment, 366
  fellowships, 375
  God's curse, 358
  group confidentiality contract, 373
  halal food, 364
  historical review of prohibition of substances in Islam, 357
  importance of enhancing spirituality in addiction services, 363–364
  influence of culture on substance use, 360–363
  Islamic concepts that may be considered in treatment process, 364–369
    accountability (*muhassaba*), 368–369
    afterlife (*akhira*), 368
    brotherhood/sisterhood (*ukhuwa*), 366–367
    family interdependence, 366
    increasing faith (*iman*), 365–366
    increasing God-consciousness (*taqwa*), 365
    intention (*niyah*), 365
    Satan (*Shaitan*), 367–368
  Islamic rituals useful in facilitating successful recovery, 369–372
    fasting, 370–371
    recitation/memorization of Qur'anic verses, 371–372
    repentance (*tawba*), 371
    ritualistic or congregational prayer (*salah*), 369–370
    supplication (*du'aa*), 370
  maintenance prescriptions, 373
  moral problem, addiction as, 362
  nonaction approach, 359
  positive addiction, 379
  problematic response for caregivers, 359
  protection of identities, 356
  punishment, mercy over, 363
  relapse prevention techniques, 368
  religio-cultural considerations for treatment settings, 372–375
    aftercare, 375
    day program, 372–373
    residential setting and detoxification units, 373–375
  religious festival holidays (*Eid*), 364
  "rewinding the tape" technique, 375
  self-pity, 371
  substance use among Muslims living in the West, 358–360
  twelve-step orientation, 375–378
  vulnerability to relapse, 379
  what Islam says about substances, 356
  why substances were prohibited, 357–358
Suicide
  attempt
    hospitalization for, 110
    overdose, 300
  bombings, 11
  contemplation, 37
  family member threat to commit, 197
  interview discussion about, 61
  prevention, 219
  prohibition of, 256
  rates, religiosity and, 15
  unsuccessful attempt, 258

T

Terrorism
  accusations, 188
  jihad and, 11
  post-9/11 world, 12
Testing, *see* Psychological testing and assessment
Theistic psychotherapy, 26
Tobacco
  difference of opinion on use of, 191
  interview discussion about, 60
  use, predictors of, 257

Traditional mental health coping and help-seeking, 33–47
  diminishing supernatural causes, 38–41
  seeking sage guidance, 41–45
  strengthening essential Islamic practices, 34–38
  suicide contemplation, 37
Trail Making test, 77

U

Unconditional positive regard, 105
University counseling centers, 213–226
  bias recognition, 223
  case study, 214–216
  confidentiality, concerns about, 215
  demand for services, 213
  family harmony, restoration of, 219
  feminist label, 218
  headdress rules, 215
  identities and labels with Muslims in counseling, 216–218
  immigration issues, 214
  intersecting identities, 217
  outreach and social justice, 220–222
  presenting issues, 218–219
  recommendations for culturally sensitive counseling, 222–223
  referral sources and help-seeking behavior, 220
  religion and coping, 219–220
  social justice advocacy, 222
  stigma, 215, 220
  "stop-hate" programs, 216

W

Water-pipe smoking, 60

Y

Youth, *see* Adolescents and emerging adults